Review and Resource Manual

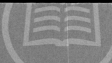

Psychiatric-Mental Health Nursing

5th Edition

D1613608

CONTINUING EDUCATION RESOURCE

NURSING CERTIFICATION REVIEW MANUAL

CLINICAL PRACTICE RESOURCE

Kim Hutchinson, EdD, RN, PMHCNS-BC, CARN

NURSING KNOWLEDGE CENTER

Library of Congress Cataloging-in-Publication Data

Hutchinson, Kim, author.

Psychiatric–mental health nursing : review and resource manual / Kim Hutchinson. -- 5th ed.

    p. ; cm.

Includes bibliographical references and index.

ISBN 978-1-935213-64-2

I. American Nurses Credentialing Center, issuing body. II. Title.

[DNLM: 1. Psychiatric Nursing--Outlines. WY 18.2]

RC440

616.89'0231--dc23

                    2015012110

The American Nurses Association (ANA) is the only full-service professional organization representing the interests of the nation's 3.1 million registered nurses through its constituent/state nurses associations and its organizational affiliates. The ANA advances the nursing profession by fostering high standards of nursing practice, promoting the rights of nurses in the workplace, projecting a positive and realistic view of nursing, and lobbying the Congress and regulatory agencies on healthcare issues affecting nurses and the public.

PSYCHIATRIC–MENTAL HEALTH NURSING REVIEW AND RESOURCE MANUAL, 5TH EDITION

JULY 2015

Please direct your comments and queries to: publications@ana.org

The healthcare services delivery system is a volatile marketplace demanding superior knowledge, clinical skills, and competencies from all registered nurses. Nursing autonomy of practice and nurse career marketability and mobility in the new century hinge on affirming the profession's formative philosophy, which places a priority on a lifelong commitment to the principles of education and professional development. The knowledge base of nursing theory and practice is expanding, and while care has been taken to ensure the accuracy and timeliness of the information presented in the **Psychiatric–Mental Health Nursing Review and Resource Manual, 5th Edition,** clinicians are advised to always verify the most current national guidelines and recommendations and to practice in accordance with professional standards of care used with regard to the unique circumstances that apply in each practice situation. In addition, the editors wish to note that provision of information in this text does not imply an endorsement of any particular products, procedures, or services.

Therefore, the authors, editors, American Nurses Association (ANA), and American Nurses Association's Publishing (ANP) cannot accept responsibility for errors or omissions, or for any consequences or liability, injury, and/or damages to persons or property from application of the information in this manual and make no warranty, express or implied, with respect to the contents of the **Psychiatric–Mental Health Nursing Review and Resource Manual, 5th Edition**. Completion of this manual does not guarantee that the reader will pass the certification exam. The practice examination questions are not a requirement to take a certification examination. The practice examination questions cannot be used as an indicator of results on the actual certification.

PUBLISHED BY

American Nurses Association
8515 Georgia Avenue, Suite 400
Silver Spring, MD 20910-3402
www.nursingworld.org

INSTRUCTIONS FOR OBTAINING NURSING CONTINUING PROFESSIONAL DEVELOPMENT (NCPD) CREDIT FOR STUDY OF *PSYCHIATRIC–MENTAL HEALTH NURSING REVIEW AND RESOURCE MANUAL, 5TH EDITION*

The American Nurses Association offers nursing continuing professional development (NCPD) credits for review and study of this manual. To obtain NCPD credit you must purchase and complete your review of the manual, pay required fees to enroll in the online module, and complete all module components by the published NCPD expiration date including disclosures, and the course evaluation. The continuing nursing education contact hours online module can be completed at any time prior to the published NCPD expiration date and a certificate can be printed from the online learning management system immediately after successful completion of the online module.

For more information about earning NCPD for this manual, visit the list of manual publications on the Nursing World website www.nursingworld.com/continuing-education.

Inquiries or Comments

If you have any questions about the content of the manual please e-mail publications@ana.org. If you have questions about the NCPD credit offered for review and study of the manual, please e-mail ananursece@ana.org.

NCPD Provider information

The American Nurses Association is accredited as a provider of nursing continuing professional development by the American Nurses Credentialing Center's Commission on Accreditation.

ANA is approved by the California Board of Registered Nursing Provider Number CEP 17219.

CONTENTS

CATEGORY I. ASSESSMENT, DIAGNOSIS, AND PLANNING

CATEGORY II. IMPLEMENTATION AND EVALUATION

Nonpharmacological Pain Management Interventions and Evaluation

Over-the-Counter, Complementary, Alternative, and Herbal Agents

Select Somatic Therapies: ECT, TMS, Brain Stimulation, VNS, Phototherapy

Nursing Theories and Theorists

Therapeutic Communication and the Nurse-Patient (Healthcare Consumer) Relationship

Written Communication and Documentation of Care

Professional Performance Standards for Psychiatric–Mental Health Nursing

Factors Affecting Scope of Practice

Psychiatric–Mental Health Professional Performance Standard 7. Ethics

Psychiatric–Mental Health Professional Performance Standard 8. Education

Psychiatric–Mental Health Professional Performance Standard 9. Evidence-Based Practice and Research

Psychiatric–Mental Health Professional Performance Standard 10. Quality of Practice

Psychiatric–Mental Health Professional Performance Standard 11. Communication

Psychiatric–Mental Health Professional Performance Standard 12. Leadership (At Every Level)

Psychiatric–Mental Health Professional Performance Standard 13. Collaboration

Psychiatric–Mental Health Professional Performance Standard 14. Professional Practice Evaluation

Psychiatric–Mental Health Professional Performance Standard 15. Resource Utilization

Patient Legal Protections

CATEGORY IV. PATIENT EDUCATION AND POPULATION HEALTH

CHAPTER 1

TAKING THE CERTIFICATION EXAMINATION

When you sign up to take a national certification exam, you will receive a packet of information from the testing agency. Review it carefully and keep it where you can refer to it frequently. It will contain information on test content and sample questions. This is critical information; review it carefully and it will give you insight into the nature of the test. The agency will also send you materials authorizing your entry into the exam. Keep these in a safe place until needed.

GENERAL SUGGESTIONS FOR PREPARING FOR THE EXAM

Step One: Control Your Anxiety

Everyone experiences anxiety when faced with the certification exam.

- ▶ Remember, your program was designed to prepare you to take this exam.
- ▶ Your instructors took a similar exam and have probably talked to students who took exams more recently, so they know how to help you prepare.
- ▶ Taking a review course or setting up your own study plan will help you feel more confident about taking the exam.

Step Two: Do Not Listen to Gossip About the Exam

A large volume of information exists about the tests based on reports from people who have taken the exams in the past. Because information from the testing facilities is limited, it is hard not to listen to this gossip.

- ▶ Remember that gossip about the exam that you hear from others is not verifiable.
- ▶ Because this gossip is based on the imperfect memory of people in a very stressful situation, it may not be very accurate.
- ▶ People tend to remember those items testing content with which they are less comfortable; for instance, those with a limited background in women's health may say that the exam was "all women's health." In fact, the exam blueprint ensures that the exam covers multiple content areas without overemphasizing any one.

Step Three: Set Reasonable Expectations for Yourself

- ▶ Do not expect to know everything.
- ▶ Do not try to know everything in great detail.
- ▶ You do not need a perfect score to pass the exam.
- ▶ The exam is designed for a beginner level—it is testing readiness for entry-level practice.
- ▶ Learn the general rules, not the exceptions.
- ▶ The most likely diagnoses will be on the exam, not questions on rare diseases or atypical cases.
- ▶ Think about the most likely presentation and most common therapy.

Step Four: Prepare Mentally and Physically

- ▶ While you are getting ready to take the exam, take good physical care of yourself.
- ▶ Get plenty of sleep, exercise, and eat well while preparing for the exam.
- ▶ These things are especially important while you are studying and immediately before you take the exam.

Step Five: Access Current Knowledge

General Content

You will be given a list of general topics that will be on the exam when you register to take the exam. In addition, examine the table of contents of this book and the test content outline, available at www.nursecredentialing.org/cert/TCOs.html.

▶ What content do you need to know?

▶ How well do you know these subjects?

Take a Review Course

▶ Taking a review course is an excellent method of assessing your knowledge of the content that will be included in the exam.

▶ If you plan to take a review course, take it well before the exam so you will have plenty of time to master any areas of weakness the course uncovers.

▶ If you are prepared for the exam, you will not hear anything new in the course. You will be familiar with everything that is taught.

▶ If some topics in the review course are new to you, concentrate on these in your studies.

▶ People have a tendency to study what they know; it is rewarding to study something and feel a mastery of it! Unfortunately, this will not help you master unfamiliar content. Be sure to use a review course to identify your areas of strength and weakness, then concentrate on the weaknesses.

Depth of Knowledge

How much do you need to know about a subject?

▶ You cannot know everything about a topic.

▶ Remember that the depth of knowledge required to pass the exam is for entry-level performance.

▶ Study the information sent to you from the testing agency, what you were taught in school, what is covered in this text, and the general guidelines given in this chapter.

▶ Look at practice tests designed for the exam. Practice tests for other exams will not be helpful.

▶ Consult your class notes or clinical diagnosis and management textbook for the major points about a disease. Additional reference books can be found online at www.nursecredentialing.org/cert/refs.html.

▶ For example, with regard to medications, know the drug categories and the major medications in each. Assume all drugs in a category are generally alike, and then focus on the differences among common drugs. Know the most important indications, contraindications, and side effects. Emphasize safety. The questions usually do not require you to know the exact dosage of a drug.

Step Six: Institute a Systematic Study Plan

Develop Your Study Plan

▶ Write up a formal plan of study.

  ▸ Include topics for study, timetable, resources, and methods of study that work for you.

  ▸ Decide whether you want to organize a study group or work alone.

  ▸ Schedule regular times to study.

  ▸ Avoid cramming; it is counterproductive. Try to schedule your study periods in 1-hour increments.

▶ Identify resources to use for studying. To prepare for the examination, you should have the following on your shelf:

  ▸ A good pathophysiology text

  ▸ This review book

  ▸ A physical assessment text

  ▸ Your class notes

  ▸ Other important sources, including: information from the testing facility, a clinical diagnosis textbook, favorite journal articles, notes from a review course, and practice tests

  ▸ Know the important national standards of care for major illnesses.

  ▸ Consult the bibliography on the test blueprint. When studying less familiar material, it is helpful to study using the same references that the testing center uses.

▶ Study the body systems from head to toe.

▶ The exams emphasize health promotion, assessment, differential diagnosis, and plan of care for common problems.

▶ You will need to know facts and be able to interpret and analyze this information utilizing critical thinking.

Personalize Your Study Plan

▶ How do you learn best?

  ▸ If you learn best by listening or talking, attend a review course or discuss topics with a colleague.

▶ Read everything the test facility sends you as soon as you receive it and several times during your preparation period. It will give you valuable information to help guide your study.

▶ Have a specific place with good lighting set aside for studying. Find a place with no noise or distractions. Assemble your study materials.

Implement Your Study Plan

You must have basic content knowledge. In addition, you must be able to use this information to think critically and make decisions based on facts.

▶ Refer to your study plan regularly.

▶ Stick to your schedule.

▶ Take breaks when you get tired.

▶ If you start procrastinating, get help from a friend or reorganize your study plan.

▶ It is not necessary to follow your plan rigidly. Adjust as you learn where you need to spend more time.

▶ Memorize the basics of the content areas you will be required to know.

Focus on General Material

▶ Most of what you need to know is basic material that does not require constant updating.

▶ You do not need to worry about the latest information being published as you are studying for the exam. Remember, it can take 6 to 12 months for new information to be incorporated into test questions.

Pace Your Studying

▶ Stop studying for the examination when you are starting to feel overwhelmed and look at what is bothering you. Then make changes.

▶ Break overwhelming tasks into smaller tasks that you know you can do.

▶ Stop and take breaks while studying.

Work With Others

▶ Talk with classmates about your preparation for the exam.

▶ Keep in touch with classmates, and help each other stick to your study plans.

▶ If your classmates start having anxiety attacks, do not let their anxiety affect you. Walk away if you need to.

▶ Do not believe bad stories you hear about other people's experiences with previous exams.

▶ Remember, you know as much as anyone about what will be on the next exam!

Consider a Study Group

▶ Study groups can provide practice in analyzing cases, interpreting questions, and critical thinking.

  ▸ You can discuss a topic and take turns presenting cases for the group to analyze.

  ▸ Study groups can also provide moral support and help you keep studying.

Step Seven: Strategies Immediately Before the Exam

Final Preparation Suggestions

▶ Use practice exams when studying to get accustomed to the exam format and time restrictions.

  ▸ Many books that are labeled as review books are simply a collection of examination questions.

  ▸ If you have test anxiety, such practice tests may help alleviate the anxiety.

  ▸ Practice tests can help you learn to judge the time you should take during an exam.

  ▸ Practice tests are useful for gaining experience in analyzing questions.

  ▸ Books of questions may not uncover the gaps in your knowledge that a more systematic content review text will reveal.

  ▸ If you feel that you don't know enough about a topic, refer to a text to learn more. After you feel that you have learned the topic, practice questions are a wonderful tool to help improve your test-taking skill.

▶ Know your test-taking style.

  ▸ Do you rush through the exam without reading the questions thoroughly?

  ▸ Do you get stuck and dwell on a question for a long time?

  ▸ You should spend about 45 to 60 seconds per question and finish with time to review the questions you were not sure about.

  ▸ Be sure to read the question completely, including all four answer choices. Choice "a" may be good, but "d" may be best.

The Night Before the Exam

▶ Be prepared to get to the exam on time.

  ▸ Know the test site location and how long it takes to get there.

  ▸ Take a "dry run" beforehand to make sure you know how to get to the testing site, if necessary.

- Get a good night's sleep.

- Eat sensibly.

- Avoid alcohol the night before.

- Assemble the required material—two forms of identification, admission card, pencil, and watch. Both IDs must match the name on the application, and one photo ID is preferred. Bring tissues, antacid chews, hard candy, and anything you might want in your pocket.

- Know the exam room rules.

  ▷ You will be given scratch paper that will be collected at the end of the exam.

  ▷ Nothing else is allowed in the exam room.

  ▷ You will be required to put papers, backpacks, etc., in a corner of the room or in a locker.

  ▷ No water or food will be allowed.

  ▷ You will be allowed to walk to a water fountain and go to the bathroom one at a time.

The Day of the Exam

▶ Get there early. If you are late, you may not be admitted.

▶ Think positively. You have studied hard and are well-prepared.

▶ Remember your anxiety reduction strategies.

Specific Tips for Dealing With Anxiety

Test anxiety is a specific type of anxiety. Symptoms include upset stomach, sweaty palms, tachycardia, trouble concentrating, and a feeling of dread. But there are ways to cope with test anxiety.

▶ There is no substitute for being well-prepared.

▶ Practice relaxation techniques.

▶ Avoid alcohol, excess coffee, caffeine, and any new medications that might sedate you, dull your senses, or make you feel agitated.

▶ Take a few deep breaths and concentrate on the task at hand.

Focus on Specific Test-Taking Skills

To do well on the exam, you need good test-taking skills in addition to knowledge of the content and ability to use critical thinking.

All Certification Exams Are Multiple Choice

▶ Multiple choice tests have specific rules for test construction.

▶ A multiple choice question consists of three parts: the information (or stem), the question, and the four possible answers (one correct and three distracters).

▶ Careful analysis of each part is necessary. Read the entire question before answering.

▶ Practice your test-taking skills by analyzing the practice questions in this book and on the NKC website.

Analyze the Information Given

▶ Do not assume you have more information than is given.

▶ Do not overanalyze.

▶ Remember, the writer of the question assumes this is all of the information needed to answer the question.

▶ If information is not given, it is not relevant and will not affect the answer.

▶ Do not make the question more complicated than it is.

What Kind of Question Is Asked?

▶ Are you supposed to recall a fact, apply facts to a situation, or understand and differentiate between options?

  ▸ Read the question thinking about what the writer is asking.

  ▸ Look for key words or phrases that lead you (see Figure 1–1). These help determine what kind of answer the question requires.

FIGURE 1–1.
EXAMPLES OF KEY WORDS AND PHRASES

▶ avoid	▶ initial	▶ most
▶ best	▶ first	▶ significant
▶ except	▶ contributing to	▶ likely
▶ not	▶ appropriate	▶ of the following
		▶ most consistent with

Read All of the Answers

▶ If you are absolutely certain that answer "a" is correct as you read it, mark it, but read the rest of the question so you do not trick yourself into missing a better answer.

▶ If you are absolutely sure answer "a" is wrong, cross it off or make a note on your scratch paper and continue reading the question.

▶ After reading the entire question, go back, analyze the question, and select the best answer.

▶ Do not jump ahead.

▶ If the question asks you for an assessment, the best answer will be an assessment. Do not be distracted by an intervention that sounds appropriate.

▶ If the question asks you for an intervention, do not answer with an assessment.

▶ When two answer choices sound very good, the best one is usually the least expensive, least invasive way to achieve the goal. For example, if your answer choices include a physical exam maneuver or imaging, the physical exam maneuver is probably the better choice provided it will give the information needed.

▶ If the answers include two options that are the opposite of each other, one of the two is probably the correct answer.

▶ When numeric answers cover a wide range, a number in the middle is more likely to be correct.

▶ Watch out for distracters that are correct but do not answer the question, combine true and false information, or contain a word or phrase that is similar to the correct answer.

▶ Err on the side of caution.

Only One Answer Can Be Correct

▶ When more than one suggested answer is correct, you must identify the one that best answers the question asked.

▶ If you cannot choose between two answers, you have a 50% chance of getting it right if you guess.

Avoid Changing Answers

▶ Change an answer only if you have a compelling reason, such as you remembered something additional, or you understand the question better after rereading it.

▶ People change to a wrong answer more often than to a right answer.

Time Yourself to Complete the Whole Exam

▶ Do not spend a large amount of time on one question.

▶ If you cannot answer a question quickly, mark it and continue the exam.

▶ If time is left at the end, return to the difficult questions.

▶ Make educated guesses by eliminating the obviously wrong answers and choosing a likely answer even if you are not certain.

▶ Trust your instinct.

▶ Answer every question. There is no penalty for a wrong answer.

▶ Occasionally a question will remind you of something that helps you with a question earlier in the test. Look back at that question to see whether what you are remembering affects how you would answer that question.

ABOUT THE CERTIFICATION EXAMS

The American Nurses Credentialing Center Computerized Exam

The ANCC examination is given only as a computer exam, and each exam is different. The order of the questions is scrambled for every test, so even if two people are taking the same exam, the questions will be in a different order. The exam consists of 175 multiple-choice questions.

▶ 150 of the 175 questions are part of the test and how you answer will count toward your score, 25 are included to refine questions and will not be scored. You will not know which ones count, so treat all questions the same.

▶ You will need to know how to use a mouse, scroll by either clicking arrows on the scroll bar or using the up and down arrow keys, and perform other basic computer tasks.

▶ The exam does not require computer expertise.

▶ However, if you are not comfortable with using a computer, you should practice using a mouse and computer beforehand so you do not waste time on the mechanics of using the computer.

Know what to expect during the test.

- ▶ Each ANCC test question is independent of the other questions.

  - ▹ For each case study, there is only one question. This means that a correct answer on any question does not depend on the correct answer to any other question.

  - ▹ Each question has four possible answers. There are no questions asking for combinations of correct answers (such as "a and c") or multiple-multiples.

- ▶ You can skip a question and go back to it at the end of the exam.

- ▶ You cannot mark key words in the question or right or wrong answers. If you want to do this, use the scratch paper.

- ▶ You will get your results immediately, and a grade report will be provided upon leaving the testing site.

Other Resources:

- ▶ ANCC website: www.nursecredentialing.org

- ▶ ANA website: www.nursesbooks.org. Catalog of ANA nursing scope and standards publications and other titles that may be listed on your test content outline

- ▶ National Guideline Clearinghouse—www.ngc.gov

FOUNDATIONAL ASPECTS OF THE BRAIN: NEUROLOGY, NEUROANATOMY, AND PATHOPHYSIOLOGY ACROSS THE LIFE SPAN

This chapter focuses on interesting developments related to the brain itself and provides an overview of the major structures and functions that affect optimal function and dysfunction. It begins with an overview of recent and revisited concepts in modern medicine, a review of normal and abnormal brain development, and basic neuroanatomy and physiology, and concludes with an appreciation for morphological effects and stress-diathesis (genetic) implications that contribute to mental pathophysiology. By reading this chapter, the reader will be introduced to new scientific developments that promote advanced understanding of mental illnesses and be pointed in the direction of exciting new frontiers in the field. With the rapidity of scientific developments, today's professional registered nurse is likely to witness a rapid succession of improvements in patient morbidity as it pertains to psychopathology. We must stay in the forefront by remaining committed to contributing, participating, and learning to do best for our patients, our communities, and our planet.

MOTHER OF FRANKENSTEIN AND OTHER ADVANCEMENTS IN BRAIN STUDIES

Have you ever held a cadaver human brain in your hands and wondered about who that person once was? Did you marvel at the sheer structure and construction of the lobes, hemispheres, and fissures? Did you find yourself considering what that person might have wanted or desired or achieved? How about their legacy that remains as a result of their being and purpose?

Have you ever physically or virtually visited the National Library of Medicine's (NLM) *Frankenstein* exhibit and contemplated 19-year-old Mary Shelley's (1797–1851) notion, macabre as it was at that time, of a recreated being that was sewn, woven, and electrically reconstructed from harvested body components and resurrected to some semblance of a life force? Are you aware that the NLM anoints Shelley as a predecessor, if you will, of modern-day transplantation (NLM, 2011)?

Fast-forward to contemporary times through all the transplantation developments of the modern era—in only the last 50 years—from the first heart transplant in 1967 in Cape Town, South Africa, to other visceral organs, corneas, fecal matter (to treat *C. difficile*), facial transplants, breast and buttock tissue implants, and wombs; among persons who are HIV positive; and to gender reassignment surgeries (Associated Press, 2014; Reardon, 2014). Very recently, researchers in Japan used cryopreserved testicle tissue to produce baby mice (Reuters Staff, 2014), thereby far expanding life-generating opportunities beyond those we'd already witnessed, such as test-tube babies and cloned sheep. On October 24, 2014, news radio reported the first transplantation of a nonbeating heart conducted in Sidney, Australia. Note that the one remaining organ yet to be transplanted is the human brain. Have you ever considered that this could be possible? Who would that brain recipient really be, really experience, and really become? Is this possible, plausible, ethical, or *what*? Suppose you were the nurse at the bedside holding the hand of the patient who received that first brain transplant. What would you think or say? Mary Shelley's Frankenstein creation received a brain; additionally, it was *electrically charged (shocked)* to its awakened state.

Perhaps actual transplantation is not an option. Enter the 21st century and the 2013 introduction of laboratory-generated cerebral organoids developed from human pluripotent stem cells, which had typically been derived from a skin cell (Brustle, 2013; Landau, 2013). These pea-sized structures made of human brain tissue resembling those of a 9- or 10-week embryo can help research scientists explore important questions about brain development, neuronal differentiation, and neurodevelopmental disease and disorders. These organoids are architecturally similar to the developing human cerebral cortex, which is cited as the most complex tissue in the animal kingdom. A promising possibility under consideration is investigating ways to directly implant stem cells into humans and allowing them to organize themselves.

This marvelously elusive and most complex structure is at the helm of our practice foci. It is the *organ brain* that holds the profound mysteries and answers to both functional and dysfunctional, adaptive and maladaptive states. It is with respect to its sheer awesomeness that we delve into this chapter to both consider and reconsider the workings of the organ brain and how our current understandings point to the mechanisms of becoming a person.

ADVANCING FIELDS OF STUDY

Since the 1990's "decade of the brain" era, to the 2000's focus on the "decade of behavior," contemporary scientific fields of study, such as psychoneuroimmunology (mind-nerves-immune system) and psychoneuroendocrinology (mind-nerves-endocrine system), have enhanced an appreciation for mind-body system integration. Some level of genetic and genomic competencies are expectations of every nurse at this time in our history because all diseases and conditions have a genetic or genomic component (ANA, 2009). In 2007 the entire human genome sequence was completed, leading to explosions in our understanding of disease and illness states. In 2012, the 1000 Genomes Project published the full sequence of 1092 genomes (The 1000 Genomes Project Consortium, 2012). A recently identified MTHFR gene, which provides instructions for making an enzyme that plays a role in processing amino acids and vitamin B folate chemical conversions, has been implicated as a possible risk factor for a number of medical and psychiatric disorders, including Asperger syndrome and autism (Genetics Home Reference, 2014).

What is clear is that no mental disorder can be explained by a single gene. Rather, psychopathology points to a variety of genetic and environmental factors, including newer understandings related to inflammatory responses associated with release of oxidative stress and free radicals (Nasrallal, 2014), leading to research involving treatments with NSAIDS and omega-3 fatty acids (still in development). Brain activity at the micro and macro levels are better understood with the advent of newer imaging techniques, such as functional magnetic resonance imaging (fMRI), magnetic resonance spectroscopy (MRS), and diffusion tensor imaging (DTI). These techniques permit examination of the *living* brain, far advancing the limitations that are imposed by *cadaver* brain analyses.

At present, with the release of funding to the National Institute of Mental Health (NIMH) in 2013, President Barack Obama's 10-year BRAIN Initiative (Brain Research through Advancing Innovative Neurotechnology; Chun, 2013) supports a sustained focus on developing technologies to advance brain mapping capabilities by aiming to map every neuron in the brain (http://brainfeedback.nih.gov/). The first 5 years is devoted to developing technologies to record, analyze, and manipulate the brain (BRAIN plan, 2014). The first round of funding awards for the BRAIN Initiative project went to the University of California at San Francisco and Massachusetts

BOX 2-1.
12 CRANIAL NERVES

- Olfactory
- Optic
- Oculomotor
- Trochlear

- Trigeminal
- Abducens
- Facial
- Vestibulocochlear

- Glossopharyngeal
- Vagus
- Accessory
- Hypoglossal

General Hospital in Boston (Brain grants, 2014). The early focus is on creating devices that stimulate areas deep in the brain, and recording brain activity for research on military personnel and veterans. With such high stakes insofar as designing studies that involve in vivo (live) participants, neuroscientists and expanding fields have much to consider from an ethical standpoint.

OVERVIEW: BASIC NEUROLOGY

An understanding of the implications of nerve impairment on optimal health is vital. Taken together with foundational knowledge of aspects of brain neurology, neuroanatomy, and pathophysiology, the psychiatric–mental health nurse can further appreciate the complex interplay between optimal and suboptimal functioning, thinking, behaving, and overall functioning. The neurological exam includes an assessment of reflexes, muscle strength, coordination, balance, and sensation. The functioning of the 12 cranial nerves provides critical information about intactness and proficiency of the gross levels of neurological function. The cranial nerves (Box 2–1) are examined by observing sense of smell, eye movements, strength of the temporal and masseter muscles, corneal reflexes, facial movements, gag reflex, and strength of the trapezia and sternomastoidal muscles.

OVERVIEW: NEUROANATOMY AND NEUROPHYSIOLOGY

The brain itself weighs approximately 3 pounds, has several billion neurons, and has tens of billions of neuronal interconnections. The largest part of the brain, the cerebrum, surrounds the older parts and can be compartmentalized into three basic components: the cerebral cortex, the cerebellum, and the brainstem. The cerebral cortex is the outer- and uppermost part of the brain; the cerebellum (or little brain) resides at the posterior region; and the brainstem is structurally continuous with the spinal cord. The brain, brainstem, and spinal cord are major structures of the central nervous system (CNS). The remainder of the nervous system, called the peripheral nervous system (PNS), is divided into the somatic branch, which is involved in voluntary motor movement, and the autonomic branch (ANS), which controls muscular and excretion activities of internal organs, blood vessels, and glands (endocrine and exocrine). The ANS branches into the sympathetic and parasympathetic tracts. The activation of the sympathetic branch results in increased heart rate, respiration, blood pressure, and energy mobilization, and decreased digestive and reproductive functions. The parasympathetic branch of the nervous system serves more homeostatic functions by maintaining heart rate, respiratory, metabolic, and digestive functions under normal conditions. You can think of the sympathetic division as the "action," or fight-flight mechanism, and the parasympathetic system as the restorative "resting state" mechanism. A person cannot remain in sympathetic stress indefinitely without wearing out physiologically, resulting in varying states of pathophysiology (illness) or dying. Optimal functioning occurs when a person has the opportunity to experience adequate and balanced parasympathetic restoration (relax, sleep).

OVERVIEW OF CORTEX FUNCTIONS

The cortex, or grey matter, is the outermost surface area of the brain, which lies directly below the protective cranium. Functional areas of the cortex serve distinctly different functions. Across the top from right to left (as if putting a headband on) lies the motor strip, located in the precentral gyrus. This band of brain tissue helps in coordinated movement; the tissue itself engages in cross-modal (across the outer surfaces) association (and deeper within surfaces). Injury to this area could result in movement disorders. Directly behind the motor strip lies the sensory strip, located in the postcentral gyrus. The five senses (auditory/hearing, visual/seeing, gustatory/tasting, tactile/touching, olfactory/smelling) provide perceptual cues to the world around us. Injury to this area may manifest as hallucinations (sensory/perceptual alterations), or be experienced in convulsive conditions. In the occipital cortex at the back of the head lie the primary structures responsible for visual acuity; the temporal cortex directly behind the sensory cortex houses auditory processes. The olfactory system plays a primitive role in triggering memories.

The outer surface of the brain is demarcated into two hemispheres (right and left), and four lobes (frontal, temporal, occipital, and parietal) which are present bilaterally, connected by a band of axons called the corpus callosum. Ascending and descending pathways carry information between the brain and spinal cord. The descending pathways traveling from the cerebral cortex to the spinal cord (corticospinal) cross to the opposite side in the brainstem. Thus an injury to the left frontal area of the brain may affect motor functioning on the right side of the body. Top-down neuronal transmission of impulses (stimuli) and cross-modal association facilitates the integration of perceptions, thoughts, and feelings into sensible wholes.

> **BOX 2-2.**
> **DISTURBANCES OF HIGHER-LEVEL COGNITIVE FUNCTIONING**
>
> ▸ **Dementia:** deterioration in intellectual and cognitive functions
> ▸ **Aphasia:** disruption of language function (frontal and temporal lobes)
> ▸ **Apraxia:** disturbance in the organization of voluntary action
>   (e.g., putting on one's clothes)
> ▸ **Agnosia:** disorganization of perception and recognition (parietal lobe)
> ▸ **Amnesia:** dysfunction of memory processes (temporal lobe)
> ▸ **Alogia:** disruption of expressive language ability; poverty of speech
>   (frontal and temporal lobes)

Terminology that refers to cortical impairment, evidenced by problems with higher-level executive or cognitive functioning, are listed in Box 2–2. Many psychiatric–mental health disorders (e.g., attention-deficit hyperactivity disorder, depression, schizophrenia) are characterized by deficits in executive and working memory functioning.

OVERVIEW OF FRONTAL LOBE FUNCTIONS

The foremost part of the cortex is the frontal lobe (*prefrontal cortex*), which is responsible for three major functions:

1. **Executive or higher-level cognitive functioning:** Refers to decision-making, planning, organization, and impulse control.

2. **Working memory:** Refers to an attentional system that can hold and manipulate information until it is transferred into long-term storage.

3. **Personality:** Develops over the early years as a function of the interplay between the brain and the environment. By late adolescence or early adulthood, the personality stabilizes and changes very little over the remaining life span. Because of the stability of personality, when persons do exhibit noticeable personality changes (e.g., becoming more outgoing, uninhibited, impulsive, socially withdrawn, apathetic), after a traumatic brain injury or concussion for example, we should be concerned about frontal lobe functioning and refer for further evaluation.

Frontal lobe syndrome and traumatic brain injuries (TBIs) are clinical conditions that may result from repeated trauma to the head, incurred from sporting injuries, combat injuries, or physical abuse. Personality changes, impulsivity, lack of initiative, and lack of spontaneity may manifest, as well as varied emotional or intellectual changes severe enough to cause major dysfunction. In addition, expressive speech (ability to articulate) results from functionality of *Broca's area*, the part of the inferior frontal cortex involved in the production of speech. Damage to this area can result in difficulty speaking and is referred to as *Broca's aphasia* (expressive aphasia).

OVERVIEW OF TEMPORAL LOBE FUNCTIONS

Hearing, interpreting language, learning and memory, and emotional responses are temporal lobe functions. Auditory hallucinations involve the temporal cortex, along with other structures of the brain. Located deep within the temporal cortices are important structures concerned with learning and memory. Primary auditory abilities and associated brain tissue projections integrate this experience with other forms of sensory information. Receptive aphasia (inability to interpret spoken language; failure to *receive* input as intended by speaker) may result from damage to *Wernicke's area*, the functional part of the posterior temporal cortex involved in the interpretation of language.

OVERVIEW OF PARIETAL LOBE FUNCTIONS

Light touch, pressure, pain, temperature, vibration, and proprioception (position sense); somatosensory modalities; and visual spatial processing are functions of the parietal lobe. The posterior portion of the parietal cortex helps us perceive and interpret spatial relationships, form an accurate body image, and learn tasks involving coordination of the body in space. Functions of the parietal lobes help with processing discrete elements into meaningful wholes (such as being able to make sense of a word or sentence that may have missing letters). When these areas become damaged, patients may develop sensory *agnosias*, defined as the impaired ability to interpret sensory information (e.g., identifying a key in one's pocket by touch, body image disturbances). Other examples of parietal dysfunction include graphomotor problems (e.g., difficulties with drawing a clock or copying a figure) and spatial difficulties (e.g., often after a cerebrovascular accident).

OVERVIEW OF OCCIPITAL LOBE FUNCTIONS

Visual acuity and visual interpretation from stimulation of the retina are functions of the occipital lobe. A visual agnosia is the inability to recognize objects by using sight. Visual hallucinations involve the visual cortex along with other brain structures. Damage to this lobe can cause visual problems in recognizing objects and written words or identifying colors. Integration of visual acuity with other sensory information through cross-modal association and projections provides for elaboration and synthesis of visual data into meaningful information.

BASAL GANGLIA: THE "BUNDLE OF NERVES"

Deep within the cerebrum are other important structures. The caudate (cravings originate here) and putamen brain structures together are referred to as the "striatum," which forms the *basal ganglia* or "bundle of nerves." The basal ganglia, very important nuclei for initiation of voluntary movement, are outside the descending corticospinal ("pyramidal") motor tracts and are thus considered *extrapyramidal*. They serve a critical role in movement. When we talk about *extrapyramidal symptoms* (EPS) involving unusual movements such as *bradykinesia* (slow movement) or *hyperkinesias* (fast movement such as ticks or tremors), we are referring to symptoms that reflect dysfunction of the basal ganglia. The nigrostriatal pathway is part of the extrapyramidal system that can be adversely affected by antipsychotic medication side effects. Parkinson disease is caused by destruction of dopaminergic neurons that project into the basal ganglia, resulting in impaired motor functioning. "Parkinsonism" is due to blockage of the same dopaminergic neurons by antipsychotics. Bradykinesia, hyperkinesia, and hypokinesia all suggest disease or damage to the basal ganglia.

THALAMUS: THE "RELAY STATION"

The thalamus is a structure that serves as a relay station between the spinal cord and cortex (where a stimulus may be interpreted). It transmits incoming sensory information to the relevant cortical areas. Similarly, it transmits descending motor information from the cortex to other areas of the brain and spinal cord. Together with the reticular activating system (RAS) in the brainstem, the thalamus helps modulate arousal levels.

HYPOTHALAMUS: THE "HOMEOSTASIS REGULATOR"

The hypothalamus serves as the master homeostatic center in the brain, regulating food and fluid intake, temperature, hunger, circadian rhythms, and the pituitary gland by way of the hypothalamic-pituitary-adrenal (HPA) axis system. In situations of perceived or actual stress, the hypothalamus responds with a cascading series of events triggered initially by the amygdala, affecting the ANS release of the neurotransmitter epinephrine (adrenalin).

CEREBELLUM: THE "GYROSCOPIC BALANCER"

The functions of the cerebellum include movement, balance, and posture. The cerebellum maintains equilibrium and works with the motor cortex and basal ganglia to control and refine movement. The cerebellum specializes in calculating the sequence of muscle contractions necessary to achieve goals in voluntary movement. When the cerebellum is dysfunctional, we may see uncoordinated and inaccurate movements such as a wide-based gait (*ataxia*), difficulties touching the finger to the nose, and difficulties maintaining balance with eyes closed (Romberg test).

LIMBIC SYSTEM: THE "PLEASURE CENTER"

The limbic system is a group of brain structures that includes the hippocampus and amygdala. The limbic system is important in regulating emotion and memory, which assures that we can recall the events of our lives along with their emotional tone. Disorders of emotion and memory involve the limbic structures and their connections.

HIPPOCAMPUS: THE "MEMORY CENTER"

The hippocampus is responsible for consolidating long-term explicit memories for facts and events. Chronically elevated levels of cortisol, as seen in many persons with depressive and anxiety disorders, appears to damage the hippocampus, and may be responsible for complaints related to learning and memory. Amnesia, defined as a severe loss of memory or learning, reflects injury to the hippocampus. Chronic marijuana use also may be responsible for memory impairments. Fortunately, the hippocampus is an area of the brain capable of generating new neurons (neurogenesis), so recovery may be possible.

AMYGDALA: THE "EMOTIONAL BRAIN"

The amygdala is a small structure located within the anterior medial portion of each temporal lobe that is important for detecting danger, recognizing emotions—especially negative ones— and recalling the emotional aspects of life events. This "emotional brain" is an important area to consider when excessive fears, emotions, and impulsivity are present.

RETICULAR FORMATION: THE "WAKE ACTIVATION CENTER"

The reticular formation, a part of the reticular activating system, is critical in activation of the normal sleep-wake cycle and circadian rhythm patterns.

BRAINSTEM: THE "AUTOMATIC LIFELINE"

The brainstem includes the pons (upper portion of the brainstem, which is connected to the thalamus), midbrain, and medulla (lower portion of the brainstem). Neurotransmitter-producing cell bodies are clustered in the brainstem with projections that travel to diffuse areas of the brain. Brainstem cells that produce several of the neurotransmitters (in following parentheses) associated with both functional and dysfunctional psychiatric symptoms, disorders, even some treatments include the *substantia nigra* (dopamine), *locus ceruleus* (norepinephrine), and *raphe nuclei* (serotonin). Specific neurotransmitters and their functions are discussed in a later section. The neurotransmitter pathways are essential for modulating motor control, memory, mood, motivation, and metabolic state.

The brainstem is also a major conduit for neuronal pathways that travel between the brain and periphery. The pons relays information between the cerebrum and the cerebellum. The medulla is the site of decussation (crossing over) of the descending pyramidal tracts, is continuous with the spinal cord, and contains both white and grey matter. A brain injury below the level of decussation will have noticeable effects on the same side of the injury. A brain injury above the level of decussation will result in peripheral impairments on the opposite side of the body.

GLIA: THE "GLUE"

The brain tissue consists of two distinct types of cells: glia and neurons. The glia are the supporting structures of the brain (like the glue), outnumbering neurons at a 10:1 ratio. In addition to providing support, they are important in guiding the migration of neurons during development and controlling the extracellular concentrations of potassium (K+) and other ions. Some glia, the oligodendrites, form the protective sheaths around the axons of neurons. This protective coating, myelin (i.e., myelin sheath), is what we refer to as white matter, whereas the uncoated neuronal cell bodies appear more gray and are referred to as gray matter. Astrocytes provide nutrients to glial cells and microglia cells remove waste from the glial cells.

THE NEURON: THE "MICROPROCESSOR CELL"

Though less numerous than glia, neurons are considered to be the more important "microprocessors" of the brain. Neurons are constructed of the cell body (soma) with its cytoplasm, nucleus, and mitochondria; the dendrite, which looks like tree branches and receives electrical impulses; and the axon, resembling a tree trunk, that carries the electrical impulse (stimulus) to the terminus where the stimulus is discharged or released into the synapse before journeying on to dendrites of the next neuron. Healthy axons are covered with myelin, a slick wax-like covering that insulates the axons and allows electrical signals (action potentials) to travel quickly down the axons, regenerating at small breaks (nodes of Ranvier) in the myelin until they reach the terminal ends for transmission to other cells.

Neurons are responsible for the majority of the communication among structures of the brain and among the brain and other body parts. Their exact number is unknown, but there are estimated to be some 100 billion neurons in the brain. Each neuron conducts impulses from one part of the body to another and each may receive input from 1 to 100,000 different axons. Collectively, more than 100 trillion connections interact. Neurons in the billions are also found in the heart and gut, lending credence to the adage that one can die from a broken heart, and connecting an understanding of the role that nerves play in many gastrointestinal symptoms. Each neuron receives input from tens of thousands of different other neurons. The complexity of these connections is nearly unfathomable.

Neurons look and act differently than other cells of the body. In common with most other cells, neurons contain a nucleus that contains DNA. All cell bodies also contain liquid cytoplasm that surrounds the nuclei, and organelles that produce necessary proteins (consider the condition of dehydration and its effect on cellular cytoplasm). Neurons exert their effects through the mechanisms of diffusion, enzymatic destruction, and reuptake (chemicals reabsorbed back from the synapse into the neuron).

SYNAPSE: THE "GAP" OR "SPACE"

The synapse or synaptic region is the area of space between neurons where the chemical neurotransmitter transfers an electrical signal to affect the postsynaptic region of the adjacent cell, thereby communicating an awareness, perception, or response in the person.

NEUROTRANSMITTERS: THE "CHEMICAL MESSENGERS"

The brain is an electrical and chemical organ. Once an electrical action potential reaches the neuron terminus of an axon, the release of neurotransmitters is activated. Neurotransmitters, produced in the brainstem, are chemicals synthesized by neurons and present in the presynaptic terminal. Once released at the terminal into the synapse, the chemical action potential diffuses across the synaptic cleft (small space between the neurons), and binds to and activates specific receptors at the postsynaptic cell. Each neurotransmitter has a specific mechanism for inactivation (enzymatic destruction) once it has activated the receptor and been released back into the synapse: it diffuses out of the synapse, gets reabsorbed into the terminal for recycling, or gets broken down by enzymes such as monoamine oxidase (MAO).

These chemical neurotransmitters travel throughout the brain's regions allowing for modulation of brain functions. Although more than 40 different neurotransmitters have been found to have CNS functions, the ones that we are most familiar with in psychiatric practice are the monoamines (Table 2–1). These include acetylcholine (ACh), dopamine (DA), norepinephrine (NE), epinephrine (E), histamine, and serotonin (5-HT). Additional CNS neurotransmitters

TABLE 2–1.
MONOAMINE AND AMINO ACID NEUROTRANSMITTERS AND THEIR FUNCTIONS

NEUROTRANSMITTER	PARTIAL LIST OF KNOWN FUNCTIONS
Dopamine	Attention and executive functioning, motivated behaviors (reward- and pleasure-seeking), addictions, mood, movement, psychosis
Norepinephrine	Arousal, concentration, learning and memory, mood, stress response
Epinephrine (adrenaline)	Peripheral activation and arousal, fight-or-flight response
Serotonin	Mood, anxiety, appetite, eating behavior, sleep
Acetylcholine	Arousal, cognition, memory, learning, contraction of skeletal muscle
Histamine	Immune responses, allergies
Glutamate	An excitatory neurotransmitter; most important for normal brain functioning
Glycine	Motor and sensory information processing
GABA	Calmness and relaxation; an inhibitory neurotransmitter

include glutamate, glycine, and gamma-aminobutyric acid (GABA). The monoamines and amino acid–type neurotransmitters can be produced right in the terminals where they will be used. Peptide types, such as beta endorphins, enkephalins, and substance P, work to modulate the sensation of pain. Protein neurotransmitters, such as beta-endorphins, are only produced in the cytoplasm of the nucleus and must be transported to the terminals. Other neuropeptides that affect overall performance and well-being include vasopressin, oxytocin, insulin, and cholecystokinin. Neurotransmitter effects result in an "exciting" or "inhibiting" receptor response, and their effects can be mediated by psychotropic medications.

At this point, it should be fairly easy see how optimal physiological functioning is intertwined with concepts from biochemistry, nutrition, and nervous system responses (sleep, rest, etc.).

BRAIN DEVELOPMENT

Brain development begins before birth. Optimal organogenesis emanates initially from the overall health of sperm and ova at conception. Nasrallal (2014) posits that the female infant possesses roughly 400 ova at birth for a lifetime, whereas male infants do not generate sperm until the onset of puberty. It is understood from data derived from the Human Genome Project that roughly 20,000 genes exist on the 23 pairs of chromosomes contributed by biological parents. A total of 50% of all the human genes (roughly 10,000) are dedicated to brain development or are expressed only in brain tissue. The remaining 50% (10,000) generates about 200 different types of organs and tissue components (Nasrallal, 2014). Subsequently, the health and wellness of the maternal internal and external environments during gestation plays a critical role in the optimization goal during fetal life. Paternal contribution to the developing fetus, however, is optimized with spermatogenesis at the point of conception. These preconception and conception ideas of environmental optimization are paramount to our understanding of postnatal human conditions, but are beyond the scope of this review manual. It is offered here as food for thought as we review anatomy, physiology, and pathophysiology of the postnatal brain, although there is recognition that maternal infections and other stressors during gestation may play an important role in the development of psychopathologies.

At birth, an infant weighs an average of only 7 pounds, yet the head is approximately one-third the size of the entire body. Even though the brain is relatively large compared to the body, it continues to develop. With the help of glial cells and growth factors, neurons continue to migrate to their terminal sites within the frontal lobes, making connections with other neurons and laying down the structures that will guide executive functioning and self-regulation. The concept of neuroplasticity refers to the ability of neural pathways and synapses in the brain to adapt to changing stimuli. Neurogenesis is the process of new brain cell generation, which takes place at the rate of approximately 700 a day (Nasrallal, 2014). Neurogenesis occurs in areas of the hippocampus. The brain continues to develop up to approximately age 25.

With aging, neuroplasticity continues providing evidence that learning, growth, and adaptation can still occur. Therefore, although processing may have slowed, we expect that older adults will maintain their viability and zest for learning. With aging we expect a general decline in the brain's physical dimensions as well as most physical systems, which can ultimately give rise to some of the psychopathology evident among elder groups. In certain neurodegenerative disorders, such as dementia, the primitive reflexes may return.

Throughout our lives, neuronal synapses are modified, solidifying memories or causing them to be forgotten. Complex mechanisms of apoptosis (appropriate cell death and elimination), neurogenesis (new neurons created in hippocampus), and neurotropic factors (specific growth and nutritional chemicals) operate in the healthy and adapting person. New neurons continue to be created in the area of the brain involved in consolidating long-term memories. Terms such as *neuroadaptation* and *neuroplasticity* describe the dynamic relationship between nature and nurture—between the brain and the environment. We have the capacity to adapt, grow, thrive, and survive. *Neurodegeneration* is an umbrella term that refers to the progressive loss of the structure and functions of neurons.

The objectives of learning basic neuroanatomy, neurophysiology, normal neuronal development, and neurodegeneration (i.e., psychopathology) include gaining an ability to identify basic structures and functions within the nervous system, identifying neurotransmitter systems that are involved in psychiatric symptoms and disorders, and understanding the rationale for selected psychopharmacological interventions that target organ brain. By knowing the basic functions of the major lobes and structures of the brain, we can understand many of the behaviors and symptoms of psychiatric and mental health disorders (National Institute of Mental Health [NIMH], 2012).

BRAIN PATHOLOGY

Pathophysiology is the disruption of normal physiological functioning that accompanies a particular syndrome or disorder. Several major theories exist regarding brain pathophysiology and its expression in selected mental disorders throughout the life span. The pathophysiology of each of the mental disorders results from some type of alteration in brain function. However, no one risk factor alone is responsible for the development of a clinically diagnosable mental disorder (Nasrallal, 2014). Rather, multiple risk factors contribute to the emergence of the disorder, with some risk factors being potentiated and others being synergistic. The average age of onset of all the adult psychiatric disorders is early adulthood; however, prodromal manifestations of some disorders may manifest in infancy, and even perhaps in utero.

Cadaver brain examination reveals neurodevelopmental anomalies, such as excessively pruned dendrites, structural or morphological atrophy, and migrational deficits that may have occurred during chromosomal strand separation and reintegration. These anomalies have cascading effects insofar as overall neurodegeneration, neuroexcitability, or neuronal inhibition.

> **BOX 2-3.**
> **HERITABILITY OF MENTAL DISORDERS**
>
> **Highest heritability**
> ▸ Schizophrenia (82%–84%) (Kendler, 2001)
> ▸ Bipolar disorder (85%–89%) (McGuffin, Rijsdijk, Andrew, Sham, Katz, & Cardno, 2003)
>
> **Medium heritability**
> ▸ Alcoholism (52%–58%) (Kendler, 2001)
>
> **Lowest heritability**
> ▸ Anxiety disorders (37%–43%) (Kendler, 2001)
> ▸ Major depression (29%–42%) (Kendler, Gatz, Gardner, & Pedersen, 2006)

GENETICS AND STRESS-DIATHESIS THEORY OF PSYCHOPATHOLOGY

The two-hit hypothesis of psychopathology cites two major factors in the etiology of mental and psychiatric disorders: (1) genetic vulnerabilities and (2) environmental stressors. Stress, itself, may trigger the production of abnormal genes, gene products, or gene expressions. Environmental stressors can be physical (e.g., viruses, other infections), or psychosocial (e.g., trauma-informed, abuse-related).

The heritability of mental disorders ranges from a low 29% for depression to as high as 89% for bipolar disorder (Box 2–3), which suggests that each mental disorder is probably associated with a number of vulnerable genes. Whether the genes that result in symptoms of mental illness will actually be outwardly expressed may depend upon environmental factors. The stress-diathesis theory of mental disorders describes contributions of genetics (diathesis) and environment (stress). The term *diathesis* describes the tendency, vulnerability, or predisposition toward psychiatric symptoms based upon genetics. Stress, in this context, refers to environmental contributions.

STRESS AND ORGAN BRAIN: THE HPA AXIS

Mental disorders are frequently comorbid with other psychopathologies. Examples include depression and anxiety (Stahl, 2008); eating disorders and depression (Stahl, 2008); and dementia and depression, anxiety, or psychosis (Kverno et al., 2008). According to the National Institute on Drug Abuse (2010), patients with mood or anxiety disorders are about twice as likely as those who do not to also suffer from a drug use disorder. The highest comorbidity appears to be with mania, with nearly 40% of affected persons having a lifetime prevalence of a co-occurring drug use disorder.

FIGURE 2–1.
HPA AXIS

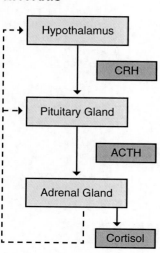

The detection of threat by the amygdala triggers the hypothalamus to set off the stress response. The stress response involves two different major pathways: the ANS and the hypothalamic-pituitary-adrenal axis (HPA axis). Activation of the ANS leads to the release of peripheral epinephrine (also called adrenalin) from the adrenal medulla. Epinephrine increases the heart rate and blood pressure and prepares us to escape the perceived danger. This response, often called the *fight-or-flight* response, is frequently accompanied by fright or anxiety. Hans Selye (1956), in his general adaptation syndrome theory, describes the *alarm, resistance, and exhaustion* stages. Activation of the fight-or-flight response is referred to as the *alarm* stage. If the stressor can be resolved, the alarm response subsides. If not resolved, the *resistance* stage is the body's continuing attempts to adapt. If adaptation fails, the eventual outcome is the stage of *exhaustion* and illness or death.

A second stress mechanism is the HPA axis (Figure 2–1). The hypothalamus releases corticotrophin-releasing hormone (CRH), which triggers the pituitary gland to produce adrenocorticotropic hormone (ACTH). ACTH stimulates the adrenal glands (on top of the kidneys) to release cortisol. Cortisol works more slowly to increase the use of glucose and decrease inflammation—both important for dealing with acute stressors. If all goes well, active coping leads to a resolution of the stressor. If the stressor is not resolved, wear and tear on the body increases with continued cortisol secretion and risk for hyperglycemia, hyperinsulinemia, hypertension, hypercholesterolemia, and eventually arteriosclerosis. A chronically elevated level of serum cortisol is a biomarker for stress. The hippocampus is particularly sensitive to cortisol, and may experience atrophy with resultant memory problems. These conditions are adaptation attempts equated with Selye's *resistance* stage.

Although the stress response is protective and adaptive, chronic activation causes increasing wear and tear on the body and eventual pathophysiology (*exhaustion* and illness or death stage) may ensue. Vulnerabilities, such as early life stressors including fetal distress, childhood trauma or neglect, significant loss, and possibly viruses or toxins, are important environmental contributors to mental disorders. Parental behaviors that might contribute to the risk for mental disorders in their offspring include poor parent–child bonding and engagement, starvation, poor nutrition, lack of vitamin D, and substance abuse.

For persons with strong genetic predispositions to develop a mental condition, it may not take much of a stressor to trigger the expression of the condition. Schizophrenia and bipolar disorder, we have seen, are the most heritable of the mental disorders. For persons who are less vulnerable to mental disorders, it may take a larger number or greater intensity of stressors to trigger the onset. Some disorders, such as posttraumatic stress disorder (PTSD) and phobias, may be triggered by exposure to extreme stress in persons with otherwise little vulnerability.

What if a pregnancy was unwanted? How might that condition transfer to the unborn child? Theories suggest that preconception health-wellness states of both mother and father may be important factors in the expression of mental illness in offspring. Can you apply these biochemical underpinnings of cortisol excessiveness to the experiences of persons who may have experienced anxiety *in utero* while gestating for 9 months during fetal periods? What of chronically violated children or adults, or those living in homeless environments? What might be the potential effects of cortisol excess on physical, emotional, and spiritual development? Do you think persons exposed to such conditions can function optimally or adequately? In some cases, yes, but how long can resistance mechanisms hold out before the human organism would succumb, exhaust, and die?

On a more positive note, how might we harness enhanced improvements in modern technology, medical science, and nursing care to foster greater resilience and hardiness for succeeding generations? For starters, let's continue to be open to learning and supporting critical advancements that hold promise for greater new beginnings and better health and well-being for all.

REFERENCES

American Nurses Association. (2009). *Essentials of genetic and genomic nursing: Competencies, curricula guidelines, and outcome indicators,* 2nd ed. Silver Spring, MD: American Nurses Association.

Associated Press. (2014). First womb-transplant baby won't be alone for long. *Winston-Salem Journal.* Retrieved from http://www.journalnow.com/eedition/mapping/first-womb-transplant-baby-won-t-be-alone-for-long/article_e265405b-2af4-55e6-a474-20ea62cb0f13.html

BRAIN grants. (2014). Seven days: 30 May–5 June 2014: Funding. *Nature, 510*(7503), 13.

BRAIN plan. (2014). Seven days: 6–12 June 2014: Policy. *Nature, 510*(7504), 193.

Brustle, O. (2013). Miniature human brains. *Nature, 501,* 319–320.

Chun, M. (2013). Straight talk with Miyoung Chan. *Nature Medicine, 19*(4), 387.

Genetics Home Reference. (2014). *Genes: MTHFR: methylenetetrahydrofolate reductase (NAD(P)H).* Retrieved from http://ghr.nlm.nih.gov/gene/MTHFR.

Kendler, K. (2001). Twin studies of psychiatric illness. Archives of General Psychiatry, 58, 1005–1014.

Kendler, K., Gatz, M., Gardner, C., & Pedersen, N. (2006). A Swedish national twin study of lifetime major depression. *American Journal of Psychiatry, 163*(1), 109–114.

Kverno, K., Rabins, P., Blass, D., Hicks, K., & Black, B. (2008). Prevalence and treatment of neuropsychiatric symptoms in hospice-eligible nursing home residents with advanced dementia. *Journal of Gerontological Nursing, 34*(12), 8–15.

Landau, E. (2013). Scientists grow mini brain from cells. *CNN U.S. Edition.* Retrieved from http://www.cnn.com/2013/08/28/health/stem-cell-brain/.

McGuffin, P., Rijsdijk, F., Andrew, M., Sham, P., Katz, R., & Cardno, A. (2003). The heritability of bipolar affective disorder and the genetic relationship to unipolar depression. *Archives of General Psychiatry, 60*(5), 497–502.

Nasrallal, H. A., & Weiden, P. J., (2014). *Psych forum: Paradigm shifts in the biology, diagnosis, and treatment of schizophrenia.* Retrieved from http://www.medscape.org/viewarticle/830903.

National Library of Medicine. (2011). *Frankenstein: Penetrating the secrets of nature.* Retrieved from http://www.nlm.nih.gov/exhibition/frankenstein/index.html.

National Institute of Mental Health. (2012). *Brain basics.* Retrieved from http://www.nimh.nih.gov/educational-resources/brain-basics/brain-basics.shtml.

National Institute on Drug Abuse. (2010). Why do drug use disorders often co-occur with other mental illnesses? *Comorbidity: Addiction and other mental illnesses.* Retrieved from http://www.drugabuse.gov/publications/comorbidity-addiction-other-mental-illnesses/why-do-drug-use-disorders-often-co-occur-other-mental-illnesses.

Reardon, S. (2014). Hopeful act: A rebel transplants organs from HIV-positive donors. *Nature Medicine, 20*(10); 1086–1088.

Reuters Staff. (2014). News & perspective: Cryopreserved testicle tissue used to produce baby mice. *Medscape.* Retrieved from http://www.medscape.com/viewarticle/827650.

Selye, H. (1956). *The stress of life.* New York: McGraw-Hill.

Stahl, S. (2008). *Stahl's essential psychopharmacology: Neuroscientific basis and practical applications.* New York: Cambridge University Press.

The 1000 Genomes Project Consortium. (2012). An integrated map of genetic variation from 1,092 human genomes. *Nature, 491,* 56–65. Retrieved from (http://www.nature.com/nature/journal/v491/n7422/full/, nature11632.html.

CATEGORY I

ASSESSMENT, DIAGNOSIS, AND PLANNING

ASSESSMENTS ACROSS THE LIFE SPAN: PHYSICAL, DEVELOPMENTAL, EMOTIONAL, MORAL, AND PSYCHOSOCIAL

This chapter compiles assessments across multiple health and wellness dimensions used by the psychiatric–mental health nurse to ensure that essential and accurate information about patient needs and strengths is obtained. The professional registered nurse considers the whole person to identify opportunities for health restoration, maintenance, growth, and adaptation. Clinical skills and tools that address physiological concerns and contributions from major psychosocial theorists are delineated.

BASIC COMPETENCIES AND PERFORMANCE SKILLS OF PSYCHIATRIC AND MENTAL HEALTH NURSES

As the most trusted healthcare provider ranked by the U.S. public (Riffkin, 2014), nurses have, and will continue to hold this distinction. "Psychiatric–mental health nursing is the nursing practice specialty committed to promoting mental health through the assessment, diagnosis, and treatment of behavioral problems, mental disorders, and comorbid conditions across the life span. Psychiatric–mental health nursing intervention is an art and a science, employing a purposeful use of self and a wide range of nursing, psychosocial, and neurobiological evidence to produce effective outcomes" (ANA, APNA, ISPN, 2014).

Basic nursing practice in the specialized area of psychiatric–mental health nursing includes the following targeted nursing tasks:

▶ Assessing mental health issues and symptoms of mental disorders, as well as the whole person (physiological, medical, spiritual, cultural, social) in diverse settings

▶ Promoting patient self-care and safety from dangerousness to self and others

▶ Using interventions to foster and promote optimal mental health

▶ Assisting patients in regaining or improving their coping abilities, and with self-care skills and activities

▶ Psychiatric rehabilitation to maximize patient strengths and prevent further disability

▶ Delivering culturally competent care

▶ Administering and monitoring psychobiological treatment regimens (e.g., prescribed psychopharmacological medications and their therapeutic, side, and adverse effects)

▶ Assisting, promoting, and monitoring patients in self-care activities

▶ Case management, counseling, and crisis care

▶ Health maintenance and health promotion

▶ Health teaching and psycho-education about coping and prevention

▶ Intake screening, assessment and evaluation of mental health symptoms, and triage

▶ Milieu therapy (providing a therapeutic environment)

▶ Communicating therapeutically

▶ Providing psycho-educational groups

▶ Providing family-centered care

▶ Collaboration with the healthcare team

▶ Engaging in professional behaviors (continuing education, ethics, research, quality initiatives)

▶ Working to decrease stigma, discrimination, and criminalization of persons with mental health problems

INTRODUCTION TO THE *SCOPE AND STANDARDS OF PSYCHIATRIC–MENTAL HEALTH NURSING PRACTICE*

The essentials of psychiatric and mental health nursing, its activities, and its accountabilities are articulated in the second edition of the *Scope and Standards of Practice: Psychiatric–Mental Health Nursing* (American Nurses Association [ANA], 2014). Psychiatric and mental health nursing is defined as "a specialized area of nursing practice committed to promoting mental health through the assessment, diagnosis, and treatment of human responses to mental health problems and psychiatric disorders" (p. 14). The *Scope and Standards* directs nursing care and delivery across six distinct practice steps and nine professional performance standards. Six nursing process practice steps for the psychiatric–mental health nurse are described in the first part of this text (Categories I and II) with eight implementation-related subsets (5a through 5h). Ten professional performance standards are covered in the latter half of this text (Categories III and IV).

The six steps of the nursing process:

1. Assessment

2. Diagnosis (nursing)

3. Outcomes identification

4. Planning

5. Implementation

6. Evaluation

PMH PRACTICE STANDARD 1. ASSESSMENT

An assessment is a systematic and continuous collection of data about the overall health of a person. The primary sources of the data are compiled from the patient interview, direct observation, labs, and other test results. Secondary sources for collateral information may include family members, other members of the healthcare team, pharmacists, employee assistance program records, emergency medical teams, law enforcement agents, supervisors, medical record reviews, caregivers, or other involved persons (e.g., school personnel and reports). Previous medical records and discharge summaries provide essential information that can point out previous events and interventions. Psychiatric–mental health nurses lend essential support to interprofessionals in comprehensive assessment data collection.

Assessment data incorporate information about the patient's past and present physical, developmental, psychological, emotional, cognitive, spiritual, interpersonal, and moral domains. Collection is systematic and continuous. Assessment data are derived through interviewing skills that seek answers to questions that may appear of a personal nature and not relative to that patient complaint or patient perception of his or her problem. It is critical that the psychiatric–mental health nurse develop therapeutic communication skills and comfort in identifying and addressing what the patient problem is; where the problem occurs (location); when the problem occurs; what triggers the problem; and what happens to the problem when something, or nothing, is done to alleviate it.

In the initial physical examination interview, we simply use open communication strategies and ask about any bothersome symptoms: "How is your (or your child's)_____?" and "What brings you here today?" Data are collected and information is documented as it pertains to

- ▶ Biographical information
    - ▹ Name
    - ▹ Age, date of birth
    - ▹ Reason for seeking health care
    - ▹ Allergies, medications, and reactions
    - ▹ Sexual orientation or preference and gender identity (LGBTQI—lesbian, gay, bisexual, transgender, queer or questioning, intersex); "Do you have sex with men, women, or both?"
    - ▹ Culture and ethnicity: "How do you identify yourself?"
- ▶ Developmental history
    - ▹ Growth and development (congenital anomalies, complications in pregnancy, milestones)
- ▶ Current medical status and history
    - ▹ Physical and neurological examination (abdominal girth, height, weight, body mass index [BMI], level of consciousness, reflexes)
    - ▹ Review of systems (ROS): head to toe; complete integumentary (skin) and pressure ulcer assessment
    - ▹ Vital signs, lab values (chemistries and electrolytes, basic metabolic rates), radiological study results (fMRI, MRI, PET scans, CT scans, DTI, MRS; see Box 3–1 for definitions)
    - ▹ Previous psychiatric episodes and treatments
    - ▹ Previous medical symptoms or illnesses and treatments
    - ▹ Current medication regimen

- ▸ Pregnancy
- ▸ Nutritional status (body mass index [BMI])
- ▸ Sleep or rest quality
- ▸ Genetic studies and results
- ▸ Recent travel outside of United States

▶ Emotional, spiritual, and psychosocial status

- ▸ Sociocultural and occupational history
- ▸ Baseline Mental Status Exam, Mini-Mental Status Exam, functional status
- ▸ Strengths and competencies
- ▸ Ability to remain safe and refrain from harming others
- ▸ Motivation, coping responses
- ▸ Relationships, spiritual beliefs, and values
- ▸ History of substance use (including tobacco: what, when last used, how much)
- ▸ Health beliefs and values

▶ Screening results

- ▸ Risk factors: falls, pain, violence and aggression, suicidal (S/I) or homicidal (H/I) ideation
- ▸ Abuse: physical, mental, domestic, sexual, emotional

▶ Diagnoses (medical and psychiatric); general functioning (impression)

▶ End-of-life and advance directives

BOX 3-1.
RADIOLOGICAL STUDIES

- ▶ **fMRI** = Functional magnetic resonance imaging measures and maps brain activity with magnetic and radio wave technology to calculate the level of oxygen uptake.

- ▶ **MRI** = Magnetic resonance imaging uses magnetic wave technology of water molecules' hydrogen nuclei to create images of brain structure.

- ▶ **PET scan** = Positron emission tomography uses nuclear medicine to produce a 3D picture and provide metabolic information.

- ▶ **CT scan** = Computer tomography provides detailed images of bony structures and some detail of soft tissue.

- ▶ **DTI** = Diffuse tensor imaging shows white matter (myelin) changes in living brains.

- ▶ **MRS** = Magnetic resonance spectroscopy provides a kind of "chemical biopsy analysis" of sections in living brains.

Components of the Physical Examination and Review of Systems (ROS)

A physical exam is routinely completed within 24 hours of admission to an inpatient psychiatric hospital or care facility. It generally proceeds from head to toe with techniques of auscultation (listening), inspection (observation), palpation (touch), and percussion (tapping). The physical examination is important to establish baseline functionality, particularly before starting any psychopharmalogic intervention. It is essential that the psychiatric–mental health nurse review all test results, the health history, and physical examination findings obtained from collaborating healthcare providers to develop an appropriate and comprehensive nursing plan of care.

While conducting a physical exam and review of systems it is important to be aware of potential medication side effects that may cloud the patient's current presentation. Abnormal findings, if present, should be evaluated in more detail to determine whether they could be contributing to psychiatric symptoms, side effects from medication, or caused by something else. The ROS documents the presence or absence of findings for each major body system (Table 3–1).

Overall level of consciousness must be assessed and monitored because the patient's consciousness and awareness responses can fluctuate. The Glasgow Coma Scale provides a standardized measure that rates eye movement, responses to painful stimuli, and verbal responses from higher numbers (more awareness and responsiveness) to lower numbers (less awareness and responsiveness). Table 3–2 displays descriptors and the scoring mechanism for the Glasgow Coma Scale (Teasdale & Jennett, 1974).

TABLE 3–1.
REVIEW OF SYSTEMS (ROS)

Neurological: cranial nerves, reflexes, sensorium, level of consciousness
Cardiovascular: vital signs, rates, rhythms, vasculature, distention
Respiratory: thorax and lungs, head and neck, hearing and vision
Hematologic: serology and chemistry
Endocrine: breasts, menarche, glands, and hormonal functions
Gastrointestinal: height, weight, BMI, appetite and nutrition, elimination, abdominal girth and sounds
Genitourinary: elimination, genitalia, reproductive organs, Tanner stage
Integumentary: temperature, flushing, tone, rash, skin, hair, nails, and evidence of lesions or bruises
Musculoskeletal: muscular tone, strength, movement, fractures, curvatures, assistive devices, pain, range of motion, gait
Immunologic: immunization status

TABLE 3–2.
LEVEL OF CONSCIOUSNESS: GLASCOW COMA SCALE

Eyes Open	Spontaneously	4
	To verbal command	3
	To pain	2
	No response	1
Command or Pain	Obeys	6
	Localizes pain	5
	Flexion: withdrawal	4
	Flexion: abnormal (decorticate rigidity)	3
	Extension (decerebrate rigidity)	2
	No response	1
Verbal Response	Oriented and converses	5
	Disoriented and converses	4
	Inappropriate words	3
	Incomprehensible sounds	2
	No response	1
TOTAL		

CRITICAL ASSESSMENT PRIORITY AREAS

Clinical Standardized (Evidence-Based) Measures: Vital Signs and Laboratory Values

Many physical imbalances or impairments can be misconstrued as symptoms of mental disorders, and vice versa. It is crucial that the psychiatric–mental health nurse recognize normal ranges for standardized measures such as vital signs and basic serum and urine chemistries. Baseline measures provide an opportunity to determine, biophysically, where the patient is at the time of collection. It provides a measure for targeting interventions that promote outcomes that return to within normal ranges.

Several factors contribute to changes in vital signs. Clinical states of anxiety or intoxication while on central nervous system stimulants result in blood pressure, pulse, and respiratory rate elevations, whereas intoxication on central nervous system depressants (e.g., narcotics) has the opposite effect. Basic clinical laboratory tests provide information to support prevention, diagnosis, or treatment of a disorder, disease, or impairment and are also used for the assessment of overall health. Specific tests may be ordered to rule out alcohol or drug abuse or other medical disorders and are critical indices to examine before confirming a psychiatric or mental illness diagnosis.

TABLE 3-3.
NORMAL RANGES: VITAL SIGNS AND CLINICAL LABS

VITAL SIGNS	LAB VALUES (FASTING)
Temperature ▸ Oral: 37° C (98.6° F) **Pulse rate (beats/min)** ▸ Infant: 120–160 ▸ Child: 75–100 ▸ Adolescent: 60–90 ▸ Adult: 60–100 **Blood pressure (mm Hg)** ▸ 1 yr: 95/65 ▸ 10 yrs: 110/65 ▸ Adolescent: 120/75 ▸ Adult: 120/80 ▸ Older Adult (over age 60): 150/90 **Respiratory rate (breaths/min)** ▸ 6 mos: 30–50 ▸ 2 yrs: 25–32 ▸ Child: 20–30 ▸ Adolescent: 16–19 ▸ Adult: 12–20	**Electrolytes (blood chemistry and basic metabolic profiles)** ▸ Na+ (sodium) 135–145mEq/L ▸ K+ (potassium) 3.5–5.1mEq/L ▸ Cl (chloride) 98–106mEq/L ▸ Mg+ (magnesium) 1.3–2.1mEq/L ▸ Ca+ (calcium; measure of parathyroid function) 8.8–10.5mg/dL **Total white blood cells with differential (neutrophils [granulocyte], eosinophils [granulocyte], basophils [granulocyte], lymphocytes [nongranulocyte], monocytes [nongranulocyte])** ▸ WBC: 4,500–10,500/mcL ▸ Agranulocytosis: WBC <2,000/mcL **Total red blood cell (RBC) counts** ▸ Male: 4.7 to 6.1 million/mcL ▸ Female: 4.2 to 5.4 million/mcL **Hemoglobin (Hgb)** ▸ Male: 12–17g/dL ▸ Female: 11–15g/dL **Hematocrit (Hct)** ▸ Male: 40%–50% ▸ Female: 37%–47% **Platelets (thrombocytes)** ▸ 150,000–400,000/mm³ **Thyroid function studies (TFS)** ▸ TSH: 2–10mIU/L **Liver function tests (LFT)** ▸ ALT (SGOT): 5–35U/L ▸ AST (SGPT): 5–40U/L ▸ Bilirubin: 0.1–1.2mg/dL **Kidney function** ▸ Creatinine clearance (CrCL: 0.5–1.5mg/dL ▸ BUN (elevated in renal disease): 5–26mg/dL **Glucose** ▸ 70–115mg/dL **HbA1C** ▸ < 5.7% **Nutrition** ▸ Serum albumin 2.6g/dL

Additional labs may include genetic testing,* therapeutic drug medication levels (lithium, valproate acid [Depakote], carbamazepine [Tegretol]), drug toxicology, T-cell levels, pregnancy, and virology.

*The MTHFR gene mutation has been identified in some persons with autism and Asperger syndrome.

Potter & Perry, 2009; James et al., 2014.

TABLE 3-4.
OVERVIEW OF PHYSICAL FINDINGS RELATED TO MENTAL DISORDERS OR TREATMENTS AND POSSIBLE ETIOLOGIES

FUNCTIONAL SYSTEM	SYMPTOMS	POSSIBLE MECHANISM
Head	Progressively severe headache (potentially affecting eyes and vision)	Hypertensive crisis due to ingested tyramine interacting with monoamine oxidase inhibitors (MAOIs)
Eyes (vision)	Nystagmus	Substance intoxication, brain lesions
	Oculogyric crisis	Neuroleptic-induced dystonia
Ears (hearing)	Diminished hearing	Poor hearing acuity may be misinterpreted as cognitive impairment in older adults
Throat and neck	High fever and sore throat	Agranulocytosis (greatest risk with clozapine [Clozaril])
	Thyroid enlargement (goiter)	Hypothyroidism
Respiratory system	Anxiety	Hyperventilation, asthma, shortness of breath
Integumentary system	Rash	Possible allergic reaction
		Risk for Stevens-Johnson syndrome (toxic epidermal necrolysis) if on lamotrigine (Lamictal)
Neurological system	Tremors	Lithium: fine-motor
		Parkinson's disease: slow-resting
		Anticonvulsants: fine-motor
	Gait and balance disturbances	Encephalopathy, intoxication, cerebellar injuries
	Disorientation, confusion	Delirium, anticholinergic toxicity, serotonin syndrome
	Weakness, numbness	Cerebrovascular events, electrolyte imbalances
	Anxiety	Drug intoxication or withdrawal, stimulants, seizures
Cardiovascular system	ECG changes	Tricyclics, anticholinergics, some antipsychotics (e.g., ziprasidone [Geodon])
	Orthostatic hypotension	Tricyclics, antipsychotics, antihypertensives
	Tachycardia	Anxiety, stimulants, anorexia
	Hypertension	Antipsychotics (metabolic syndrome)
		MAOI-induced hypertensive crisis
	Bradycardia	Beta-blockers, anorexia, Parkinson's disease
	Anxiety	Angina, congestive heart failure, mitral valve prolapse, tachycardia
	Hypercholesterolemia Hyperlipidemia	Antipsychotics (metabolic syndrome)

(CONTINUED)

TABLE 3-4.
CONTINUED

FUNCTIONAL SYSTEM	SYMPTOMS	POSSIBLE MECHANISM
Gastrointestinal (GI) system	GI distress, nausea	Lithium: recommend taking with food SSRIs: especially early in treatment
Endocrine system	Abnormal glucose metabolism	Antipsychotics (metabolic syndrome)
	Hyperprolactinemia	Antipsychotic dopaminergic blockade
	Depression	Hypothyroidism, chronically elevated cortisol (prolonged stress response)
	Anxiety	Hyperthyroidism, hypoglycemia, premenstrual syndrome
Genitourinary system	Polyuria, polydipsia	Lithium Renal disease or drugs that reduce renal clearance (e.g., NSAIDs) may increase serum concentration of drugs that are excreted by the kidneys (e.g., lithium)
	Unusual pattern of bruises or trauma	Rule out sexual or physical abuse
	Sexual dysfunction	Can be side effect of antihypertensives, antidepressants, antihistamines, or antispasmodics
	Delirium	Kidney failure Liver failure
Musculoskeletal System	Body asymmetry	Dystonias (muscle spasms as a result of Parkinsonian side effects), CVAs, lesions
	Abnormal movements: dyskinesia, dystonia, bradykinesia, akathisia	Parkinson's disease and Parkinsonism related to antipsychotic extrapyramidal side effects (EPS)
	Gait disturbances	Cerebellar dysfunction such as seen with alcoholic encephalopathy (Wernicke's disease), substance use disorders
	Swallowing problems	Parkinson's disease, advanced dementia, antipsychotic-induced dystonias
Hematological system	Easy or excessive bruising	Thrombocytopenia secondary to anticonvulsants (e.g., divalproex sodium [Depakote])

Physiological conditions that can occur as a result of psychiatric–mental health disorders or psychotropic medication use appear in Table 3–4. Regardless of the cause, many symptoms can be treated, so it is important for the nurse to identify and refer patients for a more complete physical examination or for follow-up if any abnormal physical symptoms become evident.

SUICIDE RISK ASSESSMENT

Suicide is a public health problem that is the fourth leading cause of death among persons 15 to 24, the second among those 25 to 34, the fourth among persons aged 35 to 54, and the eigth among persons 55 to 64 years (CDC, 2012c). Rates are higher among lesbian, gay, bisexual, and transgender (LGBT) youth than among non-LGBT youth. White men have highest risk, followed by Native Americans and Alaskan Natives; firearms are implicated in more than 50% of all cases. Additionally, veterans returning from deployment are identified as a highly at-risk population.

Every patient in psychiatric care must be screened for suicide risk. A critical role for the nurse is to conduct a thorough assessment to enter a clinical judgment for categorizing a patient as high, moderate, or low risk. This determination is based on the patient's overall risk factors, illness acuity, and requirement for safety implementations. If a patient acknowledges having thoughts of harming him- or herself or others, the nurse must assess the level of lethality. Lethality assessments include assessing the intent to die, severity of the ideation, availability of means, and degree of planning. If the patient appears to be acutely suicidal, immediate action is required, including hospitalization, removal of all potentially dangerous objects, and one-on-one observation. This lethality risk screening is ongoing, particularly for those who have expressed ideation and have a plan and the means to carry out the act. Additional factors may include

- ▶ Past and present suicidal ideation,
- ▶ Plan in place,
- ▶ Means available (has firearms, other weapons, ropes, strings, etc),
- ▶ Previous attempt, history of abuse or neglect,
- ▶ History of depression or other mental illness,
- ▶ Alcohol or drug abuse,
- ▶ Family history of suicide or violence; abuse or neglect,
- ▶ Physical illness,
- ▶ Feeling alone,
- ▶ Hopelessness,
- ▶ History of, or current, impulsivity,
- ▶ Depressed mood,
- ▶ Recent significant losses; poor social support; difficult home life; parental rejection or hostility,
- ▶ Population group risk factors, and
- ▶ Evidence of psychosis.

No-suicide contracts that require the at-risk patient to commit to not harming him- or herself are often included in in-patient (Shives, 2012) and outpatient care, but the evidence for their efficacy in preventing suicides is weak. Nurses should never rely on them as evidence-based implementations. Hospital policy determines the protocol for reducing the level of observation as a patient's suicide risk decreases. Generally:

▶ **High risk:** Requires continuous 1-to-1 observation between the patient and staff. This patient has a highly lethal plan with actual or potential access; is a high elopement risk; has constant suicidal ideation with a history of past attempts; is unwilling to contract for safety; voices hopelessness.

▶ **Moderate risk:** Requires check every 15 minutes. This patient is ambivalent; has plan, but no access; is a low elopement risk; may have intermittent suicidal ideation, past attempts of low lethality.

▶ **Low risk:** No precautions required; patient has no plan; 0 to 2 symptoms; rare suicidal ideation.

VIOLENCE AND ASSAULT RISK ASSESSMENT

Homicide is the second leading cause of death among 15- to 24-year-olds, and is the leading cause among 10- to 24-year-old black males; second for Native American and Alaskan Natives; third among Hispanics (Minino, 2010). Youth violence is a major public health concern. Violence toward others includes threats (verbal) and acts (physical) directed toward people, animals, or the environment. Intimate partner violence is a cyclical syndrome involving verbal threats, emotional abuse, and physical and sexual abuse. It is a negative function or destructive use of anger that is designed to punish, cause pain, and ignore the rights of others. Although people of any age can be abused, children age 4 or younger are the most vulnerable. Child abuse includes physical, sexual, and emotional abuse, and neglect.

Abuse, assault, and aggression are used to dominate, manipulate, intimidate, or control a more vulnerable other. Domestic or partner violence is the leading cause of injury to women aged 15 to 44. This age correlates to a woman's reproductive period and pregnancy itself may be a risk factor for violence perpetrated towards a woman. The perpetrator's desire to exhibit power and control can often be hidden from society. Many times, the victims are scared silent.

Basic screening assessment includes identifying past history of violence and abuse, and evidence of legal or forensic charges, which are predictors for current experience. Risk factors for perpetrators of violence and abuse include the following:

▶ Psychological

  ▸ Severe emotional deprivation or overt rejection in childhood, or parental seduction

  ▸ Exposure to violence in formative years

  ▸ Families with histories of violence, drug abuse, poverty, chronic health problems, or lack of social support

  ▸ Adults with poor boundaries

  ▸ Adults who "groom" youngsters, preying on their developmental needs for attention, support; vulnerabilities associated with desires to access material things

▶ Physiological

  ▸ Brain damage, intellectual disability, learning disabilities that impair capacity to cope with frustration

  ▸ Abuse of alcohol or other disinhibiting substances

▶ Sociocultural

  ▸ Lack of interpersonal ties

  ▸ Poor boundaries with others

  ▸ Inadequate bonding or attachments with significant others

  ▸ Learned behaviors

▶ Behavioral history

  ▸ Childhood cruelty to animals or children

  ▸ Fire-setting or similar dangerous actions (pyromania)

  ▸ Recent violent behavior toward self or others

  ▸ Recent accidents, threats, poor judgment in potentially dangerous situations

▶ Observable behavior and emotional responses

  ▸ Escalating irritability, sensitivity, or hostility

  ▸ Altered states of consciousness, substance abuse

  ▸ Emotions: severe anger (rage) or fear (panic)

  ▸ Active psychotic symptoms with paranoid ideation

DOMESTIC, PARTNER, AND INTIMATE ABUSE, ASSAULT, AND VIOLENCE

As nurses, we recognize family violence patterns ranging from those that originate early in life such as failure to thrive (manifestation of infantile depression or poor parent-child bonding?) and shaken baby syndrome (maladaptive parenting or discipline?) through domestic violence (personal boundary violations; rape, incest) to elder abuse and neglect. Does caregiver role strain play a role in sandwich-generation households (parents raising and caring for their children as well as their parents)? Domestic or intimate violence refers to an escalating, and usually persistent, pattern of abuse in which a person in an intimate relationship controls a vulnerable person or persons through force, intimidation, threat of violence, control of finances or any combination thereof. The three most common categories of domestic violence involve child abuse, intimate partner abuse, and elder abuse.

Vulnerable population groups include children, women aged 15 to 44 (reproductive age), frail older adults, persons with mental illnesses or cognitive impairments, and persons with mental delays (children and adults) and physical disabilities. Women are more at risk for abusive behavior, particularly during pregnancy and the period immediately after a separation (Stuart, 2009). Intimate partner abuse in heterosexual relationships tends to be gender-related, with more women being victimized; the majority of spousal or intimate partner perpetrators are men. However, intimate partner abuse also occurs in gay relationships where it is not gender-related; both abuser and victim are of the same sex. Domestic violence is a serious event in which the victim can be physically injured, psychologically traumatized, or neglected. More pregnant women die as victims of domestic violence than from any other cause.

Perpetrators of domestic and intimate violence come from all walks of life, socioeconomic strata, educational levels, races, ethnicities, and occupations. They are more likely to have grown up in an abusive household, been exposed to community or peer group violence, or both. Most perpetrators have low self-esteem and dependent personalities. They tend to lack impulse control and frequently view their victim as their property. Poverty, stress, and cultural values supportive of violence as a way of controlling behavior contribute to the development of abusive behaviors. Alcohol and other substance abuse is frequently a precipitating factor, although not the cause of domestic violence. Perpetrators can be paid caregivers or long-term care personnel as well as family members or persons with legal authority to make healthcare or financial decisions for the abused. Domestic abuse can take many forms:

▶ Emotional: Systematic degradation of a person's self-worth in the form of verbal attacks, controlling or limiting the victim's rights, isolating the victim from social contacts, and destroying the victim's personal property or pets.

▶ Physical: Intentional infliction of bodily harm through punching, beating, kicking, burning, shoving, twisting hair or limb, withholding food, or forcing compliance through actual or threatened physical force. Physical abuse also includes denying the victim food, fluids, or sleep. Indicators can include dislocations, fractures, burns, abrasions on limbs or torso consistent with strap or rope marks, bruising (particularly bilateral bruising to the arms or inner thighs), evidence of repeated bruising without medical cause, or traumatic loss of teeth or hair.

▶ Psychological indicators: Requires further exploration when children display sudden changes in school performance; present as overly compliant, passive, withdrawn, or demanding without reason; runs away or doesn't want to go home; describes the relationship with parent or caregiver as negative; displays inability to concentrate that cannot be attributed to a physical or psychological cause; reports physical or sexual abuse by a parent or caregiver; or refuses to change clothes for gym periods.

▶ Sexual: Forcing sex on an unwilling person, unsolicited sexual intimacy (fondling breasts or buttocks, or genital contact without penetration), indecent exposure, or forced exposure to sexually explicit material or unusual sex practices. It also includes sexual behaviors with a person who is unable to give valid consent (e.g., a minor, a person with cognitive impairments). Use of a child for pornography or other sexually exploitive activities is sexual abuse. Sexual abuse can consist of not revealing a sexually transmitted disease and failing to take precautions to safeguard the other person. Women with disabilities may be at greater risk.

The most common form of sexual abuse of children is incest—sex with a family member. Possible indicators requiring further exploration with children include

  ▸ Unusual incidence of urinary tract infections,

  ▸ Bruises, itching, rawness in the perineal area or inner thighs,

  ▸ Nightmares, fear of going to bed,

  ▸ Changes in behavior, extreme mood swings, withdrawal,

  ▸ Unusual interest or highly developed knowledge in sexual matters,

  ▸ Enuresis; encopresis, and

  ▸ Presence of a sexually transmitted disease.

▶ Neglect: The most common form of child and elder abuse; can be active or passive. Active neglect refers to the intentional disregard by caregivers and others for the physical, emotional, or financial needs and welfare of a child, disabled or cognitively impaired adult, or frail older adult. It can include withholding of care or finances, or failure to provide adequate supervision needed by the victim. Passive neglect is not intentional; the caregiver may not be able to provide appropriate care or supervision because of his or her own disability, lack of resources, lack of maturity, or ignorance. The following are possible indicators of child or frail older adult neglect:

  ▸ Is consistently dirty or has a distinct body odor

  ▸ Lacks appropriate clothing for the weather

  ▸ Doesn't have lunch or lunch money

  ▸ Lacks adequate medical or dental care, medications, or eyeglasses

  ▸ Appears apathetic, or afraid something is happening to her or him

  ▸ Lack or inappropriate supervision of a child's leisure and adolescent sexual activities

  ▸ Abuses alcohol or other drugs

  ▸ Child frequently absent from school

  ▸ Not in approved age-appropriate car seat

  ▸ Left alone; unattended

There is a predictable cycle to spousal or intimate partner abuse. Without treatment, it always repeats.

▶ Tension-building (escalation or buildup) phase: Tension rises with minor abuses; the victim tries to appease the perpetrator.

▶ Explosion (acute battering) phase: The abuser inflicts physical injury, psychological harm, or both.

▶ Honeymoon phase: The abuser is remorseful and apologetic, promising that the abuse will not happen again. Undoing, a common defense mechanism, may be observed with "promises to never do it again."

Later, the tension-building phase reappears and the cycle repeats (Dugan & Hock, 2006).

Children who are abused may need to be removed from the home or placed temporarily with a relative to prevent further episodes of abuse. Educate the abused child about self-protective strategies and remind him or her that the abuse was not his or her fault. Treatment approaches for children should reflect the child's developmental level.

For adults who are abused, help to identify and explore a safe environment in which the victim has safe alternatives should she or he need them (e.g., a shelter, staying with a friend or relative). Develop a safety plan that details the steps the adult victim should take in case of abuse, including collecting of important papers, money, and phone numbers. Educate adult victims of abuse, and explore and correct misperceptions that the victim provokes the perpetrator to become abusive.

If the problem-based assessment indicates a risk for violence, or if any unusual or unexplained bruising or injuries are present (bite marks, burns, evidence of neglect, history or presence of multiple fractures in various stages of healing, frequent incidence of urinary tract infections), further action is required.

Although no single injury informs the nurse that physical abuse has occurred, the nurse should look for patterns of injury or more than one indicator related to the possibility of physical and other forms of abuse. Abuse should be suspected when injuries are not explainable, family members provide different explanations, or the explanation does not fit the observed injuries. A history of similar injuries, multiple visits to the Emergency Department, and a delay between the onset of injury and seeking medical care should raise suspicion. Always believe a patient who reports abuse.

Referral to have a rape kit collected by a Sexual Assault Nurse Examiner (SANE), if available, is prudent. SANEs are experts in history-taking, physical and emotional assessment, recognition, and documentation of trauma response and injury—experts at collecting and managing forensic evidence. SANEs also provide emotional and social support during the courtroom testimony if required by the judicial system (see www.iafn.org for more information).

The nurse has a *duty to warn* and protect any potential victim of physical violence. Specific reporting guidelines are incorporated into state laws. The nurse must report any suspected child abuse to Child Protective Services. Though not mandatory in all states, the nurse can also contact Adult Protective Services to report suspected abuse of older adults or vulnerable adults. In most states, professionals are protected from breach of confidentiality in reporting suspected child or elder abuse and neglect. In a court of law, the judgment about reporting of child or elder abuse or neglect will be made on the basis of these published guidelines, and what a reasonable and prudent nurse would do in a similar situation.

Treatment of the victim begins with the assessment. Interview the alleged victim alone. Believe the abuse claim. Validate the person's feelings. Document signs of abuse and encourage treatment (children entering treatment for depression, anxiety, or eating disorders often have underlying abuse issues requiring assessment). Additionally, the nurse is legally obligated to report gunshot wounds, knife wounds, or other injury that may have resulted from various illegal or unlawful acts.

PAIN ASSESSMENT

The Joint Commission (TJC) provides pain management standards (2012) requiring that every patient be routinely assessed for pain, that pain assessment be documented, and pain managed for each patient. Specifically, these standards call for healthcare providers to

- ▶ Recognize the right of patients to appropriate assessment and management of their pain,

- ▶ Screen for the existence of pain, and assess for pain in all patients,

- ▶ Record results of the assessment in a way that facilitates regular reassessment and follow-up,

- ▶ Establish standards for regular monitoring and intervention,

- ▶ Educate relevant providers in pain assessment, management, and reassessment,

- ▶ Establish policies and procedures that support appropriate prescribing and ordering of pain medications,

- ▶ Ensure that pain does not interfere with participation in rehabilitation,

- ▶ Ensure staff competency in pain management,

- ▶ Educate patients and their families about the importance of effective pain management,

- ▶ Include patients' needs for pain management in the discharge planning process, and

- ▶ Collect data to monitor the appropriateness and effectiveness of pain management (pain control performance improvement plan).

The American Pain Society (APS) (Department of Veterans Affairs, 2000) has identified pain as the fifth vital sign, suggesting that it should be assessed with each evaluation of the standard four vital signs (temperature, pulse, respiration, and blood pressure). The difference in pain evaluation is that, because it is a symptom, only the patient can advise you of its existence and intensity, both verbally and nonverbally. In assessing for pain, it is important to ask questions about

- ▶ Onset and duration,

- ▶ Location,

- ▶ Character of the pain (sharp, dull, burning, persistent, changes with movement, direct or referred),

- ▶ Intensity, using a 0 to 10 numerical rating scale, with 0 being no pain and 10 being unbearable pain,

- ▶ Personal beliefs about pain and its management, fears about disease progression or adverse side effects,

▸ Exacerbating and relieving factors,

▸ Responses to current and past treatment,

▸ Patient's emotional state (secondary gain?), and

▸ History of substance dependence (crossover tolerance).

The International Association for the Study of Pain for Nursing (ISAP, 2014, p. 1) describes seven principles that guide the pain curriculum for nurses:

1. "Pain is viewed as a biopsychosocial phenomenon that includes sensory, emotional, cognitive, developmental, behavioral, spiritual, and cultural components.

2. Pain may be acute, persistent, or a combination of acute or chronic.

3. Pain must be assessed in a comprehensive and consistent manner using valid and reliable assessment tools.

4. Patients have a right to the best possible pain management. Pain assessment and management are integral aspects of nursing care and should involve patients and their families.

5. Pain assessment and management should be recorded in a clear and readily accessible manner.

6. Patient and family education about pain and its management are essential components of nursing care.

7. Nurses are essential members of the pain management team."

Pain is what the patient says it is. The experience of pain can be acute or chronic. Even when pain medication is essential to successful treatment, behavioral interventions can result in reduced pain intensity and improvement in physical and psychosocial functioning.

Although chronic pain is typically a less intense sensory experience for patients than acute pain, it can be extremely debilitating as a physical and psychological experience for both patients and their families. In addition to the physical aspects of pain, chronic pain can compromise quality of life, as well as personal and professional relationships. Pain issues can be exacerbated by other psychosocial and behavioral factors. McCaffery (2001) notes that pain can exacerbate or cause symptoms of anxiety and depression.

Chronic pain is a risk factor for mood and substance disorders, as well as sexual dysfunction. Historically, pain has been underrecognized and undertreated. Unrecognized or undertreated pain may result in psychiatric symptoms such as anxiety, depression, and agitation. If pain is present, a complete assessment should be conducted. The **ABCDE** mnemonic approach includes screening, assessment, and treatment.

▶ Ask about pain regularly. Assess pain systematically.

▶ Believe the client and family in their report of pain and what relieves it.

▶ Choose pain control options appropriate for the client, family, and setting.

▶ Deliver interventions in a timely, logical, and coordinated fashion.

▶ Empower clients and their families. Enable them to control their course to the greatest extent possible.

The Wong-Baker **FACES** scale (1988) can be used from age 3 and up. Patients are asked to point to the facial expression that best describes the pain intensity:

▶ 0 = no hurt (smiling, happy face)

▶ 10 = hurts worst (sad, crying face)

NUTRITION ASSESSMENT

Patient reports of weight loss or gains above or below 15% of expected weight for age and height require physical and mental work-ups to differentiate between medical and psychiatric causes. Recent weight loss may suggest depression (with loss of appetite) or thyroid disease (hyperthyroidism). Recent weight gains could suggest side effects of medications or other metabolic problems.

The U.S. Department of Agriculture (USDA) (2010) provides evidence-based dietary guidelines that promote health and reduce risk for major chronic diseases. The www.choosemyplate.gov website provides specific diet and physical activity recommendations.

Obesity is associated with many health risks, including hypercholesteremia, hyperlipidemia, type 2 diabetes, heart disease, stroke, hypertension, osteoarthritis, sleep apnea, and some forms of cancer. Poor diet and sedentary lifestyle contribute to obesity. The heritability of obesity is equivalent to that of height (Bear, Connors, & Paradiso, 2006) and, as with all the mental disorders, more than one gene is involved. Obesity can result from a variety of disorders that cause hormonal imbalance, including hypothyroidism, hypercortisolism, primary hyperinsulinism, pseudohypoparathyroidism, and acquired hypothalamic problems (e.g., tumors, infections, traumatic syndromes). There may also be some psychosocial and emotional components involved, such as an unconscious desire to be less desirous to sexual or relationship overtures. This complex factor may be present in eating disorders on both ends of the spectrum (overeating to anorexia).

Concern has been voiced regarding the risk of metabolic syndrome in patients who are taking atypical antipsychotics. *Metabolic syndrome* includes the following signs: abdominal obesity, dyslipidemia, raised blood pressure, insulin resistance with or without glucose intolerance, proinflammatory state, and prothrombotic state. Persons with metabolic syndrome are at risk for premature coronary heart disease.

Because many of the psychotropic medications can cause weight gain and increase the risk for metabolic syndrome, it is especially important that we monitor weight and body mass index (BMI) before initiating and during treatment. BMI can be calculated based on weight and height, and BMI calculators and charts are readily available for both adults and children on websites such as the Centers for Disease Control and Prevention (http://www.cdc.gov/nccdphp/dnpa/healthyweight/assessing/bmi/index.htm) or National Heart, Lung, and Blood Institute (http://www.nhlbi.nih.gov/health/educational/lose_wt/BMI/bmi_tbl.htm). The normal range of BMI for adults is between 18.5 kg/m2 and 24.9 kg/m2, with 25–29.9 kg/m2 indicating overweight and anything over 30 kg/m2 indicating obesity. To assess a patient's nutritional status, determine these factors:

▶ Personal information: Age, activity level, cultural background, socioeconomic status, personal preferences, use of alcohol or illegal drugs, supplements, prescriptions

▶ Body mass index (BMI): Can be calculated from height and weight

▶ Whether body weight is within norms for gender, age, and height, or is 15% or more above or below expected weight, requiring further work-up

▶ 24-hour food history or diary

▶ Fluid intake: Calculate nutritional intake from food diary kept for 3 to 7 days and compare it with the 2010 USDA guideline values to determine whether dietary habits are adequate.

▶ Knowledge of nutrition

The American Academy of Pediatrics recommends exclusive breastfeeding for about 6 months, followed by continuation of breastfeeding as complementary foods are introduced for 1 year or longer as mutually desired by mother and infant. (American Academy of Pediatrics, 2012). Caution is issued if the mother is on psychotropic medications or is HIV-positive. Infant caloric needs are higher in first 6 months of life because of rapid brain growth and development (approximately 108 kcal/kg body weight). Intake can decrease in second 6 months (98 kcal/kg of body weight). The USDA (2010) recommends that for toddlers age 2 and older, nutrient-dense food (variety) can increase and total intake can decrease as activity increases to balance appropriate overall weight gain with growth.

Physical activity reduces the risk for development of chronic diseases in adulthood. The basic recommendation (USDA, 2010) is to engage in at least 30 minutes of moderate-intensity physical activity on most days for adults, 60 minutes or more for children and for adults who need more intense weight management strategies.

FALL RISK ASSESSMENT

Falls are one of the major sources of injury among older adults, as well as among patients of all ages. The Joint Commission (TJC, n.d.) offers strategies to reduce the risk of patient harm from falls. Hospitals and long-term-care facilities are required to implement and evaluate fall-reduction programs. Many of the psychiatric drugs can cause sedation and, therefore, increased risk for falls. The Edmonson Psychiatric Fall Risk Assessment tool (Edmonson, Robinson, & Hughes, 2011) can be used to evaluate a patient's fall risk potential. Other risks for falls include the following:

▶ Age over 60; history of falls, smoking, or alcohol or drug abuse

▶ Mental status: lethargic, confused or disoriented, unable to understand directions, impaired memory or judgment

▶ Physical conditions: acute illness, dehydration, vertigo, unsteady gait, problems affecting weight-bearing joints, weakness, paresis or paralysis, seizure disorder, impaired vision, impaired hearing, slow reaction times, diarrhea, urinary frequency, incontinence, urgency, nocturia, orthostatic hypotension, stroke, musculoskeletal disorders, and Parkinson's disease

▶ Medications: diuretics, antihypertensives, central nervous system depressants (e.g., benzodiazepines, alcohol), medications that increase gastrointestinal motility (e.g., laxatives), selective serotonin reuptake inhibitors (SSRIs), antipsychotics, hypoglycemic agents, anticonvulsants, mood stabilizers

▶ Use of ambulatory devices (indicates problem with walking): cane, crutches, walker, wheelchair, geri-chair, braces

SEXUAL HEALTH ACROSS THE LIFE SPAN

Genesis

Humans are sexual beings from birth. Sexual expression and satisfaction is a normal and healthy experience. At birth, gender is signalled initially by putting either a pink or a blue cap on the infant's head. Cap color is determined by visual recognition of male versus female genitalia.

At each age and stage, humans contend with issues related to sexuality. Infants initially explore their bodies because learning at this stage progresses by way of sensory and motor explorations. The male infant finds his penis and the female infant finds her vulva and clitoral areas. The toddler or preschooler focuses attention to excretion and related body parts, while negotiating strong and different feelings for parents of both sexes (Oedipal and Electra complex described by Freud for example). The school-aged population desires interaction primarily with same-sex peers, and questions concerned with gender assignment (male versus female) may arise and may feel discordant with the child's personal perception of self. Adolescents, with powerful hormonal surges, may find themselves openly questioning their sexuality as they gain comfort with secondary sex characteristics similar to adult bodies; body image issues surface because adolescents may be lanky, clumsy, and a little uncomfortable in their own rapidly changing bodies. The adolescent is clarifying gender identity, and may engage in exploration of sexual orientation. The average age for menarche (menses) is 12; for nocturnal emissions and ejaculation between 12 and 14. Sexuality and expression continues throughout adulthood and the middle age years; adults continue to develop intimacy and sexuality. Older adults, with declining health and hormonal changes, still may engage in healthy sexuality; sex is still possible.

What if an infant is born with ambiguous genitalia, or genitourinary anomalies? Patients with genitourinary morphological and structural problems are often closely followed by urologists and surgeons. Consultation with psychiatry and psychiatric services may come in later ages (i.e., puberty and beyond) if mood, anxiety, or substance use disorders develop secondary to coping issues. Anecdotal and patient history reviews reveal that greater than 50% of children, adolescent, adults, and older adults have experienced sexual assault or abuse, which may also create a need for psychiatric or mental health services.

The three phases of sexual response—libido, arousal, and orgasm—all have distinct and relatively nonoverlapping neurotransmitter functions (Stahl, 2008). Each stage can be affected by mental disorders or their psychopharmacologic treatments. Depression and anxiety are commonly associated with sexual dysfunction. Manic episodes may result in increased libido and sexual behavior. Of the neurotransmitter systems that we have discussed (Chapter 2) in relation to the mental disorders, dopamine and the brain reward pathways are thought to play a role in

> **BOX 3–2.**
> **SEXUALITY ACROSS THE LIFE SPAN**
>
> ▸ **Infants:** Initial body exploration
>
> ▸ **Toddler and Preschooler:** Gender identity formation
>
> ▸ **School Age:** Interest in same-sex peer group; increased need for privacy
>
> ▸ **Adolescent:** Onset of secondary sex characteristics; exploration of sexual orientation; body image issues
>
> ▸ **Adult:** Continuing development of intimacy and engagement in sexual behaviors
>
> ▸ **Middle Age:** Declining hormones; menopause; andropause in men (approximately ages 48–52)
>
> ▸ **Older Adults:** Declining health and hormones; healthy sex and sexuality still possible and of interest.

increasing libido or sexual desire. Serotonin has a negative influence, and norepinephrine a positive influence, on sexual arousal and orgasm. When we consider that most of the psychotropic drugs affect these three neurotransmitter systems, it is not surprising that sexual dysfunction is often an unwanted side effect of treatment, and therefore a possible cause for a patient's nonadherence to prescribed regimens.

Assessment of sexual health is crucial across the life span because we are sexual beings from birth, and a host of physical and mental health issues can cause diminished sexual response requiring health teaching, prevention, and intervention. Medication side effects for many of the major categories of drugs (antihypertensives, antidepressants, antihistamines, antispasmodics, sedative-hypnotics, alcohol, diuretics, and narcotics) are known to have some degree of diminishing effects on libido. The population of patients over the age of 50 is one of the fastest-growing groups for contracting HIV (human immunodeficiency virus), yet this group is often overlooked because healthcare providers fail to elicit sexual histories because of their age. Like adolescents, adults need accurate education about sexual issues that may be of a sensitive nature. Box 3–2 outlines the interplay between age and sexual health concepts:

NICOTINE (TOBACCO) USE ASSESSMENT

Ask all new patients, "Do you use nicotine or nicotine products?" "Do you chew or snuff tobacco"? (If you just ask about smoking, you might miss the chewing, snuffing, and electronic cigarette [vaping] users of nicotine). It is important for the nurse to identify smoking status and nicotine use, not only because of its known deleterious effects on health but because most healthcare and public environments have instituted "no tobacco" policies in clinical settings.

The nurse recognizes that this current public policy initiative has implications for persons who may be dependent upon tobacco or other nicotine products (Hutchinson & Cagle, 2010). The Fagerstrom Test for Nicotine Dependence (Heatherton et al., 1991) is an evidence-based clinical screening tool designed to help determine the potential severity of nicotine withdrawal from smoked and smokeless tobacco varieties. Cotinine is a byproduct of nicotine use that can be measured by way of serum analysis. This metabolite is mainly excreted by the liver, and secondarily by way of the kidneys and lungs.

SUBSTANCE USE SCREENING

Increasingly, use and abuse of and experimentation with novel substances are appearing among substance abusers. Newer chemicals and substances seen include WET (marijuana laced with formaldehyde), K2 ("spice"), K3, bath salts, and freon inhalation. Indicators pointing to suspected use include impaired mental status and impaired cognitive presentations.

The CAGE questionnaire (Ewing, 1984) (Box 3–3) is a simple 4-item screening tool that detects alcohol (or other substance) problems. A person scoring 1 on the screening should be further assessed for substance problems and a person scoring 2 or more is considered to be positive for a substance disorder.

The Clinical Institute Withdrawal Assessment, Alcohol revised (CIWA-Ar), (Sullivan et al., 1989) is an instrument that helps in the assessment of alcohol withdrawal symptomology and serves as a guide treating the condition. During detoxification from alcohol, CIWA-Ar scores are determined every 30 minutes until the scores are reduced to less than 10 for three consecutive assessments or for 4 hours.

BOX 3–3.
CAGE SCREENING QUESTIONNAIRE

1. Have you ever felt the need to **C**ut down on your drinking (drug use)?
2. Have you ever felt **A**nnoyed by criticism of your drinking (drug use)?
3. Have you ever felt **G**uilty about your drinking (drug use)?
4. Have you ever taken a drink (drug) first thing in the morning (**E**ye-opener) to steady your nerves or get rid of a hangover?

Scoring: 2 or more "yes" responses indicates a substance disorder; 1 "yes" requires further assessment.

STANDARDIZED ASSESSMENT AND SCREENING TOOLS USED IN PSYCHIATRIC PRACTICE

Screening tools have also been developed for many mental health conditions. The goals of screening and diagnosis differ. Screening is the identification of persons who might have a particular problem. In screening, false positives are possible, but the ultimate goal is to detect all persons at risk for a particular disease, disorder, or condition and refer them for further analysis and diagnosis. Diagnosis is the process of identifying the correct reason for the symptoms so treatment can begin. Diagnoses need to be accurate, so false positives are not acceptable.

A variety of standardized scales are in the public domain. The use of standardized measurement tools is essential for assessing baseline patient presentations and for identifying the quantity and quality of change in patient response to specific implementations. Standardized psychometric rating scales can help add more specificity to findings of symptoms and can be used to evaluate responses to treatment. They allow us to make evidence-based care a continuous part of everyday practice. Use standardized measures whenever possible. They provide a common language for assessment that can be clearly communicated between care providers. Box 3–4 lists examples of some measurement tools that are currently used in practice and are available in the public domain. This is not a complete list; there are many additional measures available that have application in different populations, with different diagnoses, and appropriate for different settings. The psychiatric–mental health nurse needs to become familiar with these and other measures or rating scales and how to administer them and interpret their results.

The Brief Psychiatric Rating Scale (BPRS; Overall, 1988) is an 18-item scale measuring positive symptoms, affective symptoms, and general psychopathology. It can be applied on observation of the patient and can be used to monitor outcomes of treatment.

The Abnormal Involuntary Movement Scale (AIMS; Guy, 1976) is useful for quantifying the presence of extrapyramidal side effects (EPS) in patients who are taking antipsychotics. The presence and severity of each potential abnormal movement is rated from none to severe when directed to perform the following actions as directed with fluidity and control and without evidence of jerking or spasticity:

- ▶ Sitting, standing, walking
- ▶ Opening and closing mouth and sticking out tongue
- ▶ Rapid finger-thumb tapping
- ▶ Passive flexion and extension of the arms without evidence of muscle rigidity.

The Mini-Mental State Exam (MMSE) provides objective indicators of current mental status and is scored on a scale between 0 and 30 points. Normal scores range between 25 and 30 points. Patients scoring a total of 24 or lower should be further evaluated for medical (dementia, delirium) or substance-related problems.

BOX 3-4.
SELECT LIST OF STANDARDIZED RATING AND MEASUREMENT SCALES USED IN PSYCHIATRIC PRACTICE

All listed tools are in the public domain and can be used in clinical practice. These are only examples. Many other measurement scales are available.

General Symptom Measures
▸ Brief Psychiatric Rating Scale (BPRS)
▸ Positive and Negative Syndrome Scale (PANSS)
▸ Yale-Brown OCD Scale
▸ Sheehan Disability Scale (SDS)
▸ Quality of Life Enjoyment and Satisfaction Questionnaire
▸ Young Mania Rating Scale
▸ McGowan Risk Assessment for Violence
▸ Mental Status Examination (MSE)

Pain
▸ Wong-Baker FACES Rating Scale (1 least pain to 10 worst pain)

Alcohol Withdrawal
▸ Clinical Institute Withdrawal Assessment, Alcohol revised (CIWA-Ar (Sullivan, et al., 1989))

Opioid and Narcotic Withdrawal
▸ Clinical Opioid Withdrawal Scale (COWS)
▸ Clinical Institute Narcotic Assessment (CINA)

Activity Level
▸ Iowa Connors Rating Scale—rates selected behaviors

Abnormal Movements
▸ Abnormal Involuntary Movement Scale (AIMS)
▸ Barnes Akathisia Rating Scale

Nutrition Status
▸ Body Mass Index (BMI)
▸ Mini Nutritional Assessment (MNA)

Assessments Specific for Infants, Children, and Adolescents
▸ Apgar score for neonates
▸ Denver Developmental Screening Test II (DDST II) for infants and toddlers
▸ Home and environment, education and employment, eating, activities, drugs, sexuality, suicide/depression, safety (HEEADSSS) for adolescents (Klein et al., 2014)
▸ Tanner staging

Cognitive Functioning
▸ Mini Mental State Examination (MMSE)
▸ Montreal Cognitive Assessment (MOCA)

Suicidality
▸ Columbia-Suicide Severity Rating Scale (C-SSRS); adult and child versions

Depression
▸ Hamilton Rating Scale for Depression (HAM-D; Hamilton, 1960)
▸ Cornell Scale for Depression in Dementia (CSDD; Alexopoulos et al., 1988)
▸ PHQ-9 for depression (Pfizer Inc., 1999)
▸ Beck Depression Inventory (BDI I and II; adult and adolescent versions) (Beck, 1979; Steer, Ball, Raneeri, & Beck, 1997)
▸ EPDS (Edinburgh Postnatal Depression Screening); can also be used prenatally
▸ Children's Depression Rating Scale
▸ Geriatric Depression Scale
▸ Montgomery-Asberg Depression Rating Scale (MADRAS)

Nicotine Withdrawal
▸ Fagerstrom Test for Nicotine Dependence (FTND), 6-item scale to measure the potential severity of nicotine withdrawal

Anxiety
▸ Hamilton Anxiety Scale
▸ Multidimensional Anxiety Scale for Children (MASC)

TABLE 3-5.
MINI MENTAL STATE EXAMINATION (MMSE)

MEASURE	SCORE (POINTS)
Orientation	Max = 10
▸ Year, season, date, day, month.	
▸ State, county, town, hospital, floor (1 points given for each correct reply).	
Registration	Max = 3
▸ Have patient name three observed objects (1 point given for each correctly named or registered).	
Attention and Calculation	Max = 5
▸ Count back from 100 serially by 7 (93, 86, 79, 72, 65) or spell the word "world" backwards (1 point given for each series subtracted correctly or each letter spelled in reverse).	
Recall	Max = 3
▸ Correctly name (recall) the three objects "registered" earlier (1 point given for each correctly remembered).	
Language	
▸ Name items (show a pencil and a watch, for example).	Max = 2
▸ Repeat: "No ifs, ands, or buts."	Max = 1
▸ Carry out 3-stage command: "Take paper in your right hand; fold it in half; place it on the table."	Max = 3
▸ Read this sentence (which is written on a piece of paper): "Close your eyes."	Max = 1
▸ Write a sentence. Sentence must contain a noun and a verb.	Max = 1
▸ Copy overlapping pentagons	Max = 1

Adapted from M. Folstein, S. Folstein, & P. McHugh, 1975, "Mini-Mental State": A practical method for grading the cognitive state of patients for the clinician, *Journal of Psychiatric Research*, 12, 189–198.

The Mental Status Exam (MSE) is a *subjective* report of the patient's current mental state as observed by the nurse. Assessment of mental status is a continuous part of the nursing process. When MSE findings are reported, they consist of what the nurse observed *at the time* of the interaction, not before and not after. Box 3–5 describes the components of the MSE. Physical observation of the patient is part of the MSE. The Mental Status Examination is a component of the psychiatric and neurological exam and is an ongoing assessment tool.

BOX 3-5.
COMPONENTS OF THE MENTAL STATUS EXAM

Appearance and Behavior

▶ Overall appearance related to age, culture

▶ Hygiene and grooming

▶ Style, appropriateness of clothing to age, weather, occasion

▶ Posture and mannerisms

▶ General behavior (impulsivity, passive, hostile, fearful)

▶ Motor behavior (e.g., pacing, lethargic, catatonic)

▶ Attitude toward clinician and willingness to cooperate

Mood and Affect

▶ Mood: internal feelings that influence behavior (e.g., depressed, suspicious, elated, euthymic): "How do you feel?"

▶ Affect: emotional expression variation; found in face, voice, use of body movements (e.g., flat, guarded, inappropriate, blunted, restricted, labile, full range, depressed, overreactive, stable): How does the person look? Are mood and affect congruent or not?

Thought Processes

▶ Continuity and organization of ideas

   ▶ Problems with word-finding

   ▶ Processing of abstract ideas

   ▶ Blocking, unexpected thought stoppage

▶ Flow and rhythm: slowed or racing thoughts

▶ Logical coherency of ideas

▶ Amount: excessive speech or poverty of speech

▶ Language or meaning deficits

Processing Deficits: How is the Patient Understanding?

▶ Clanging: choice of words based on similar sounds, not associated ideas

▶ Echolalia: repetition of other people's words or phrases

▶ Neologisms: creation of new words that do not make sense

▶ Word salad: disorganized, senseless progression of words

▶ Perseveration: tedious repetition of the same words or ideas regardless of stimuli

▶ Flight of ideas: ideas are not logically connected; abrupt changes in topic

▶ Loose associations: limited or no logical progression between words or ideas

   ▶ Circumstantial: excessive and unnecessary detail, eventually answering the question

   ▶ Tangential: never returns to the point or answers the question

▶ Thought-blocking: interruption or delay in thought processing, not related to lack of concentration, distraction, or anxiety

Thought Content: What is the Patient Saying?

▶ Suicide: plan, opportunity, means?

▶ Homicide: victim, realistic plan?

▶ Delusions: fixed, false beliefs

▶ Phobias: intense, unreasonable fears

▶ Obsessions: intrusive, repetitious

(continued)

BOX 3-5.
CONTINUED

Delusional Thinking: What is the Patient Thinking?

Delusions: false beliefs that cannot be dislodged by logic or contradictory evidence; not congruent with normative culture or religious beliefs

▶ Of reference: other people's thoughts, words, or actions refer to self

▶ Persecution: other people have malevolent intentions toward self, or are conspiring against the person

▶ Religious: unrealistic special relationship with God

▶ Nihilistic: destruction of self, world, or body part

▶ Grandiose: special, gifted, powerful, or important without factual support

Perception: How is the Patient Seeing and Experiencing the World?

▶ Depersonalization: feeling detached or as if he or she is an outside observer of his or her own mental processes or body

▶ Illusions: false perceptions; misinterpretation of some stimuli

▶ Déjà vu or flashbacks: "I've been here before!"

▶ Hallucinations: differ among the medical and psychiatric disorders; no stimuli, but person perceives something through one or all the five senses

  ▶ Delirium: may be accompanied by visual or aural hallucinations or both

  ▶ Dementia: visual hallucinations are common with Lewy body dementia.

  ▶ Depression with psychotic factors: mood-congruent (e.g., hearing people whisper criticisms in depression)

  ▶ Seizures or brain injury: visual, auditory, tactile, gustatory, olfactory

  ▶ Schizophrenia: generally auditory, may be mood-incongruent (person may seem euthymic but hear command to harm another person [command hallucination]); bizarre hallucinations such as hearing a conversation among several people are suggestive of schizophrenia

  ▶ Dementia: visual hallucinations are common with Lewy body dementia

  ▶ Substance-related intoxication or withdrawal: any kind; depends on the drug

Sensorium and Cognition: How is the Patient Sensing and Remembering the World?

▶ Memory recall: immediate, recent, remote

▶ Orientation to person, time, and place

▶ Concentration: serial 7s (keep educational level in mind)

▶ Abstract thinking

▶ Disturbances suggest organic dysfunction due to meds, substance abuse, neurodegenerative or neurocognitive disorder

Judgment: How Does the Patient Make Decisions?

Realistic decision-making based on:

▶ Current level of knowledge

▶ Realistic understanding of options

▶ Resources

▶ Strengths and limitations

Insight: How Does the Patient Connect Thoughts, Experiences, and Understanding?

▶ Extent of patient's awareness of his or her problem

▶ Willingness to look at his or her role in maintaining symptoms

▶ Awareness of behavioral consequences and lifestyle changes needed for coping

AGE-APPROPRIATE PHYSICAL AND DEVELOPMENTAL HISTORY AND EXAMINATIONS IN SPECIAL POPULATIONS

Fetus, Neonate, Infant

Early signs of childhood disorders may manifest as problems with language skill development, communication; display of stereotypic behaviors and gestures; difficulty with play activities; or development of enuresis, encopresis, or sensory or perceptual abnormalities. Many disorders can be diagnosed as early as age 2, but the full range of signs and symptoms may not present until later. Early diagnosis can lead to early interventions; however, there is a paucity of good, accurate screening tools available. A few screening tools and assessments are presented below.

Factors that negatively affect fetal optimization include in-utero exposure to maternal TORCH infections, maternal HIV or AIDS, and maternal substance use. Perinatal infections account for 2% to 3% of all congenital anomalies, with generally mild effects on the mother and potentially serious effects on the fetus. Knowledge of these diseases provides the nurse with critical information regarding pregnancy assessment, as well as treatment guidance and opportunities to teach prevention. *TORCH* (Stegman & Carey, 2002) is the acronym given to different maternal infections with organisms that cross the placental barrier (**T**oxoplasmosis, **O**thers [syphilis, varicella-zoster, parvovirus B19], **R**ubella, **C**ytomegalovirus [CMV], and **H**erpes; Table 3–6).

TABLE 3–6.
TORCH INFECTIONS AND FETAL/INFANT EFFECTS

Toxoplasmosis	Mother and infant are asymptomatic at birth. 15% of infected infants die; 85% show severe psychomotor retardation. Today, women are screened for antibodies during the first prenatal visit.
Syphilis	Hepatomegaly, jaundice, hemolytic anemia, and other blood dyscrasias at birth; pregnancy complications, including potential for stillbirth, low birth weight
Varicella-Zoster (chickenpox)	Low birth weight, microcephaly, cortical atrophy, chorioretinitis, skin scarring, localized muscle atrophy, encephalitis, hypoplasia of an extremity
Parvovirus B19 (fifth disease)	Presence of mild rash, slapped-face appearance (erythema infectiosum)
Rubella (German measles)	Most infected fetuses develop rubella in the first trimester, before 10 weeks. With cell division slowed by the disease, 50% will show slowed growth and fewer cells than normal.
Cytomegalovirus (CMV)	Most common cause of perinatal infection. Mother asymptomatic; infant can have birth deformities, seizure disorders, blindness. Most problems show up between 3 to 7 years and include lowered IQ, deafness, motor defects, and learning disabilities.
Herpes	There is no definite link between herpes and any congenital disease, but when the mother has genital herpes, prematurity, spontaneous abortion, and certain congenital anomalies can be associated. If the mother has open lesions in the birth canal and the infant is grossly contaminated, there is a 30%–50% infection rate for infants delivered vaginally.
Hepatitis B	Most infants are asymptomatic.

HIV AND AIDS ASSESSMENT: LIFE SPAN PERSPECTIVES

Additional maternal factors that negatively affect the developing fetus include congenital acquired immunodeficiency syndrome (AIDS) and bioneurodevelopmental compromises that result from maternal substance use. AIDS is an infectious disease caused by the human immunodeficiency virus (HIV), which attacks the T-lymphocytic white blood cells and the CD4 immune cells. Many children have become infected either in the womb or during delivery. It is possible for a woman to be unaware that she has been infected by the virus until her infant develops AIDS. A few may have become infected later through breastfeeding transference. Some children may have become infected because of sexual abuse. Nurses, parents, and other caregivers who have close contact with HIV-infected children or adults, such as sharing beds and eating utensils, are NOT at high risk for transmission of HIV.

Infants who are infected with HIV suffer frequent infections and diarrhea, and fail to thrive and gain weight. Enlarged lymph glands, spleen, liver, and salivary glands are common, and many children have delayed development, perhaps because of brain damage from the virus.

Diagnosis of HIV infection is made by way of assay measures that quantify the number of antibodies that the body has developed in its attempt to fight the HIV virus. It takes 2 weeks to 3 months for the antibodies to show up in the HIV test. During this time, a person can transmit the virus to others, including the fetus. Three different responses to HIV testing are:

1. The person may have no symptoms of illness but can still transmit the virus to others.

2. Infected persons may develop HIV disease and have symptoms less severe than those of AIDS, including loss of appetite, weight loss, fever, night sweats, diarrhea, skin rashes, tiredness, lack of resistance to infections, or swollen lymph nodes. These symptoms can be caused by other diseases, so expert diagnostics are required to identify HIV disease.

3. Opportunistic infections such as *Pneumocystis jiroveci* pneumonia (PJP; formerly called *Pneumocystis carinii* pneumonia or PCP) and Kaposi's sarcoma that would not otherwise be able to get a foothold take advantage of the AIDS patient's compromised immune system. Opportunistic infections are usually the cause of death for the AIDS patient.

SUBSTANCE USE AND RISK FOR DEVELOPMENTAL DISABILITY

According to Shepard's Catalog (1995), there are more than 2,000 drugs, chemicals, and other physical and biological teratogenic agents that may adversely affect the newborn's development. Such effects to the mother and newborn may include chromosomal abnormalities, nonchromosomal congenital abnormalities and defects, low birth weight, altered fertility patterns, spontaneous abortion, developmental disabilities, behavioral disorders, childhood malignancies, and fetal, neonatal, or childhood death. Tobacco smoke, carbon monoxide, nicotine, alcohol, and polycyclic aromatic hydrocarbons can all adversely affect the fetus by causing increased bleeding during pregnancy, long-term birth disorders, spontaneous abortion, and rupture of the membranes. Drugs such as opiates, barbiturates, anesthetics, sex steroids, and food additives can produce developmental disabilities, congenital heart defects, and fetal death.

FETAL ALCOHOL SYNDROME (FAS)

Alcohol is a legal substance and is readily available to all populations, despite the imposition of legal age limitations. When pregnant mothers drink excessive amounts of alcohol during pregnancy, physical and mental defects may develop in the fetus. Alcohol passes through the placenta to the fetus soon after the mother drinks, and the fetus gets the same amount as the mother, but the fetal organs are immature and do not break down the alcohol as quickly as the mother's, so the blood level of alcohol in the fetus will be higher.

Women who drink 3 or more ounces of pure alcohol each day frequently give birth to babies who have FAS. This amount of alcohol is equivalent to six cans of beer, six mixed drinks, or six 4-ounce glasses of wine. Two to five drinks a day can also damage the fetus and produce some of the signs of FAS, called fetal alcohol effects (FAE). Some women can drink heavily throughout pregnancy and have children with no signs of FAE or FAS.

Neonates with FAS have a characteristic appearance, are unusually small at birth, and don't usually catch up as they get older. Their eyes are usually small and widely spaced, and they have a short, upturned nose and small, flat cheek. They may suffer from a variety of organ malfunctions, especially of the heart. Most neonates with FAS have small brains and are mentally delayed to some degree. Many are poorly coordinated, have short attention spans, and exhibit behavioral problems. FAS is one of the most common known causes of birth defects producing intellectual and developmental delays. It is the most common preventable cause.

In the United States, one of every 750 newborns has FAS, approximately 5,000 babies per year—comparable to the number of children born with Down syndrome each year. Drinking alcohol during pregnancy also can increase the risk of miscarriages, stillbirth, and death in early infancy. Heavy drinkers are 2 to 4 times more likely than nondrinkers to have a miscarriage between the 4th and 6th months of pregnancy.

TABLE 3-7.
EFFECTS OF SUBSTANCES ON MATERNAL, FETAL, AND NEONATAL WELL-BEING

SUBSTANCE	ROUTES	MATERNAL EFFECTS	FETAL EFFECTS	LABOR EFFECTS	NEONATE EFFECTS	DEVELOPMENTAL EFFECTS
Alcohol	Drink, inhale vapors	Acute withdrawal, sedation, inebriation, organ damage (heart, liver, stomach)	Fetal alcohol effect (FAE) and fetal alcohol syndrome (FAS): growth deficiency, microcephaly, stillbirth, decreased birth weight, joint and facial anomalies, genito-urinary anomalies, cardiac anomalies	Acute withdrawal, transient muscular hypotonia	Acute withdrawal with sedation, seizures, poor feeding	Developmental delay, hyperactivity, low IQ
Amphetamines and stimulants	Snort, IV, drink, heat and inhale vapors, pipes	Dilated pupils, euphoria, excitation, loss of appetite, increased blood pressure and heart rate, insomnia	Intrauterine growth retardation, bilary atresia, transposition of great vessels	Tremors, hypertonicity, poor suck rate, high-pitched cry	Long-term effects not known	
Barbiturates	Oral	Habituation, sedation	Delivery sedation	Tremors, hypertonicity, poor suck rate, high-pitched cry	Long-term effects not known	
Caffeine	Oral	Irritability, headaches	Spontaneous abortion, stillbirth	Decreased birth weight	Long-term effects not known	
Tobacco and nicotine	Smoke, inhale vapor, chew, patches	High tar and nicotine cigarettes cause some heart and lung problems	Decreased birth weight and head size	Jitteriness, poor feeding	Lower scholastic scores, increased risk for sudden infant death syndrome (SIDS)	

SUBSTANCE	ROUTES	MATERNAL EFFECTS	FETAL EFFECTS	LABOR EFFECTS	NEONATE EFFECTS	DEVELOPMENTAL EFFECTS
Cocaine	Smoke, inhale, free base	Stimulation, tachycardia, hypertension, heart attack	Increased spontaneous abortion, congenital anomalies; abruptio placentae, cerebral infarction	Tremors, hypertonicity, muscle weakness, seizures	Developmental delay, 4%–15% increased rate of SIDS	
Heroin	IV, IM, snort, smoke	Habituation, sedation	Small for gestational age	Withdrawal symptoms, tremors, hypertonicity, poor feeding, diarrhea, seizures, irritability	5%–10% increased rate of SIDS	
Marijuana, cannabis, THC	Smoke, ingest	Sedation, hallucinations	Before conception: chromosome changes, decreased sperm counts, memory impairment	Bleeding problems	Sedation, tremors, habituation, excessive response to light	Long-term effects not known; psychosis
Phencyclidine (PCP)	Smoke, inject	Hallucinations, agitation, nystagmus	Delivery agitation	Irritability, microcephaly, uncoordinated fine motor skills, sensory input problems	Long-term effects not known	

It is important to recognize that maternal contribution to fetal-neonate optimization is fairly clear. Optimal organogenesis emanates from the overall health of the mother; future scientific developments may illuminate additional information relative to paternal sperm and genetic contributions and ultimate fetal outcomes. Table 3–7 outlines known adverse effects on maternal, fetal, and neonatal well-being when used during pregnancy.

NEONATAL ASSESSMENT

The transitional period for the newborn is considered to be the first 24 hours of life. Assessment of neurological intactness involves obtaining 1- and 5-minute Apgar scores (named for its inventor, Virginia Apgar, whose name is also used as a mnemonic in which APGAR = **a**ppearance/skin coloration, **p**ulse/heart rate, **g**rimace/reflex irritability and cry, **a**ctivity/muscle tone, and **r**espiration/breathing effort). Two points are available in each of the five categories, so obtainable scores are between 0 and 10 total, with 10 being the best possible score. Neonate screening is further accomplished through analyses of blood specimens to detect disorders that lead to developmental problems.

Normal birth weight averages 6 to 8 pounds (2.7 to 3.6 kg), with the head approximately one-third the size of the body. At birth, neonates normally display characteristics that include grasping, rooting, sucking, startle or Moro reflex, and Babinski reflex (toes spread apart when the sole of the foot is touched). The Babinski reflex disappears by about 1 year of age; the others by about 4 months. By around 2 weeks of age, the infant prefers the mother's voice and has the ability to discriminate colors, smells, and tastes. Although development proceeds a bit differently for each person, on average, other physical milestones include balancing the head (4 months); walking and grasping small objects (12 to 16 months); running and further refinements of purposive speech and language skills (2 years); jumping, dancing, and drawing or copying simple objects (3 years); skipping (age 5); and riding a bike (age 6). Development proceeds in a progressive manner that is orderly and predictive, emanating from cephalic (head) to caudal (tail). Deviations in developmental sequence, therefore, may indicate an anomaly. Birth weight should double by 6 months of age and triple by 1 year.

INFANT AND TODDLER ASSESSMENT

The Denver Developmental Screening Tool II (DDST-II) is used to assess functional abilities of the infant and toddler across four domains: 1. fine and gross motor abilities (can grasp small ball; small raisin); 2. language skill acquisition and communication abilities (begins with hard consonant sounds); 3. personal and social skill abilities (recognizes consistent caregivers); and 4. adaptive abilities (can reach for specific items). Childhood disorders may manifest as delays or problems in any of these areas and may be evident as early as age 2. Full range of delay or problems may not be present until age 3 or later. There is a lack of good screening tools for this population; however, early diagnosis can lead to early interventions. General characteristics pointing to sequential development attainment are listed below:

- ▶ Newborn: can express pleasure
- ▶ 2 weeks of age: prefers mother's voice; can discriminate colors, smells, tastes
- ▶ 2 to 4 weeks of age: whole face smiles and laughs
- ▶ 4 months: can balance head
- ▶ 6 months: can sit
- ▶ 8 months: stranger anxiety develops
- ▶ 10 months: can creep, be pulled to feet; has crude prehensile grasp
- ▶ 12 months: can walk with help and grasp a small pellet
- ▶ Age 1: speaks in 1-word sentences—"Cookie!"
- ▶ Age 2: speaks in 2-word sentences—"Want cookie!" can run with ease but not great skill; can copy a circle; displays anger when autonomy is threatened; guilt and remorse (moral development)
- ▶ Age 3: can stand on 1 foot, dance, jump, and build a tower of 10 cubes; can copy a cross; attempts to control emotions
- ▶ Age 2 to 4 years: vocabulary increases rapidly
- ▶ Age 5: can skip and copy a square
- ▶ Age 6: can ride a bike with automatic ease

ADOLESCENT ASSESSMENT

The major emotional tasks of adolescents include separating from family, achieving a sense of identity, achieving body mastery, and controlling powerful sexual and aggressive urges. Not until late adolescence or early twenties is the development of the brain (and personality) complete. The average age of puberty for females is from 10 to 14 years, with menarche around age 11; puberty for males is from 10½ to 17½ years. During puberty, most adolescents experience a growth spurt and develop secondary sex characteristics. It is important, therefore, for the nurse to determine whether the adolescent is engaged in sexual activity. The sexual history assessment may be obtained through direct, matter-of-fact questioning: "Are you sexually active?" A positive response can be followed with the question: "Do you have sex with boys, girls, or both?" (CDC, n.d.). Additional questions are required to learn whether the adolescent knows what behaviors constitute sexual activity, whether the sexual relationship is consensual and monogamous, and whether the adolescent practices safe sex every time. The nurse should explain to the adolescent that patients are asked these questions to determine whether the nurse needs to plan for prevention or problem-oriented interventions. The manner in which the psychiatric–mental health nurse presents questions of a sensitive nature is critical for demonstrating the degree of openness appropriate to and available in the therapeutic relationship.

The HEEADSSS 3.0 assessment is a tool for gaining information regarding particular issues of concern when working with adolescent populations; the areas covered are **h**ome and environment; **e**ducation and employment; **e**ating; **a**ctivities; **d**rugs; **s**uicide; **s**exuality; and **s**afety.

ADVANCED AGE ASSESSMENT

As people advance in age, physical systems also change. Table 3–8 reviews common changes associated with aging.

TABLE 3–8.
CHANGES IN PHYSICAL SYSTEMS ASSOCIATED WITH AGING

PHYSICAL SYSTEMS	CHANGES WITH AGING
Neurological	▶ Decreases in neurons and some neurotransmitters
	▶ Brain becomes smaller and lighter
	▶ Vision and hearing loss
Endocrine	▶ Changes in production of most hormones; change in function may not occur
Respiratory	▶ Decline in respiratory muscle strength and control of breathing
Cardiovascular	▶ Stiffening of heart and blood vessels
	▶ Decline in cardiac output
	▶ Decreased ability of heart and vessels to adapt to stress
Gastrointestinal	▶ Decreased hepatic blood flow may decrease drug clearance
Genitourinary	▶ Decreased size of kidneys
	▶ Decreased renal blood flow
	▶ Decline in creatinine clearance rate
	▶ Erectile dysfunction in approximately 67% of men by age 70 (Stahl, 2008)
Musculoskeletal	▶ Decline in muscle mass, with increasing weakness
	▶ Bone loss
Integumentary	▶ Increased dryness of skin
	▶ Increased thinning and decreased elasticity in skin
	▶ Wrinkles and age spots from excessive sun exposure
Hematologic	▶ Decreased ability of bone marrow to produce rapid increases in red blood cells after blood loss

NEURODEGENERATIVE DISORDER ASSESSMENT: DEMENTIA AND DELIRIUM

Persons who score below the normal range on the MMSE (Table 3–5) and, upon further assessment, do not appear to have substance use problems should be further assessed to rule out delirium (acute problem onset) or dementia (insidious progressive problem). A recent report of the Alzheimer's Foundation (Powers, Ashford, & Peschin, 2008), recommends early detection and treatment of dementia. Unrecognized dementia reduces the autonomy of affected persons and increases their risks for harm from a variety of causes, including participation in other potentially harmful activities (e.g., driving), nonadherence to prescribed medication regimens, and other difficulties with activities of daily living. Patients who score within the impaired range of the MMSE and are also disoriented and confused may have delirium and should be referred for further evaluation.

PSYCHIATRIC DIAGNOSIS: INFANCY, CHILDHOOD, AND ADOLESCENTS

The *Diagnostic Classification of Mental Health and Developmental Disorders of Infancy and Early Childhood* (National Center for Infants, Toddlers, and Families, 2005) is a classification system used to diagnose and assess disorders among infants and children birth to 3 years old. Some of the most commonly noted behavioral problems are excessive crying, excessive fearfulness, feeding problems, separation and attachment difficulties, and sleeping problems.

In the book *Psychiatric Examination of Children* (1981), Simmons describes the areas commonly covered in a mental status exam of children and adolescents. The mental status exam should take place in a relaxed environment, without rush and stressors such as phone calls or interruptions. Toys, games, dolls, cars, puppets, and so on, should be visible and available in the exam room because their presence tends to lower the child's anxieties and they are very useful during the assessment, particularly when verbal communication is difficult. Simmons recommends the following areas for inclusion:

▶ Appearance: description of the physical size, manner of dress, hygiene, posture, and any obvious handicaps

▶ Mood or affect

▶ Orientation and perception: description of the child's concepts of time and ability to perceive who and where he or she is

▶ Defense (coping) mechanisms: description of major defenses the child uses to cope with anxiety

▶ Neuromuscular integration: description of the child's ability to mobilize in a coordinated fashion and to execute gross and fine motor movements

▶ Thought processes and verbalizations: description of the child's thoughts. Are they formed in a logical, cohesive, and secondary process, or are flights of ideas, loose associations, and primary process thoughts present? Is the child preoccupied or having hallucinations or delusions?

▶ Fantasy: description of the child's ability to fantasize and know the limits of fantasy. This gives data about wish fulfillment, dreams; use drawings, play.

▶ Superego: description of the child's value system, ability to discern right from wrong, and ability to respond to limit-setting

▶ Concept of self: description of the child's level of self-esteem, self-image, and self-ideal; object relations and identifications

▶ Awareness of problems

▶ Estimated intelligence quotient (IQ): description of the child's general fund of information for his or her age and other age-appropriate tasks

PSYCHIATRIC DIAGNOSIS: ADULTHOOD

The *Diagnostic and Statistical Manual of Mental Disorders,* Fifth Edition (DSM5; APA, 2013) is the classification system that represents the latest scientific thinking for the criteria and organizational structure of mental disorders. This latest version is based on advancements in the understanding of underlying vulnerabilities and characteristic symptoms of mental disorders and includes a developmental life span approach. Additional disorders have been described in this edition, and certain disorders are described under more representative headings that are more comprehensive than in previous editions. For example, Neurodevelopmental Disorders is a new heading that includes autism spectrum disorders, intellectual disorder, attention-deficit/hyperactivity disorder, and tic disorders such as Tourette's syndrome. Additionally, substance-related disorders are now covered under the heading Substance Use and Addictive Disorders and include gambling disorder as the only behavioral addiction. Obsessive-compulsive disorder has been found to involve distinct neurocircuits; therefore, it no longer falls under the Anxiety Disorder heading, and new problems, such as skin-picking disorder, now fall under the Anxiety Disorder heading. The psychiatric–mental health nurse needs to be familiar with these disorders and their criteria because symptom management is the goal of both nursing and medical implementations. The psychiatric–mental health nurse decisively works to identify nursing diagnoses for each identified physical and psychiatric problem that has been diagnosed. Medical psychiatric diagnoses fall within the purview of the psychiatrist and psychiatric–mental health nurse practitioner. The full scope of the DSM5 is beyond the scope of this text; however, the complete list of diagnostic headings and subsets are listed below for convenience:

- ▶ Neurodevelopmental Disorders

- ▶ Schizophrenia Spectrum and Other Psychotic Disorders

- ▶ Bipolar and Related Disorders

- ▶ Depressive Disorders

- ▶ Anxiety Disorders

- ▶ Obsessive-Compulsive and Related Disorders

- ▶ Trauma- and Stressor-Related Disorders

- ▶ Dissociative Disorders

- ▶ Somatic Symptom Disorders

- ▶ Feeding and Eating Disorders

- ▶ Elimination Disorders

- ▶ Sleep-Wake Disorders

- ▶ Sexual Dysfunctions

- ▶ Gender Dysphoria

- ▶ Disruptive, Impulse Control and Conduct Disorders

- ▶ Substance Use and Addictive Disorders

- ▶ Neurocognitive Disorders

- ▶ Personality Disorders

- ▶ Paraphilic Disorders

- ▶ Other Disorders

GLOBAL ASSESSMENT OF FUNCTIONING (GAF)

The DSM5's Global Assessment of Functioning (GAF) scale provides an objective rating used by psychiatrists and psychiatric nurse practitioners for estimating overall psychosocial functioning that augments the psychiatric diagnosis. The GAF is a useful metric for documenting baseline functioning and tracking progress with treatment interventions. The GAF measurement is generally coded for the period of time surrounding the evaluation, although an estimate is sometimes made about previous periods of time for comparison (e.g., the last year).

TABLE 3-9.
DSM5 GLOBAL ASSESSMENT OF FUNCTIONING BY SYMPTOM SEVERITY AND LEVEL OF FUNCTIONING

CODE	SYMPTOM SEVERITY	LEVEL OF FUNCTIONING
91–100	No symptoms	Superior functioning
81–90	Absent or minimal symptoms	Good functioning
71–80	Transient and expectable reactions to psychosocial stressors	No more than slight functional impairment in social, occupation, or school settings
61–70	Mild symptoms	
	Generally functioning pretty well, with some difficulties	
51–60	Moderate symptoms	Moderate difficulty in functioning
41–50	Serious symptoms (e.g., suicidal ideation)	Serious impairment in functioning
31–40	Some impairment in reality testing or communication	Major problems in functioning
21–30	Behavior influenced by delusions or hallucinations or serious impairment in communication	Inability to function in almost all areas
11–20	Some danger of hurting self or others or gross impairment in communication	Major problems in functioning, occasionally fails to maintain hygiene
0–10	Persistent danger of severely hurting self or others	Inability to maintain minimal personal hygiene or commits serious suicidal act with clear expectations of death

The scale ranges from 1–10 ("persistent danger of severely hurting self or others") to 91–100 ("superior functioning in a wide range of activities, life's problems never seem to get out of hand, is sought out by others because of his or her many positive qualities"). Patients with a GAF of 30 or less are unable to care for themselves ("behavior is considerably influenced by delusions or hallucinations, inability to function in almost all areas"), warranting hospitalization, some measure of court-decreed intervention, or both. The GAF is determined by the scale range (see Table 3–9) that matches the person's symptom severity or the level of functioning (e.g., social, occupational, school), whichever is worse.

GENERAL AGE-APPROPRIATE FUNCTIONAL-LEVEL SURVEY ACROSS THE LIFE SPAN

The general survey involves observing the patient for age-appropriate appearance, behaviors, and developmental milestones. We also observe the patient's interactions with family members, or others if present.

TABLE 3–10:
OBSERVATION OVERVIEW OF GENERAL FUNCTIONING ACROSS THE LIFE SPAN

Neonates and Infants	Observe parent–infant interactions, feeding, nutritional state, and cry
Early Childhood	Observe mood, nutritional state, speech, cry, facial expression, apparent emotional and chronologic age, skills, parent–child interactions, separation, tolerance, affection, and discipline
Late Childhood	Observe orientation to time and place; factual knowledge; language and number skills; motor skills used in writing, tying laces, buttoning, and drawing
Adult	Observe orientation to time and place; factual knowledge; language and number skills; motor skills used in writing, tying laces, buttoning, and drawing
Older Adults	Observe for use of adaptive devices such as hearing aids, canes, walkers, wheelchairs, or elevated commodes. Note ambulatory strength and balance. How are older adults coping with end-of-life issues?

PSYCHOSOCIAL AND ENVIRONMENTAL PROBLEMS

Psychosocial and environmental problems judged to be significant stressors may contribute to clinical disorders. Stress may arise from any of the following life situations:

- ▶ Primary support group: death of group member, health problems, abuse, dysfunction

- ▶ Social environment: death of friend, inadequate, living alone, discrimination

- ▶ Education: illiteracy, academic problems, inadequate school environment, discord with teachers or fellow students

- ▶ Occupation: unemployment, job dissatisfaction, job change, discord with boss or coworkers

- ▶ Housing: homelessness, inadequate housing, unsafe neighborhood

- ▶ Economic: extreme poverty, inadequate finances, low income, insufficient welfare support

- ▶ Healthcare access: inadequate or unavailable care, inadequate transportation or health insurance

- ▶ Other: exposure to disasters, war, or disharmony with nonfamily caregivers

ASSESSMENT OF PSYCHOLOGICAL, EMOTIONAL, AND SPIRITUAL HEALTH, GROWTH, AND DEVELOPMENT: THEORIES FROM THE FIELD OF PSYCHOLOGY

Theories of Freud, Piaget, and Erikson suggests neurological influences as the infant develops skills and cognition. Evidence is derived from observing reactions of infants to caregivers during the first 2 years of life. Patterns of terrifying experiences in infancy (perhaps even during the intrauterine period) may flood the amygdala, resulting in connections in memory circuits leading to hyperarousal states. These neural connections may be modifiable through subsequent life experiences.

Freud's Psychoanalytic Theory

Although psychoanalytic approaches developed by Sigmund Freud are no longer regularly used in today's managed care environment, many of the concepts remain relevant knowledge for psychiatric and mental health nurses. Psychoanalytic theory was initially developed by Freud (1949) and is based on the premise that most behavior is unconsciously motivated and has meaning (although the meaning may be unconscious). Psychoanalytic theory proposes that helping people trace these unconscious contributors to current behavior patterns and relationships enables them to better understand their dysfunctional patterns of relating and correct their behavior. Anxiety reduction is the goal. Freud also described the structure of personality and developed the psychosexual stages of personality development.

Freud's Personality Structures

Freud believed that behavior is heavily influenced by unconscious motivation and anxiety. He was the first theorist to introduce the concept of the unconscious, which he contended was key to understanding hidden mental processes that govern behavior. Therapeutic interventions are designed to help the client bring into conscious awareness those unconscious conflicts that the client is still acting on in the present. Freud was also the first theorist to describe transference, countertransference, and resistance. These psychological processes, along with defense mechanisms, can sabotage a relationship, which often occurs without the person having any real recognition of why he or she is feeling and reacting to the other in a manner that has little to do with the reality of the current situation. In fact, the issues of transference, countertransference, and resistance discussed in the therapeutic impasse section are Freudian concepts that have considerable relevance in today's therapeutic environment.

TABLE 3–11.
SIGMUND FREUD'S STAGES OF PERSONALITY DEVELOPMENT

Freud's Stages of Personality	
Id (present at birth)	Refers to primitive drives or instinctual energy—those associated with raw pleasure, hunger, sex, and aggression. The id operates according to the "pleasure principle," expecting immediate gratification of these drives without thought to the reality of a situation. "I want it NOW!"
Ego (develops at 4 to 6 months of age)	The part of the personality in contact with reality. The ego's primary function is to mediate between the instinctual impulses and the environment. The ego functions as a mediator to protect the person from acting solely on instinctual primitive drives, while providing a reality check for superego rigidity. Sometimes referred to as the personality's "executive function," the ego is associated with a person's higher cognitive functions of thoughtful reflection and learning. "I want it NOW, but I can wait until after lunch!"
Superego (develops at 3 to 6 years of age)	Emerges later, representing morality and the ethical standards of society. The superego evolves when the child has the capacity to identify with and internalize the prohibitions and demands of parent figures, primarily in response to rewards and punishments. The superego consists of two elements: conscience, which prevents people from doing morally wrong actions, and ego ideal, which motivates people to perform at higher moral levels. The superego can be in conflict with the id and ego as it fulfills its functions of inhibiting the expression of id impulses, persuading the ego to substitute moralistic goals for realistic ones, or strives for perfection. "I want that person's pocketbook, but I shouldn't take it."

Freud defined the personality as consisting of three major systems—the id, the ego, and the superego—which he believed are in frequent conflict. Discordant interaction among the three systems can lead to maladjusted behavior. Internal conflicts create anxiety, which occurs when the ego cannot successfully mediate between the id and the superego. The ego uses mostly unconscious defense mechanisms to protect the person from experiencing anxiety.

Freud's Psychosexual Stages Theory of Personality Development

Freud explained personality development conceptually in terms of *psychosexual stages*. He maintained that a child's personality evolves naturally through a variety of age-related, sequential stages of development, each focused on a primary erogenous zone (body part). If the child successfully negotiates the associated life issues at the appropriate stage, personality develops normally. If these life issues are not successfully resolved during the appropriate developmental stage because of parental overindulgence or frustration, a person becomes "fixated" at that psychosexual developmental stage. This fixation will significantly affect his or her adult personality in negative ways. Freud did not describe stage development in adulthood, most likely because people he assumed that one's psychological development stopped when one's physical development did, upon reaching late adolescence or early adulthood. Freud's five stages of psychosexual development are identified in Table 3–12.

TABLE 3–12.
FREUD'S FIVE PSYCHOSEXUAL STAGES OF DEVELOPMENT, TASKS, AND DEFENSES

STAGE	AGE RANGE	ZONE	DEVELOPMENTAL TASK	DEFENSE (MENTAL) MECHANISMS AND EXAMPLES
Oral	Birth to 18 months	Mouth	Establishing trusting dependence	**Substitution** (displacement): thumb- and nipple-sucking activity; satiety

The erogenous zone in the oral stage is the mouth, which infants and toddlers use first to explore their world, and then to communicate through words. Fixation behaviors include alcoholism, overeating, overdependence on others, other hand–mouth behaviors. Successful stage attainment is noted in an ability to establish trusting dependence expressed through resolution of passive and aggressive impulses.

Anal	18 months to 3 years	Anus	Development of self-control; feelings of autonomy	**Introjection:** standards of cleanliness and toilet training **Projection:** places blame for failure onto others **Displacement** (substitution): child becomes angry at parents, destroys toys, etc.

In the anal stage, the anus is the child's most sensitive erogenous zone, as the toddler learns to control elimination of body wastes through toilet training. Unsuccessful resolution of the anal stage can result in a personality "fixation" on obsessive behaviors and problems with authority figures. Successful stage attainment is noted in the development of self-control and feelings of autonomy expressed through resolution of retentive and expulsive impulses.

Phallic	3 to 5 years	Genital area	Establishing sexual role identity	**Repression:** forgetting infantile fears (e.g., a boogey man) **Reaction Formation:** Behaves in extra-brave manner to maintain repression of fears **Identification:** Boy with mother; girl with father

The phallic stage represents the most critical psychosexual conflict in Freud's developmental model. Here the erogenous zone is the **genital** region as the child begins to explore sexual differences between girls and boys. The conflict is labeled the ***Oedipus complex*** in boys and the ***Electra complex*** in girls. These complexes lead, according to Freudian theory, to normal differentiation of male and female personalities. Fixation at this psychosexual stage of development can result in uncertainty about one's identity as a male or female and affect a person's capacity to engage in a close, loving relationship. Successful stage attainment is noted in establishment of sexual role identities and beginning resolution of the Oedipal and Electra complexes.

(CONTINUED)

TABLE 3-12.
CONTINUED

STAGE	AGE RANGE	ZONE	DEVELOPMENTAL TASK	DEFENSE (MENTAL) MECHANISMS AND EXAMPLES
Latency	6 to 12 years	None; sexual drive is dormant	Group identification	**Identification:** with schoolteachers, scout leaders, peers of same sex in clique formations, gangs **Displacement** (substitution): of attitudes toward parents or to authority figures outside the home **Compensation:** for mediocre academic achievement by excelling in sports
Freud did not consider the latency stage to be a psychosexual stage of development but rather a period of dormancy, in which the child's libidinal energy is repressed and diverted into asexual activities such as athletics, school activities, and same-sex friendships. Successful stage attainment is noted in an ability to establish group identification and resolution of the Oedipus and Electra complexes.				
Genital	12 to 15 years	Genital area	Development of social control over instincts	**Identification:** with peers **Repression:** of sexual impulses and hostility **Sublimation:** of sexual energy in sports and artistic endeavors
The genital stage focuses on the **genitals** as the primary erogenous zone. As the adolescent develops mature sexual characteristics, his or her sexual interests focus on the opposite sex. Successful negotiation of life issues associated with the genital phase form the central foundation for mature sexual relationships. Successful stage attainment is noted in an ability to develop social control over instincts and sexual expression.				

Erikson's Theory of Psychosocial Development

Erik Erikson furthered Freudian theory and described personality development through eight *psychosocial stages*, essentially extending the concept that people continue personality development challenges. So in contrast to Freud, Erikson maintained that personality development does not end with adolescence (genital stage), but continues onward from birth through death. Erickson additionally broadened Freud's conceptualization of personality development to include social and cultural influences on psychosocial personality development.

According to Erikson, the *epigenetic* stages of personality development are present at birth, but will unfold according to a planned, sequential, age-related schema that incorporates cultural and social values. Each stage is characterized by a particular psychosocial crisis involving a specific developmental task that builds on previous stages, and points the way for subsequent stages. This task must be achieved for a healthy transition to the next phase of development. While, ideally, the ego should sequentially resolve the appropriate psychosocial crisis for each developmental stage, Erikson proposed that task outcomes of stage development are not fixed. They can be modified by later positive experiences or challenges to the ego. Erikson also identified a specific virtue or strength associated with each developmental stage.

Erikson's Eight Stages of Man

A student of Freudian theory, Erikson reconceptualized and extended concepts to ages beyond adolescence. Eriksonian theories looked at life stages from birth through older adulthood. Thus, he endorsed an understanding that people continue to develop toward meeting new challenges and demands throughout the life span. Erikson's eight stages are reviewed below:

Stage 1: Trust vs. Mistrust (Birth to 1 year)

▶ Corresponds to Freud's oral stage of development

▶ Virtue or strength: hope

▶ Quality of the primary caregiver relationship has a profound effect on the child's ability to balance trust with mistrust

▶ Needs must be met for basic core of trust to develop

▶ Emotional needs: security in being loved, fed, kept warm, etc.; consistency for predictable trust; dependability of the feeding person to define one's identity as a separate person

▶ Frustrations: weaning

▶ Successful achievement: developing trust in relationships, ease in feeding, depth of sleep, relaxation and movement of bowels, allows primary caretaker out of sight without undue anxiety or rage

▶ Nonachievement: unable to trust others, suspicious, withdrawn into schizoid and depressive states

Stage 2: Autonomy vs. Shame and Doubt (1 to 3 years of age)

▶ Corresponds to Freud's anal stage of development

▶ Virtue or strength: willpower

▶ Child learns sense of self; self-consciousness is associated with doubt

▶ Mastering skills involving the learning of control over bodily functions, holding on and letting go, what is the child's and what is someone else's; where the child begins and ends is primary

▶ Learning limits and what is permissible in the environment helps develop important skills related to the will

▶ Task is for the child to learn these things and parent to teach these things successfully and without excessive shame or doubt

▶ Autonomy: sense of rightful dignity and lawful independence

▶ Shame: self-consciousness; one is visible and not ready to be visible; being "shamed" leads to repressed rage and defiance

▶ Doubt: brother of shame; fear of being attacked or overpowered

▶ Emotional needs: to make decisions, learn control over bodily functions, explore the physical world, learn limits, learn what is permissible; freedom from excessive shame and permission to express resentment

▶ Frustrations: development of sphincter control

▶ Successful achievement: developing an internal locus of control; feels adequate; expresses some self-control without loss of self-esteem; good will and pride; sense of justice

▶ Nonachievement: develops external locus of control; feels inadequate; low self-esteem; secretiveness; feelings of persecution

Stage 3: Initiative vs. Guilt (3 to 6 years of age)

▶ Corresponds to Freud's phallic stage of development

▶ Strength or virtue: purpose

▶ Guilt: sense of badness

▶ Task of identification with same-sex parent to make oneself endearing to opposite-sex parent

▶ Child takes initiative in creating play roles observed in the adults around him or her

▶ Child begins to take on social role identification consistent with his or her gender; natural sexual curiosity needs to be satisfied; questions about where babies come from and masturbation are normal

▶ Parents have to teach children what is appropriate without inflicting sense of badness about themselves, sex, or their bodies

▶ Emotional needs: to test, to find out what's wrong, to learn control over body functions, to satisfy sexual curiosity, to differentiate reality from fantasy, to have adequate parent figures for identification, to be permitted resentment

▶ Frustrations: arrival of new sibling, physical threats in relation to genital play

▶ Successful achievement: purposeful, positive behaviors; feeling guilty appropriately; loving; relaxed; bright in judgment; energetic; task-oriented

▶ Nonachievement: sees own behavior as bad; experiences a high level of guilt; hysterical denial; paralysis; inhibition; psychosomatic disease; self-righteousness; moralistic surveillance; overcompensatory showing off

Stage 4: Industry vs. Inferiority (6 to12 years of age)

▶ Corresponds to Freud's latency stage of development

▶ Strength or virtue: competence

▶ Development of multiple skills, which creates the sense of industry and accomplishment

▶ Experience success and failure; feelings of inadequacy and inferiority occur when competence cannot be achieved

▶ Manual and social dexterity (locomotor skill refinements)

▶ Need good role models outside the family (e.g., teachers, scout leaders)

▶ To avoid a sense of inferiority, child must be exposed to multiple arenas to discover his or her best skills

▶ "Hero worship" and same-sex crushes are common

▶ Emotional needs: to develop confidence through social, manual, mental dexterity; to experience success in competition; to experience failure in order to learn realistic limitations and compensations; and to have adequate adults to identify with

▶ Frustrations: separation from home

▶ Successful achievement: feels competent; enjoys work or school; able to problem-solve; productive; task completion skills; steady attention; perseverance; manipulation of tools

▶ Nonachievement: feels inferior; may withdraw or act out; mediocrity; self-restriction; conformity

Stage 5: Identity vs. Role Confusion (12 to 18 years of age; puberty and adolescence)

▶ Corresponds to Freud's genital stage of development

▶ Strength or virtue: fidelity

▶ Most important stage according to Erikson

▶ "Who am I? How am I different and separate from my family of origin? What is my role in society?"

▶ Emancipation from parents and development of independence; muscular coordination

▶ Definition of sexual identity and role; straight, gay, popular, sexy

▶ Gangs and cliques prevail; need for sense of belonging

▶ Developing a personal philosophy of life, morals, and values

▶ Emotional needs: to be allowed emancipatory rebellion against parents; to develop some independence to define sexual identity and role; to develop durable, sustaining relationships outside the family; to be a needed member of a group who makes worthwhile contributions; socially constructive work

▶ Frustrations: biological readiness for sexual expression versus cultural convention and need for more emotional maturity

▶ Successful achievement: incorporates beliefs and values taught earlier; variety of roles well established; idealistic; integrative (integrates identity with libido; aptitudes with opportunity); confident

▶ Nonachievement: has problems with many roles (social, vocational, interpersonal); delinquency problems; psychotic episodes; doubt; over-identification with heroes; cliques and crowds important

Stage 6: Intimacy vs. Isolation (young adulthood)

▶ Strength or virtue: love

▶ Builds on a sense of identity by expanding it to include relationships with others

▶ Mate selection

▶ Development of mutually satisfying relationships through marriage and friendships

▶ Starting a family and keeping relationship commitments

▶ Experiencing a sense of intimacy with partners, friends, companions

▶ Successful achievement: establishes mature and intimate relationships; makes commitments; sacrifices; compromises; work productivity; satisfactory sexual relationships

▶ Nonachievement: tends toward isolation; fearful of intimacy; self-absorbed; distancing behaviors; character problems

Stage 7: Generativity vs. Stagnation (middle adulthood)

▶ Strength or virtue: nurturance and care

▶ Creating meaningful work

▶ Establishing and guiding the next generation

▶ Contributing to the betterment of society

▶ Coping with life changes—midlife crisis, which creates the need for new meanings and purpose

▶ Stagnation: self-absorption

▶ Socializing vs. sexualizing in human relationships

▶ Successful achievement: develops family; guides next generation; productivity and creativity

▶ Nonachievement: feels useless and unneeded; egocentric focus; regression to an obsessive need for pseudo-intimacy; personal impoverishment; self-love; lack of faith

Stage 8: Ego Integrity vs. Despair (maturity/older adulthood)

▶ Strength or virtue: acceptance and wisdom

▶ Life review as the person looks back on his or her life

▶ Feeling life has meaning and one has made a meaningful, vital contribution = integrity

▶ Feeling life has had little meaning and reflecting on perceived failures = despair

▶ Can accept death as a part and completion of life

▶ Successful achievement: acceptance of "good" and "bad" aspects of life; positive self-concept; assurance of order and meaning; new and different love for one's parents; emotional integration; fellowship with others; acceptance of leadership

▶ Nonachievement: sees past life as a failure; negative self-concept; fear of death; sense time as too short; disgust

Jean Piaget's Theory of Cognitive Development

Jean Piaget's theory of cognitive development is perhaps the best-known theory in cognitive developmental psychology. Piaget was a Swiss child psychologist who believed that learning was an active, dynamic process comprising four successive developmental stages of adaptation leading to increasingly complex levels of organization (principle of equilibrium). Piaget (1990) proposed that a child's physiological and psychological maturation *together with the social environment* played a significant role in a child's cognitive development. Thus, interaction with the social environment plays an important role in the development of intellectual competence. Piaget proposed that children develop cognitive structures, which he labeled *schemas*, to help them learn about and understand their environments. These schemas create increasingly complex understanding through complementary processes that Piaget termed *assimilation, accommodation,* and *organization.*

▶ **Assimilation** is the process of using and transforming environmental data so it can be placed in preexisting cognitive structures. *Example:* Infant is able to transfer the same sucking schema used to suck from the breast to suck successfully from a bottle.

▶ **Accommodation** is the process of developing a new mental schema, which the infant uses when the new information does not fit into established cognitive structures. In this case, the schema itself changes to accommodate the new information. *Example:* Infant needs to modify the sucking schema developed by sucking on the breast or bottle to learn to drink from a glass.

▶ **Organization** is the natural process by which the child learns to organize information into related, interconnected structures.

Piaget, a Swiss psychologist, studied his three children in developing his theory of how we learn to know what we know (i.e., gain cognition). Developmental delays observed in a child's cognitive development sometimes are associated with meeting physical maturation milestones and educational expectancies. In addition to psychosocial benchmarks, areas of concern can include "attention and activity regulation; speech and language; play; motor skills; bladder and bowel control; and scholastic attainments, particularly in reading, spelling, and mathematics" (Goodman & Scott, 2005, p. 5). Piaget conceptualized four major stages, each building upon the previous, in developing cognition. The four stages are outlined in Table 3–13 below.

TABLE 3-13. PIAGET'S FOUR STAGES OF COGNITIVE DEVELOPMENT

1. Sensorimotor stage (infancy)	Child learns about the environment through motor activity. Knowledge of the world (environment) takes place through direct physical interactions and experiences with touching and feeling objects. Physical mobility allows the child to explore and gain new intellectual knowledge. Peek-a-boo game-playing helps the infant learn the concept of *object permanence*—the idea that persons or objects in the environment still exist in reality, although temporarily out of sight.
2. Pre-operational stage (toddler and early childhood)	Child begins to incorporate the use of symbols as language use emerges and the child is able to express thoughts verbally. The child acquires representational skills and mental imagery emerges through exercises in magical thinking. However, thinking occurs in a nonreversible manner; thought processes are predominantly egocentric and concrete so the child is only able to think about things from his or her perspective.
3. Concrete operational stage (elementary school age; approximately 7 years through early adolescence)	Child demonstrates more complex thinking skills through manipulation of symbols associated with concrete objects, and is able to classify objects using a variety of criteria. The child is able to take into account more than one perspective, but is not able to consider all the logically possible outcomes. As concrete operational thinking develops, the child is able to conduct mental activities that are reversible, such as combining, subtracting, dividing, sorting, or seeing the connection between a nickel and two dimes representing the same 25 cents as a quarter.
4. Formal operational stage (adolescence and adulthood)	A significant cognitive shift allows for the logical use of symbols related to abstract concepts. Children in the formal operations stage can formulate hypotheses and reason theoretically, without referring to concrete objects. They can think through and problem-solve issues at an abstract level. They have the capacity to appreciate a wide range of viewpoints. Not all adolescents or adults reach the formal operation stage.

Lawrence Kohlberg's Moral Development Theory

Lawrence Kohlberg (Kohlberg, Levine, & Hewer, 1983) developed a sequential model of moral development comprised of three levels: pre-conventional, conventional, and post-conventional; and six stages of moral reasoning. This theory extends Freud's superego development stage.

TABLE 3–14. LAWRENCE KOHLBERG'S MORAL DEVELOPMENT THEORY

Preconventional (2 to 12 years)

Stage 1.	Obedience- and punishment-driven. Moral reasoning and decision-making are based solely on the consequence that taking one action over another entails. There is no recognition of the needs or rights of others. Commonly found in children.
Stage 2.	Self-interest–driven. Moral reasoning and behavior are based on the person's perception of what is best for him- or herself in the situation. Beginning token awareness of the needs of others, but only in relation to how it would benefit oneself.

Conventional (adolescent and adult)

Stage 3.	Interpersonal accord– and conformity-driven. Moral reasoning and decision-making reflect the person's perception of the social approval or disapproval of a moral action. The person evaluates the rightness or wrongness of a behavior according to the dictates of personalized social approval, and acts accordingly.
Stage 4.	Authority and social-order obedience-driven. Moral reasoning and decision-making begin to transcend individual interpretations of the meaning of behavior. There is awareness and acceptance of more universal ideas of what is right and wrong. Kohlberg suggests that most people's moral reasoning rests at stage four.

Postconventional **or Principled** (adulthood)

The postconventional or principled level incorporates differences in individual values with social understandings, resulting in a broader and deeper examination of the rightness or wrongness of value-laden behaviors.

Stage 5.	Social contract–driven. Moral reasoning and decision-making reflect a self-determining understanding of different values and opinions measured against social laws. The person is able to draw moral conclusions about behaviors based on what is best for the general well-being of all concerned in a particular situation.
Stage 6.	Universal ethical principles–driven. Moral reasoning and decision-making are based on abstract reasoning of what is justice in a particular situation. The person acts because something is morally right in and of itself, and not in relation to the expectations of others or of accepted social values. Most people do not achieve Stage 6 of moral reasoning.

Sullivan's Interpersonal Psychodynamic Theory

Harry Stack Sullivan (Evans, 1996) considered the interpersonal relationship as the keystone of therapeutic intervention. Hildegard Peplau patterned her theoretical approach to nursing interventions with psychiatric patients on Sullivan's theory. Sullivan's theoretical model focused on anxiety as being a consequence of faulty social interactions. People begin to develop personifications of self and others as the "bad me," the "good me," and the "not me" based on interpersonal interactions with important people in their lives. The *good* me represents those aspects of self that people like about themselves and are willing to share with others. The "good me" produces very little anxiety. The "bad me" represents the parts of self that a person does not like and is reluctant to share with others. The "bad me" creates anxiety. The "not me" represents those aspects of self that are so anxiety-provoking that the person does not consider them to be a part of him- or herself. This part of self exists primarily in the unconscious. People cope with the anxiety produced by undesired traits through *selective inattention*. The basic anxiety a person faces is the fear of rejection by important significant others. Sullivan's description of *parataxic distortion* refers to a person's fantasy perception of another person's attributes; for example, describing a new love relationship as "a perfect match" without considering important personality differences.

Maslow's Hierarchy of Needs Theory

Abraham Maslow (1970) theorized a hierarchy of needs, beginning with a drive to fulfill the most basic physiologic needs first before they can fully advance to the next level. As each need level is satisfied, the person is able to move on to the next higher level. Maslow's theories are optimistic, humanistic, and idealistic. The focus is on what is right for people, not what is wrong. Maslow conceptualized people as resourceful while we journey toward becoming all that we can be. Satisfaction of lower level needs propels people in fulfilling personal potential. Maslow is one of the 1969 founders of the *Journal of Transpersonal Psychology*, which laid foundation for a new field referred to as positive psychology.

Maslow referred to the first four levels as *deficit need levels*, meaning that if these needs are not met, the person is not able to realize his or her full potential because attention is directed toward meeting lower needs. For example, a person deprived of food or water cannot focus on finding friends or feeling a sense of community because she or he is coping with basic survival needs. The needs hierarchy, elevating from most basic needs to the more esoteric needs, is usually represented by pyramidal figures like the one in Figure 3–1.

FIGURE 3–1.
MASLOW'S HIERARCHY OF HUMAN NEEDS

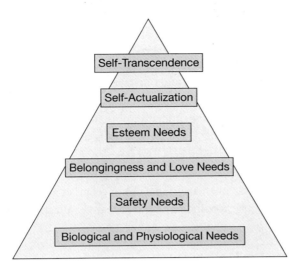

TABLE 3–15.
MASLOW'S HIERARCHY OF NEEDS THEORY:
LOWEST (MOST BASIC) TO HIGHEST LEVEL NEEDS

Physiologic Needs	Air, food, water, sex, rest, sleep, and avoiding pain
Safety and Security Needs	Stable, safe environment; job security; sufficient financial assets to live with at least minimum comfort
Love and Belonging Needs	Friends, supportive family, sense of community; sense that others care for you
Esteem Needs	Need for the respect of others and of self, which includes feelings of confidence and achievement
Self-Actualization Needs	A growth motivation need, which can only be addressed when the deficit needs are taken care of satisfactorily. Self-actualized people are not perfect; they respect themselves and have a healthy respect for others.
Self-Transcendence Needs	The need to help others reach self-actualization. It considers the "greater good (Koltko-Rivera, 2006; McLeod, 2014)."

Adapted from Maslow, 1970; McLeod, 2014; Koltko-Rivera, 2006.

Attachment Theory

John Bowlby (1958) describes a theoretical approach related to emotional attachments. He proposed that attachment behaviors are innate, instinctive responses occurring between primary caregiver and child. It is possible to observe attachment behaviors in infants, such as smiling, crying, and clinging. Children learn early in life to discriminate between loving, constant caregivers who are sensitive to their needs and others in their environment. Both primary caregiver and child play an active role in seeking proximity and contact with each other. These early experiences create internal working models important in the development of later social relationships. As the child matures, he or she is able to seek other satisfying attachment figures in his or her environment if early attachments have been favorable experiences. The capacity to form reciprocal affectionate bonds with others has an important effect on a person's emotional life. Maternal deprivation, or loss or threat of loss of important attachment figures, is a significant factor in the development of psychopathology, such as reactive attachment disorder (RAD).

Advance Directives for Mental Health

Some mental disorders present as episodic flare-ups with periods of unimpaired capacity in between (e.g., bipolar disorder). During a period of unimpaired capacity, the patient may legally initiate an advance directive for mental health care, which is designed to give specific written or oral instructions about treatment, and may appoint a power of attorney for health care. The advance directive is a legal document providing specific instructions about such matters as where the patient should be hospitalized, treatment desires, and the name of the healthcare agent charged to make healthcare decisions in the event of the person's incapacity. This agent must follow the directions given by the patient in his or her period of competency. The National Resource Center on Psychiatric Advance Directives (www.nrc-pad.org and http://myplanmylife.com/resources.cfm) provides information for psychiatric and mental health nurses and for persons with mental illnesses.

Advance directives documentation improves communication of the patient's desires to the mental health team. It allows a patient to

▶ Register refusal for receiving certain psychiatric interventions, such as ECT and psychotropic medications,

▶ Specify conditions under which these interventions are acceptable,

▶ Appoint a trusted surrogate decision-maker, a person authorized to give consent on the patient's behalf, and

▶ Register willingness to participate in research studies.

End of Life

Elisabeth Kübler-Ross (1969), who was well-known for her work with terminally ill patients, identified five developmental stages associated with the dying process. Kübler-Ross's book *Death and Dying* is still considered the classic work in thanatology. Her research findings showed little variation in the basic patterns from person to person, regardless of differences in religious or cultural background. She claimed that most dying patients go through five developmental stages from the time they receive a terminal diagnosis to the time of their actual death. These stages are not prescriptive; not all patients go through the full sequence of stages, and many people fluctuate between the different stages. Kübler-Ross postulated five stages:

1. **Denial:** "No, not me." The person feels shocked and refuses to believe what is happening. Some people stay in denial throughout their illness and, unless it interferes with appropriate treatment, denial is not necessarily a bad thing. It helps sustain hope for some people.

2. **Anger:** "Why me?" As denial subsides and the person acknowledges a terminal diagnosis, anger can emerge. In this stage, patients can be irritable, demanding, critical of others—particularly caregivers, family, even God. As with other forms of anger, it often covers anxiety.

3. **Bargaining:** "Yes me, but…." In this stage, the person tries to strike a bargain with God or the universe, asking for more time, as in "Just let me live until my son graduates."

4. **Depression:** "Yes, me." In this stage, the person can experience feelings of hopelessness and helplessness, and can be consumed with the impact of the impending death. The difference between this stage and the acceptance stage is that the person is still working through the finality of death.

5. **Acceptance:** "Yes, me, and I am ready." In this stage, the person accepts the inevitability of death, and begins to actively prepare to leave this world. The patient is likely to become more detached from others in the environment and to complete unfinished business.

Dugan (2004) suggests that Kübler-Ross's efforts to portray the human experience of receiving a terminal diagnosis and coping with a significant loss—namely, the ultimate loss of self—is largely responsible for the subsequent development of end-of-life care as an important field in medicine today. The End of Life Nursing Education Consortium (ELNEC) offers Train-the Trainer courses for nurses wishing to improve end-of-life care in the United States, administered through American Association of Colleges of Nursing (AACN) and the City of Hope National Medical Center.

End-of-Life Assessment Across the Life Span

The end of life, often more closely contemplated as a reality for older adults, may be a reality for some families at the beginning of life. However, as people live longer and more treatment options become available for persons with life-threatening conditions, mental health issues related to the end of life at any age take on more relevance.

The nurse, as advocate, is often the caregiver that becomes aware of the need for a family meeting to discuss end-of-life care issues. The nurse may facilitate family decision-making, particularly about palliative or hospice care; encourages the patient and family to develop an advance directive; and provides pain management and comfort care. Communication strategies include:

- Identifying patient goals and expectations of care and treatment
- Avoiding euphemisms for words such as "death" and "dying"
- Being specific when using words such as "hope" and "better"
- Listening to and honoring patient and family preferences, values, and cultural beliefs

If patients and families are dealing with a chronic illness, some level of emotional preparedness may have developed in the anticipation of death. Anticipation allows the emotional work to begin before the actual death occurs. Important processes the nurse can facilitate for dying patients and their families are helping members reminisce and recall milestones; inquiring about spiritual or religious beliefs and needs; allowing for expressions of sadness; and assisting in transition from hope for recovery to hope for a peaceful, dignified death. For child and adolescent mental health, alert the school nurse or counselor to help children experiencing or anticipating a death in the family.

Palliative Care

Palliative care recognizes dying as a normal part of the life process. Interventions are intended to relieve suffering while preserving the highest quality of life for patients of all ages. The World Health Organization (WHO, 2002) describes palliative care as "an approach that improves the quality of life of patients and their families facing the problems associated with life-threatening illness through the prevention and relief of suffering by means of early identification and impeccable assessment, and treatment of pain and other problems—physical, psychosocial, and spiritual."

This specialized type of care addresses the health needs of patients with life-threatening disorders and conditions such as congenital or neonatal anomalies, HIV or AIDS, congestive heart failure, cancer, emphysema, neurodegenerative disorders, end-stage diabetes, and renal failure. Patient comfort is the primary treatment goal of palliative care, with the focus on the relief of pain, stress, and symptoms (e.g., shortness of breath, nausea, fatigue, confusion) associated with terminal illness. A team approach is used to address patient and family needs, including pain, management of clinical complications, and modifications to the care plan as the patient's condition changes. It is provided from the time a serious, life-threatening, or terminal diagnosis is given, throughout the trajectory of the terminal illness and actual death, and after the death to help families cope with their loss. Interventions are tailored to meet the individualized needs of patients and families; offer professional support, information, and care during the progression of the patient's illness; integrate the physical, spiritual, and psychological components of patient care and support; and provide grief and bereavement counseling to families after the death of their family member.

Bereavement and Grief

Bereavement is the time after a loss during which a person expresses grief. Persons experiencing loss can include friends and intimate partners, as well as family members. Four phases of bereavement in uncomplicated grief are typically recognized (National Cancer Institute, 2014):

- ▶ **Shock and numbness:** Survivors find it difficult to believe the death; they feel stunned and numb.

- ▶ **Yearning and searching:** Survivors experience separation anxiety and cannot accept the reality of the loss. They try to find and bring back the lost person and feel ongoing frustration and disappointment when this is not possible.

- ▶ **Disorganization and despair:** Survivors feel depressed and find it difficult to plan for the future. They are easily distracted and have difficulty concentrating and focusing.

- ▶ **Reorganization:** When a person dies or a significant loss occurs, there may be several losses, each of which can trigger mental, physical, social, emotional, or spiritual reactions.

George Engel (1964) described grief and grieving as a subjective, personal, physical, emotional, and spiritual response to the death of something or someone important to a person. Although grief is a universal experience, each person grieves in a unique way; there is no single right way to grieve. There is no set timetable for reaching the subsequent stages of grieving, nor are the stages of grief distinct—they overlap and people can revisit previous stages. Intense emotions are normal during the grieving process. Feelings about the loss can come in waves, striking most often when the person is alone or at night. Grief therapy is designed to help people identify and cope with blockages in the grieving process, such as unfinished business with the deceased, previous unresolved losses, and insecurity about ability to reestablish relationships without the deceased. Some patients require medication as well.

Most grief reactions are self-limiting and the person begins to integrate the meaning of the lost relationship with having a life beyond the relationship as a necessary part of life's journey. *Complicated grief reactions* represent extreme reactions to grief in the form of prolonged, intense grief or emotional apathy that interferes with functioning. Variables thought to influence the emergence of complicated grief include:

- ▶ Sudden, untimely, or unexpected loss
- ▶ Suicide or homicide
- ▶ Limited social network that the person can call upon
- ▶ Significant cumulative losses
- ▶ Strong ambivalence (love-hate feelings) toward the relationship
- ▶ Overly close, intense relationship

Symptoms of complicated grief include:

- ▶ Absence of, or delayed, grief
- ▶ Inability to form new relationships
- ▶ Persistent feelings about the lost relationship
- ▶ Avoiding any reminders of the lost relationship
- ▶ Acute anxiety or agoraphobia related to being alone
- ▶ Sleeplessness and significant changes in eating habits
- ▶ Difficulty carrying out normal routines
- ▶ Extended bitterness, numbness, or detachment about life
- ▶ Symptoms of depression, anxiety disorders, posttraumatic stress disorder, or substance use disorder related to the lost relationship

Children may have more problems with grief because of more limited life experiences, concerns about who will care for them, and limited ability to work through their grief verbally. Depending on their stage of development, children may also believe they "caused" the death because of their behavior. Grief in children reflects their personalities, developmental stages, and meaning of the lost relationships. It is often expressed behaviorally as anger or avoidance behaviors, as though the loss had not occurred. Nightmares, significant changes in eating habits, concerns about health, school problems, or difficulties in peer relationships can reveal a child's grief. Developmental differences also appear in grieving:

▶ Infants and toddlers: Unaware of the permanence of death, may keep looking for the lost person; may appear unresponsive or lethargic, lose weight or interest in feeding

▶ Preschoolers: Aware of the physical death, but see it as reversible; thoughts about the death may involve magical thinking, including thinking they contributed to the person's death; grief gets expressed behaviorally with sleep and eating disturbances, frequent crying or temper tantrums, clinging behavior

▶ School-age children: Beginning awareness of the permanence of death; may ask questions about where the person goes or what happens after death; school behaviors may reflect aggressive or destructive responses, sudden outbursts, or clinging behavior

▶ Adolescence: Conceptually aware of the permanence of death; express grief in words and behaviors indicative of losing someone important (e.g., anger, sadness, lack of energy); loss of a parent during adolescence is difficult because of the adolescent need to work through a transitional period of separation from the parent

Children who experience death or divorce of a parent, especially around the ages of 4 to 6 and 12 to 14, are more at risk for the development of depression later in life. Children should be allowed to attend memorial services, see the grave site, and ask questions about the deceased if they wish to do this. They need to have questions responded to honestly in age-appropriate language, and with empathy.

Children need proactive support from the adults in their environment to work though the grieving process, at the time of the loss and periodically during their childhoods and adolescence, especially for nodal events such as graduation, starting a new school, or making a move. Some schools have grief groups and peer support for children and adolescents who have lost significant persons in their lives.

REFERENCES

Adubato, S. (2004). Making the communication connection. *Nursing management, 35*(9), 33–35.

Alexopoulos, G, Abrams, R., Young, R., & Shamoian, C. (1988). Cornell Scale for Depression in Dementia. *Biological Psychiatry, 23,* 271–284.

Arnold, E., & Boggs, K. (2007). *Interpersonal relationships in nursing, 5th ed.* Philadelphia: Elsevier.

American Academy of Pediatrics. (2012). Breastfeeding and the use of human milk. Retrieved from http://pediatrics.aappublications.org/content/early/2012/02/22/peds.2011-3552.full.pdf+html.

American Nurses Association, American Psychiatric Nurses Association, International Society of Psychiatric Nurses (2014). *Scope and standards of practice: Psychiatric–mental health nursing, 2nd ed.* Silver Spring, MD: Author.

American Psychiatric Association. (2013). *Diagnostic and statistical manual of mental disorders, 5th ed.* Arlington, VA: American Psychiatric Publishing.

Bear, M., Connors, B., & Paradiso, M. (2006). *Neuroscience: Exploring the brain, 3rd ed.* Baltimore: Lippincott Williams & Wilkins.

Beck, A. T. (1979). *Cognitive therapy and the emotional disorders.* New York: Penguin Books.

Bowlby, J. (1958). The nature of the child's tie to his mother. *International Journal of Psychoanalysis, 39,* 350–373.

Boyd, M. A. (2008). *Psychiatric nursing: Contemporary practice, 4th ed.* Philadelphia: Lippincott Williams & Wilkins.

Centers for Disease Control and Prevention. (n.d.). *A guide to taking a sexual history.* CDC Publication: 99–8445. Retrieved from http://www.cdc.gov/std/treatmentSexualHistory.pdf.

Centers for Disease Control and Prevention. (2012a). About parvovirus B19. *Parvovirus B19 and fifth disease.* Retrieved from http://www.cdc.gov/parvovirusB19/about-parvovirus.html.

Centers for Disease Control and Prevention. (2012b). Varicella. *Vaccines and immunizations.* Retrieved from http://www.cdc.gov/vaccines/pubs/pinkbook/varicella.html.

Centers for Disease Control and Prevention. (2012c). *Understanding suicide: Fact sheet.* Retrieved from http://www.cdc.gov/violenceprevention/pdf/suicide_factsheet_2012-a.pdf.

DeHert, M., Correll, C. U., Bobes, J., Cetkovich-Bakmas, M., Cohen, D., Asai, I., & Leucht, S. (2011). Physical illness in healthcare consumers with severe mental disorders. I. Prevalence, impact of medications and disparities in health care. *World Psychiatry 10*(1), 52–77.

Department of Veterans Affairs (2000). *Take 5: Pain: The 5th vital sign, revised edition.* Washington, DC: Author.

De Santos, M., De Luca, C., Mappa, I., Spagnuolo, T., Licameli, A., Straface, G., & Scambia, G. (2012). Syphilis infection during pregnancy: Fetal risks and management. *Infectious Diseases in Obstetrics and Gynecology.* Retrieved from http://dx.doi.org/10.1155/2012/430585.

Dugan, D. (2004) Appreciating the legacy of Kübler-Ross: One clinical ethicist's perspective. *American Journal of Bioethics, 4*(4): W24–28.

Dugan, M. K., & Hock, R. (2006). *It's my life now: Starting over after an abusive relationship or domestic violence, 2nd ed.* New York: Brunner-Routledge.

Edmonson, D., Robinson, S., & Hughes, L. (2011). Development of the Edmonson Psychiatric Fall Risk Assessment Tool. *Psychosocial nursing and mental health services, 49*(2): 29–36.

Engel, G. (1964). Grief and grieving. *American journal of nursing, 64*(9), 93–98.

Erikson, E. H. (1963). *Childhood and society, 2nd ed.* New York: W. W. Norton & Company.

Evans, F. B. (1996). *Harry Stack Sullivan: Interpersonal theory and psychotherapy.* London: Routledge.

Ewing, J. A. (1984). Detecting alcoholism: The CAGE Questionnaire. *Journal of the American Medical Association, 252*: 1905–1907.

Folstein, M., Folstein, S., & McHugh, P. (1975). Mini-Mental State: A practical method for grading the cognitive state of patients for the clinician. *Journal of Psychiatric Research, 12*, 189–198.

Goodman, R., & Scott, S. (2005). *Child psychology (2nd ed.).* Hoboken, NJ: Wiley-Blackwell.

Guy, W. (1976). CDEU: Assessment manual for psychopharmacology (DHEW Publication No. 76–338). Washington, DC: Department of Health, Education, and Welfare, Psychopharmacology Research Branch.

Hamilton, M. (1960). A rating scale for depression. *Journal of Neurology, Neurosurgery and Psychiatry, 23*, 56–62.

Heatherton, T. F, Kozlowski, L. T, Frecker, R. C., & Fagerstrom, K. O. (1991). The Fagerstrom Test for Nicotine Dependence: A revision of the Fagerstrom Tolerance Questionnaire. *British Journal of Addiction, 86*, 1119–1127.

Hutchinson, K. & Cagle, J. (2010).Abstract: No tobacco: A strategy for inpatient care settings. *Journal of the American Psychiatric Nurses Association, 16*(6), 373.

International Association for the Study of Pain (2014). *IASP curriculum outline on pain for nursing.* Retrieved from http://www.iasp-pain.org/Education/CurriculumDetail.aspx?ItemNumber=2052.

James, P. A., Oparil, S., Carter, B. L., Cushman, W. C., Dennison-Himmelfarb, C., Handler, J., …Ortiz, E. (2014). Evidence-based guidelines for the management of high blood pressure in adults: Report from the panel members appointed to the eighth Joint National Committee (JNC 8). *Journal of the American Medical Association; 311*(5): 507–520. doi: 10.1001/jama.2013.284427.

The Joint Commission. (n.d.). *Speak up: Reduce your risk of falling.* Retrieved from http://www. jointcommission.org/assets/1/18/Speakup_falls_brochure.pdf.

The Joint Commission. (2012). Facts about pain management. Retrieved from http://www.jointcommission. org/pain_management/.

Klein, D. A., Goldenring, J. M., & Adelman, W. P. (2014). HEEADSSS 3.0: The psychosocial interview for adolescents updated for a new century fueled by media. *Contemporary Pediatrics.* Retrieved from http://contemporarypediatrics.modernmedicine.com/contemporary-pediatrics/content/tags/ adolescent-medicine/heeadsss-30-psychosocial-interview-adolesce?page=full.

Kohlberg, L., Levine, C., & Hewer, A. (1983). *Moral stages: A current formulation and a response to critics.* Basel, NY: Karger.

Kneisl, C. R., & Trigoboff, E. (2009). *Contemporary Psychiatric–mental health nursing, 2nd ed.* Upper Saddle River, NJ: Prentice Hall.

Koltko-Rivera, M. E. (2006). Rediscovering the later version of Maslow's hierarchy of needs: Self-transcendence and opportunities for theory, research, and unification. *Review of General Psychology, 10*(4): 302–317.

Kübler-Ross, E. (1969). *On death and dying.* New York: Macmillan.

Maslow, A. (1970). *Motivation and personality, revised edition.* New York: Harper & Row.

Maslow, A. H. (1943). A theory of human motivation. *Psychological Review, 50*(4), 370–396.

McLeod, S. (2014). Maslow's hierarchy of needs. *Simply Psychology.* Retrieved from http://www.simplypsychology.org/maslow.html.

McCaffery, M. (2001). Overcoming barriers to pain management. *Nursing 31*(4), 18.

Minino, A. M. (2010). Mortality among teenagers aged 12–19 years: United States, 1999–2006. NCHS Data Brief No. 37. May 2010.

National Cancer Institute. (2014). Grief, bereavement, and coping with loss. Retrieved from http://www.cancer.gov/cancertopics/pdq/supportivecare/bereavement/HealthProfessional/page3.

National Center for Infants, Toddlers, and Families. (2005). *Diagnostic classification of mental health and developmental disorders of infancy and early childhood.* Washington, DC: Zero to Three Press.

Overall, J. (1988). The Brief Psychiatric Rating Scale (BPRS): recent developments in ascertainment and scaling. *Psychopharmacology Bulletin, 24,* 97–99.

Pfizer Inc. (1999). *Patient health questionnaire (PHQ-9).* Retrieved from http://www.uspreventiveservicestaskforce.org/Home/GetFileByID/218.

Piaget, J. (1990). *The child's conception of the world.* New York: Littlefield Adams.

Potter, P., & Perry, A. (2009). *Fundamentals of nursing, 7th ed.* St. Louis: Mosby Elsevier.

Powers, R. E., Ashford, J. W., & Peschin, S. (2008). *Memory matters. Screening approaches to increase early detection and treatment of Alzheimer's disease and related dementias, and recommendations for national policy.* New York: Alzheimer's Foundation of America.

Riffkin, R. (2014). Americans rate nurses highest on honesty, ethical standards. Retrieved from http://www.gallup.com/poll/180260/americans-rate-nurses-highest-honesty-ethical-standards.aspx.

Shepard, T. H. (1995). Catalog of Teratogenic Agents (Shepard's Catalog). *Children's Environmental Health Network.* Retrieved from http://cehn.org/catalog_teratogenic_agents_shepards_catalog.

Shives, L. R. (2012). *Basics of psychiatric–mental health nursing, 8th ed.* Philadelphia: Lipincott Williams & Wilkins.

Stahl, S. (2008). *Stahl's essential psychopharmacology: Neuroscientific basis and practical applications, 3rd ed.* New York: Cambridge University Press.

Simmons, J. E. (1981). *Psychiatric examination of children, 3rd ed.* Philadelphia: Lea & Febiger.

Steer, R.A., Ball, R., Raneeri, W.F. & Beck, A. (1997). Further evidence for the construct validity of the Beck Depression Inventory-II with psychiatric outpatients. *Psychological Reports, 80*; 443–446.

Stegmann, B. J., & Carey, J. C. (2002). TORCH infections. Toxoplasmosis, other (syphilis, varicella-zoster, parvovirus B19), rubella, cytomegalovirus (CMV), and herpes infections. *Current Women's Health Reports, 2*(4):253–258.

Stuart, G. W. (2009). *Principles and practice of psychiatric nursing, 9th ed.* Philadelphia: Mosby.

Sullivan, J., Sykora, K., Schneiderman, J., Naranjo, C. A., & Sellers, E. M. (1989). Assessment of alcohol withdrawal: The revised Clinical Institute Withdrawal Assessment for Alcohol scale CIWA-Ar. *British Journal of Addiction, 84,* 1353–1357.

Teasdale, G. & Jennette, B. (1974). Assessment of coma and impaired consciousness. A practical scale. *Lancet 2*, 7872:81–4.

Townsend, M. C. (2009). *Psychiatric mental health nursing: Concepts of care in evidence-based practice* (6th ed.). Philadelphia: FA Davis.

U. S. Department of Agriculture. (2010). *Dietary guidelines for Americans.* Retrieved from http://www.cnpp.usda.gov/sites/default/files/dietary_guidelines_for_americans/PolicyDoc.pdf.

Vuckovich P. (2003). Psychiatric advance directives. *Journal of the American Psychiatric Nurses Association, 9*(2), 55–59.

Wong, D., & Baker, C. (1988). Pain in children: Comparison of assessment scales. *Pediatric Nursing, 14*(1): 9–17.

World Health Organization. (2002). *Palliative care definition.* Retrieved from www.who.int/cancer/palliative/definition/en.

CHAPTER 4

PROBLEM IDENTIFICATION, NURSING DIAGNOSES, AND PLANNING ACROSS THE LIFE SPAN

This chapter reviews the most common problems (psychiatric diagnoses) that compromise optimal functioning across populations. Common psychiatric disorders and criteria are presented in the *Diagnostic and Statistical Manual of Mental Disorders,* 5th edition (DSM5; American Psychiatric Association [APA], 2013) and are presented for quick reference. In practice, the DSM5 is important for determining accurate diagnoses, which helps in determining appropriate medication and treatment regimens. The psychiatric and mental health nurse pursuing certification should have a good working knowledge and understanding of clinical presentations that help to substantiate particular diagnoses, serve as baseline indications at initial presentations, and provide targeted markers for determining effectiveness of interventions.

EUSTRESS AND DISTRESS

It should be noted that experiences of stress undergird the expression of many medical or psychological pathologies. In fact, stress is linked to "turning on" pathophysiological expressions. As discussed in chapter 2, one of the theories linking to psychopathology is environmental stressors, which may take the form of infections, traumas, or abuses. As it stands, many medical conditions mimic psychiatric symptoms. And no wonder; we are talking about the condition as it presents in one organism, a person who is not separated into fragmented body components. Each system of the body may express dysfunction, which may or may not be rooted in our psychological and emotional selves. Table 4–1 considers particular medical conditions that may be comorbid with certain psychological problems.

TABLE 4-1.
PHYSICAL AND PSYCHOLOGICAL PRESENTATIONS: CHICKEN OR EGG?

Cardiovascular	▶ Migraine
	▶ Essential hypertension
	▶ Angina
	▶ Tension headaches
Musculoskeletal	▶ Rheumatoid arthritis
	▶ Low back pain
	▶ Multiple sclerosis: anxiety, depression, euphoria, ataxia, muscle weakness, diffuse neurological signs with exacerbations and remissions
Respiratory	▶ Hyperventilation
	▶ Asthma
Endocrine	▶ Hyperthyroidism
	▶ Diabetes
	▶ Impotence
	▶ Frigidity
	▶ Premenstrual syndrome
	▶ Cushing's syndrome: depression, insomnia, emotional lability, mania, psychosis
	▶ Adrenocortical insufficiency: lethargy, depression, psychosis, delirium, anorexia, nausea, vomiting
	▶ Hyperthyroidism: nervousness, irritability, insomnia, pressured speech, fear, impending death, anxiety disorders, psychosis, heat intolerance, diaphoresis, tremor
	▶ Hypothyroidism: lethargy, depression, anxiety disorders, paranoia, psychosis, cold intolerance, dry skin, apathy
	▶ Hyperglycemia: anxiety, agitation, delirium, acetone breath
Neurological	▶ Tumor: judgment, seizures, loss of speech, or smell
	▶ Frontal lobe syndrome: mood or personality changes and irritability
Integumentary	▶ Neurodermatitis
	▶ Eczema
	▶ Psoriasis
	▶ Pruritus
Immunology	▶ AIDS: depression, personality changes, impaired memory, mutism, progressive dementia, mania, delirium
Gastrointestinal	▶ Anorexia
	▶ Peptic ulcer
	▶ Irritable bowel syndrome
	▶ Colitis
	▶ Obesity
	▶ Thiamine deficiency: confusion, confabulation, decreased concentration, neuropathy, Wernicke-Korsakoff's psychosis
	▶ Vitamin B12 deficiency: irritability, pallor, dizziness, ataxia, fatigue

TRAUMA-INFORMED CARE

Trauma is an overwhelming event that affects feelings of safety, creates a sense of helplessness, and continues to affect ones perception of reality. The World Health Organization (2014) notes that exposure to trauma and stress at a young age, in addition to genetics, nutrition, perinatal infections, and exposure to environmental hazards can cause mental disorders. Trauma-informed care models provides an important framework that focuses nurses to an understanding of impacts to the brain amygdala and stress hormone activation that results from trauma exposure.

Otto Rank's (1957) psychoanalytical speculation posited that our first experience with trauma occurred during the trauma of birth, reflected in recovery-based language expressions such as wanting to feel "new born" or "born again." Even earlier, consider the fetal environment during organogenesis and its effect on optimal neurological development. Did the mother-to-be have an optimal or non-optimal natal time frame? How might experiences of fear, abuse, and safety compromise the developing neonate? How about considering how historically laden trauma experienced by ancestors (slavery, Holocaust, genocide) actually may have altered the DNA structure within previous generations? Young infants and children who witness, or are victims of violence and violent acts experience triggered amygdala and HPA hormonal storms that may rewire the brain to heightened sensitivity. Impaired resilience and increased sensitivity to stress triggers to offspring may result. Manifestations may be apparent with observations of sleep disorders, learning and behavioral difficulties, or development of other traumatic anxiety disorders (see *Anxiety Disorders* on page 117). Sources estimate that 70% of U.S. adults have experienced some type of traumatic event at least once in their lifetimes with 20% going on to develop post-traumatic stress disorder (http://www.nurseptsdtoolkit.org/_/moreInfo/3.php).

Stress is understood as a normal life occurrence that is to be expected. The goal, therefore, is to identify how to cope with stress by engaging in adaptive responses rather than not coping, by engaging in maladaptive responses. A basic application of understanding stress is awareness that each patient experiences some level of stress by virtue of entering the unknowns involved in hospitalization or engagement with a healthcare provider. Personal control is often either given up or shared with a healthcare provider who is perceived as powerful and able to detect problems that people may be very sensitive about. By the same token, the nurse also experiences some level of stress and anxiety in patient encounters because of similar unknowns. With this reality out and on the table, it is paramount that the educated nurse take responsibility for setting a tone of trust-building though acceptance, openness, expressed concern, and compassion.

As discussed in chapter 2 in reference to the HPA axis, Hans Selye (1956) brought forth a theoretical explanation for stress as it is experienced, describing three stages of alarm, resistance, and exhaustion. Consider the tenets of Stuart (2009) regarding a model of stress adaptation. Stuart's stress adaptation model requires the psychiatric–mental health nurse to work with the patient to identify biological, psychological, environmental, legal, ethical, sociocultural, and other risk factors that trigger a stress response in the patient. Any factor is a stressor if the patient perceives it to be so. The cognitive meaning, the affective feeling, the behavioral response, as well as the genetic predisposition of the patient-precipitant relationship are factors that will determine the patient's ultimate coping resources. These strengths and coping resources are drawn from a person's personal abilities, level of social support, material assets, and belief system. The nurse will explore these resources in planning care for the patient, as addressed later in this chapter. Criteria for diagnosing psychopathology are found in the *Diagnostic and Statistical Manual of Mental Disorders,* 5th edition (DSM5; APA, 2013).

PSYCHIATRIC-MENTAL HEALTH PRACTICE STANDARD 2: NURSING DIAGNOSIS

Several diagnostic classification systems exist for identifying problems and specific directions of care for mental disorders. The resource for developing nursing diagnoses was developed by the NANDA International (NANDA-I). The NANDA-I classification system (NANDA International, n.d. a) was developed by nurses to identify problems treatable by nurses. NANDA-I nursing diagnoses, unlike DSM5 (APA, 2013) diagnoses, identify the patient's response to health problems, not the medical diagnosis. They are based upon the conceptualization of the human response to actual or potential health problems from the unique nursing perspective. The diagnosis is based upon an analysis and synthesis of collected data and the recognition of functional patterns and trends. Nursing diagnoses allow for recognition of emergent and urgent problems, patterns, and trends in comparison with normal standards. Diagnoses provide for prioritization; highest priorities are addressed first. An accurate diagnosis guides the direction of treatment and evaluation of care outcomes (NANDA International, n.d. a, n.d. b). A partial list of NANDA-I–approved diagnoses that might apply to patients with mental disorders are listed in Box 4.1.

Once problems have been identified and nursing diagnoses made, the psychiatric–mental health nurse plans and implements nursing care addressing priorities for treatment. The highest priority is given to conditions that, if untreated, could result in harm. These would include conditions that involve basic survival needs or safety needs related to suicidal or homicidal ideation (SI or HI) or threat of harm from others (e.g., domestic violence, child or elder abuse). Intermediate priority is given to nonemergent, non–life-threatening, but distressing, painful, or dysfunctional symptoms (e.g., hallucinations, agitation). Lower priority is given to issues that are not specifically related to the illness or prognosis (e.g., occupational, social stressors). Maslow's hierarchy of needs can be used to conceptualize the priorities for care planning.

The nursing care plan specifies, by priority, the diagnoses, short-term and long-term goals and expected outcomes, and interventions, including the what, when, where, how, and who. When available, current, evidence-based practice guidelines, clinical pathways, or clinical algorithms can be used. When new or unusual care needs arise, the nurse is advised to use current research to identify evidence-based approaches. In planning for safe and effective quality care, the Joint Commission (2015) establishes annual Behavioral Health Care National Patient Safety Goals:

BOX 4.1. SELECT LISTING OF NANDA-I NURSING DIAGNOSES

- Anxiety (mild, moderate, severe, panic)
- Adjustment, impaired
- Confusion (acute, chronic)
- Coping (ineffective, readiness for enhanced, compromised family, defensive)
- Denial, ineffective
- Decisional conflict
- Family processes (dysfunctional, interrupted, readiness for enhanced)
- Fatigue
- Fear
- Grieving (anticipatory, dysfunctional)
- Health maintenance, ineffective
- Health-seeking behavior
- Hopelessness
- Identity, disturbed personal
- Loneliness, risk for
- Memory, impaired
- Noncompliance; nonadherence
- Nutrition, altered; more or less than body requirements
- Pain (acute, chronic)
- Parenting (enhanced readiness, impaired, risk for impaired)

- Posttraumatic syndrome or risk
- Rape trauma syndrome
- Relocation stress syndrome or risk
- Role performance, ineffective
- Self-care deficit (bathing, dressing, feeding, etc.)
- Self-esteem (chronic low, situational low, risk for low)
- Self-mutilation or risk for
- Sensory perception, disturbed or altered
- Sexual dysfunction
- Sexuality pattern, disturbed
- Sleep pattern, disturbed
- Social interaction, impaired
- Social isolation
- Sorrow, chronic
- Spiritual distress, risk; readiness for
- Suicide risk
- Thought process disturbed or altered
- Trauma, actual or risk
- Violence, risk for other- or self-directed
- Wandering

- Identify persons served correctly. Use at least two ways to identify individuals served. for example, use the individual's name and date of birth. This is done to make sure that each individual served gets the correct medicine and treatment.

- Use medications safely. Record and pass along correct information about a patient's medicines. Find out what medicines the patient is taking. Compare those medicines to new medicines given to the patient. Make sure the patient knows which medicines to take when they are at home. Tell the patient it is important to bring their up-to-date list of medicines every time he or she visits a doctor. Prevent infection. Use the goals to improve hand cleaning.

- Identify patient safety risks. Find out which individuals served are most likely to try to commit suicide.

PSYCHIATRIC–MENTAL HEALTH PRACTICE STANDARD 3: OUTCOMES IDENTIFICATION

Outcomes identify the desired results for improvements in patient functionality and well-being that are demonstrated from interaction with nurses and the healthcare environment. Guidelines are constructed to lay out consistency of elements, and they can be measured along several dimensions: clinical, functional, satisfaction, and financial.

Outcomes are clear statements indicating what "will" happen for patients as a course of clinical care. Regardless of the dimension, each outcome considers these guidelines:

▶ Patient and family-centered: focuses on diagnosis; suited to patient or population of interest

▶ Singular: separate goals for each identified problem or need

▶ Mutual: agreed upon by patient, family, or both and nurse, team, or healthcare providers

▶ Measurable, reliable, valid: describes quality, quantity, severity, frequency (standardized assessment tools and scales)

▶ Time-limited: set short- and long-term goals

▶ Realistic: attainable to provide a sense of accomplishment; sensitive to changes within or between persons

▶ Evidence-based: algorithms, practice guidelines, clinical pathways

▶ Cost-effective

Specific outcomes criteria in keeping with Psychiatric–Mental Health Practice Standard 4: Planning will be presented with each psychiatric problem presented in this chapter.

TABLE 4–2.
OUTCOME DIMENSIONS

Clinical Outcomes	Health status, relapse, recurrence, readmission, number of episodes, symptomatology, coping responses, high-risk behaviors, incidence reports
Functional Outcomes	Functional status (e.g., Global Assessment of Functioning or GAF), social interaction, activities of daily living (ADLs), occupational abilities, quality of life, family relationships, housing arrangements
Satisfaction Outcomes	Satisfaction with treatment, treatment outcomes, treatment team and organization, patient satisfaction measures
Financial Outcomes	Cost, revenue, length of stay, use of resources

MAJOR PSYCHIATRIC MENTAL HEALTH PROBLEMS

Psychotic (Thought) Disorders

Pathogenesis: Theories

Scientific research has determined that subtle prodromal symptoms of schizophrenia may be present from early childhood. They can include delayed language development and asymmetrical use of major muscles of the body. These early findings have led researchers to the hypothesis that schizophrenia is a neurodevelopmental condition. In other words, the brains of persons who develop schizophrenia may not develop normally. It has been hypothesized that the early migration of neurons in brain development may be faulty, resulting in abnormal connections (migrational defects), or excessive, inadequate, or improper pruning of synapses or neurons. It is also hypothesized that maternal flu infection or iron deficiency, as well as substance use by the person, increase the risk for development of psychotic-inducing disorders.

Neurodegeneration theories describe the process of pruning away unnecessary connections in the brain going awry, resulting in destruction of too many neurons and their connections. A process called *excitotoxicity* (Stahl, 2008) has been used to describe the potential self-destruction of neurons resulting from too much glutamate and excitatory neuronal activity. Support for a neurodegenerative mechanism in schizophrenia comes from monozygotic twin studies showing that affected twins tend to have enlarged ventricles of the brain in comparison to their healthy twin siblings. Ventricular enlargement is due to atrophy of the brain tissues, creating more space for fluid in the ventricles.

The pathophysiology of schizophrenia is also characterized by abnormal neurotransmission. Abnormally elevated levels of dopamine in the limbic system are thought to be responsible for positive symptoms (hallucinations, delusions, abnormal speech, and abnormal behavior). Because dopamine is essential for learning, memory, and motivation, the negative symptoms (amotivation, apathy, and anhedonia) and cognitive impairment may reflect lower-than-normal levels of dopamine in the prefrontal cortex. Although dopamine is the neurotransmitter most associated with schizophrenia, researchers are learning that other neurotransmitters, such as glutamate, may also have important roles.

Schizophrenia Syndrome

The experience of psychosis is evident in many subtypes of schizophrenia, pointing to a clearer understanding of what is now referred to as *schizophrenia syndrome*. Nasrallal and Weiden (2014) posit the following occurrences that precipitate increased risk for the development of schizophrenia syndrome:

- ▶ Childhood traumas
- ▶ Paternal age older than 45
- ▶ Migration from another country
- ▶ Pregnancy and delivery complications
- ▶ Urbanicity
- ▶ Winter birth (vitamin D deficiency)
- ▶ Antibodies to one's own N-nitrosodimethylamine (NDMA)
- ▶ Glutamate toxicity

Readers should view the Nasrallal & Weiden (2014) webinar listed in the references for details pertaining to these recent developments.

The average age of onset for schizophrenia, a major psychotic disorder, usually start between ages 16 and 30 with men experiencing symptoms a little earlier than women. Although it is rare, children can develop the disorder, and most of the time, people do not get schizophrenia after age 45 (National Institute of Mental Health, 2015). Support for the neurodevelopmental theory comes from the observation that during the late adolescence, when most people develop full access to the frontal executive functions of the brain, persons with schizophrenia start to demonstrate disordered thinking.

The date of onset is defined by a 6-month period of positive symptoms; however, the prodrome period leading up to the first acute episode may last days to years before the diagnosis. Family members often can look back after the diagnosis of schizophrenia and identify a period of altered behavior leading up to the first major episode of psychosis. During this time, an adolescent may withdraw from family or friends, use drugs, and exhibit changes in motivation and school performance. Subtle delays in language and motor skills may even have been present early in life.

The three major symptom categories of schizophrenia that reflect brain abnormalities are the positive symptoms, negative symptoms, and cognitive dysfunction (diminished executive functioning and working memory). Evidence of delusions, hallucinations, and disorganized behaviors are the hallmarks that define "positive" symptoms, whereas "negative" symptoms include tendencies to withdraw from others, lack of motivation or concern about appearance, and anhedonia. Usually continuous social and occupational dysfunction for at least 6 months is present. In fact, according to Nasrallal and Weiden (2014), the abuse of phencyclidine (PCP, a veterinary anesthetic) perfectly mimics the symptoms of schizophrenia syndrome. Two or more of the following symptoms must have been present for a significant portion of time during a 1-month period for a diagnosis of schizophrenia:

▶ Positive symptoms

  ▸ Delusions

  ▸ Hallucinations

  ▸ Disorganized speech

▶ Negative symptoms

  ▸ Disorganized behavior

  ▸ Withdrawal, apathy, alogia, amotivation

Schizophrenia can be further differentiated according to predominance in symptomology:

▶ Paranoid type

▶ Disorganized type

▶ Catatonic type

▶ Undifferentiated type

After an acute episode of psychosis, recovery to previous levels of functioning may be incomplete, often characterized by the persistence of negative symptoms (severe and persistent mental illness or SPMI). Because it afflicts young adults, this devastating and chronic illness can be characterized as the "Alzheimer's disease of the young."

Additional classifications of psychotic disorders are listed in Box 4–2. The specific criteria for each are not addressed in this text. The psychiatric–mental health nurse needs to understand the overarching signs of psychosis itself (delusions and hallucinations) as the focus of psychiatric and nursing interventions.

BOX 4–2.
PSYCHOTIC AND THOUGHT DISORDERS: SCHIZOPHRENIA SYNDROME

▶ Schizophrenia
▶ Schizophreniform disorder
▶ Schizoaffective disorder
▶ Brief psychotic disorder
▶ Delusional disorder

Mood Disorders

Pathogenesis: Theories

Monoamine Dysregulation Theory

Monoamines are the neurotransmitters that include serotonin (5HT), norepinephrine (NE), and dopamine (DA). The hypothesis that depression is caused by a reduction or deficit in one or more of the monoamines forms the basis for treating with the traditional antidepressants. Cerebral blood flow is diminished and hippocampal volume is decreased (Rosedale et al., 2013). The actual mechanism of depression is probably more complicated, involving the monoamine receptors and other cellular events, including the regulation of gene expression (Stahl, 2008).

Dysregulation of the HPA Axis Theory

A second hypothesis about the pathophysiology of depression involves the stress response systems, in particular, the hypothalamic-pituitary-adrenal-axis (HPA axis). The HPA axis appears to be the main site where genetic, hormonal, and environmental influences converge in mood disorder etiology. In the autonomic and complex interplay between thoughts, emotions, and behaviors, when a person perceives stress, a circular biofeedback loop activates that stimulates the hypothalamus to secrete corticotropin-releasing hormone (CRH). This hormone stimulates the pituitary gland to release arenocorticotropic hormone (ACTH). This systemically circulating hormone activates the adrenal glands (atop the kidneys) to release the hormone cortisol. Circulating cortisol results in activation of the "fight-or-flight" response. All senses become hyperalert, blood is physiologically shunted from the digestive system out to skeletal muscles, pupils become dilated, respiration deepens and becomes more rapid, and cardiac output increases. These neurophysiological responses can be represented as the physiological resistance stage, outlined by Hans Selye (1956), when the person is taxing multiple organ systems while simultaneously evoking homeostatic balance. When stressors remain high for long periods of time (such as a state of homelessness, being in a combat zone, living in terrorizing or traumatizing environments) with concomitantly high cortisol levels, major biochemical, physiological, anatomical, and psychological damages may ensue.

Early life stressors, such as the loss of a parent, trauma, or neglect, have been shown to produce lasting effects on the HPA axis, leading to chronic difficulty in managing stress and chronically elevated levels of cortisol. The support for this hypothesis of depression is that persons with major depressive disorder often present with hypercortisolemia, resistance of cortisol to suppression by dexamethasone, blunted ACTH responses to corticotrophin-releasing hormone (CRH) challenge, and elevated CRH concentrations in the cerebrospinal fluid (CSF).

Vitamin D Deficiency Theory

Recent evidence suggests that vitamin D, which exerts neurological benefits on cognition, memory, and mood, may be deficient among persons who develop mood disorders (Farrington, 2013).

Classifications of Mood Disorders

Disorders of mood can include depression (unipolar disorder) or bipolar disorder, or the less acute but long-lasting dysthymic and cyclothymic variations.

The distinction between unipolar depression and bipolar depression is important because the two disorders require different treatments. Bipolar depression is more likely to have a heritable (genetic) component than unipolar depression, and a person with bipolar disorder is more likely to have had previous symptoms, treatments, or hospitalizations. Depression can occur at any age, including the first and last years of life. *Failure-to-thrive* (FTT) in infants, a clinical condition often requiring pediatric hospitalization, may be indicative of infantile depression. Geriatric failure-to-thrive (GFTT), seen among some older adults, may also have roots in mood disorders. The average ages of onset for the development of mood disorders are listed below.

> **BOX 4-3. MOOD DISORDERS**
>
> ▸ Disruptive mood dysregulation disorder
> ▸ Dysthymia
> ▸ Seasonal affective disorder (SAD)
> ▸ Postpartum depression
> ▸ Adjustment disorder
> ▸ Bipolar I
> ▸ Bipolar II

▸ Disruptive mood disorder dysregulation

  ▸ Can occur at any age (infantile failure-to-thrive; geriatric failure-to-thrive)

  ▸ Generally between 20 and 50 years

  ▸ Mean age of onset: 40 years

▸ Bipolar disorder

  ▸ Childhood (5 to 6 years) to age 50

  ▸ Mean age of onset: 21 to 30 years

Mood dysregulation can co-occur with other medical illnesses, such as cardiovascular disease, Parkinson's disease, neurodegenerative and neurocognitive disorders, traumatic brain injuries, hypothyroidism, and cancer, as well as with life stressors. Although the average age for diagnosing bipolar disorder is in the late 20s or early 30s, many of the symptoms, including impulsivity and difficulty controlling emotions, can be present as early as age 4 or 5. These early symptoms of bipolar disorder are often misdiagnosed as attention-deficit hyperactivity disorder (ADHD). Mood disorders can be triggered by upsetting life events, life transitions, physical transitions or illness, and chronic stress. Remember, assessment of mood states is determined by subjective affirmation by the patient. The nurse or clinician cannot merely look at the patient's affect and infer mood. Therapeutic communication skills (reviewed later) guide the psychiatric nurse in eliciting mood states, and then considering congruence (agreement) between mood and affect.

Disruptive Mood Disorder Dysregulation

The diagnosis of disruptive mood disorder dysregulation (formerly referred to as major depressive disorder) is evident by symptoms in the affective, behavioral, cognitive, and emotional domains of functioning as outlined below:

▶ Affective

  ▸ Hopelessness

  ▸ Worthlessness and despair

  ▸ Apathy

  ▸ Anhedonia

  ▸ Emptiness

  ▸ Feelings of excessive guilt

▶ Behavioral

  ▸ Psychomotor retardation or agitation

  ▸ Verbal communication decreased

  ▸ Hygiene and grooming decreased

  ▸ Social isolation

▶ Cognitive

  ▸ Confusion

  ▸ Indecisiveness

  ▸ Diminished ability to think or concentrate

  ▸ Self blame

  ▸ Suicidal ideation

  ▸ Recurrent thoughts of death

▶ Physical

  ▸ Body slowdown

  ▸ Sleep disturbances

  ▸ Weight loss or weight gain

  ▸ Insomnia or hypersomnia

  ▸ Fatigue or loss of energy

Dysthymic Disorder

As opposed to persistent, or chronic depression, in dysthymic disorder, people experience a depressed mood for most of the day more days than not, for at least 2 years. This describes people said to be in a "blue funk," akin to Oscar the Grouch on *Sesame Street*. Persons with this mood dysregulation rarely present for psychiatric intervention.

Adjustment Disorder

Life changes can precipitate mood dysregulation, which may also be referred to as situational depression, or a primary stress response syndrome. Acknowledgement of some precipitant (e.g., recent divorce, change in school, off to military) that has occurred in the last 3 months or so may lead to this diagnosis.

Seasonal Affective Disorder

Some people experience depression during fall and winter, returning to normal moods in spring and summer. The fall-winter experience may be related to reduced natural light from sunshine that is evident in some parts of the world. Light inhibits the production of melatonin, a hormone that affects mood and induces sleep.

Postpartum Depression

Postpartum depression ("baby blues") within the first 10 days postpartum that lasts at least 2 weeks is experienced by upwards of 70% of new mothers. The phenomenon is thought to be related to rapid fluctuations in hormones that occur around the perinatal period (before and after birth). Early recognition is critical for the health of both mother and infant. Untreated episodes may progress to an emergency situation of postpartum psychosis that could lead to infanticide.

NANDA-I: Mood Disorders

▶ Risk for suicide related to:

  ▸ Feelings of hopelessness, helplessness, or worthlessness

  ▸ Anger turned inwards

  ▸ Reality distortions

▶ Low self-esteem related to:

  ▸ Learned helplessness

  ▸ Significant losses

  ▸ Cognitive distortions leading to negative self-image

▶ Dysfunctional grieving related to:

  ▸ Real or perceived loss

  ▸ Bereavement overload (not adequately dealing with losses)

▶ Social isolation related to:

  ▸ Negative self-perception

  ▸ Egocentric behaviors

Bipolar I and II Pathogenesis: Monoamine Dysregulation Theory

Bipolar manic episodes may involve the same neurotransmitter systems as depression, with problems related to overactivity rather than underactivity. Elevated levels of serotonin (5HT), norepinephrine (NE), and dopamine (DA) in areas of the brain regulating mood and behavior could explain symptoms such as irritable or expansive mood, pressured speech, flight of ideas, decreased sleep, and increased goal-directed activity. *Sensitivity* and *kindling* are two terms that have been used to describe neuronal activity in bipolar disorder. Early in the course of the illness, mood episodes may be triggered by significant stressors. Over time, the brain appears to become sensitized to stress and much less stress is necessary to trigger an episode. The neurons respond to slight provocations like kindling wood for fire: a small spark and the kindling catches fire immediately.

Bipolar I disorder is characterized by episodes of severe mood swings, from mania to depression. Bipolar II disorder is a milder form, characterized by milder episodes of hypomania that alternate with depression. Both mood disorders can occur in children and adolescents. Mixed featured types may include the presence of psychosis or rapid cycling (cyclothymia—four or more episodes with a 12-month period). Observable symptoms that may be noted by the nurse include

▶ Expansive, cheerful mood,

▶ Irritable when wishes unfulfilled,

▶ Flighty, rapid flow of ideas,

▶ Inflated self-esteem,

▶ Decreased need for sleep,

▶ Distractibility,

▶ Increase in goal-directed activity,

▶ Excessive involvement in pleasurable activities,

▶ Lacking depth of personality and warmth,

▶ Increased libido or sexual promiscuity,

▶ Irresponsible financial management,

▶ Loquacious (more talkative than usual),

▶ Continuous high elation,

▶ Emotional lability: rapid changes,

▶ Fragmented, racing, and disjointed thoughts,

▶ Extreme hyperactivity,

▶ Delusions, hallucinations (psychotic features),

▶ Increased, disorganized, and incoherent speech,

▶ Flamboyant dress, and

▶ Grandiosity and inflated sense of self.

NANDA-I: Bipolar Disorders

▶ Risk for injury

▶ Risk for violence (self or other directed)

▶ Disturbed thought processes

▶ Disturbed sensory perception

▶ Nutritional deficiency

▶ Impaired social interaction

NANDA-I for Suicide, Homicide, Aggression, Abuse, Assault

▶ Risk for suicide, homicide, aggression, abuse, or assault

▶ Hopelessness

▶ Ineffective coping related to negative role-modeling

▶ Risk for violence to others related to childhood environment of violence

Psychiatric–Mental Health Practice Standard 4: Planning

Improvement outcomes for all patients with mood disorders:

▶ The patient will experience no harm or injury.

▶ The patient does not display physical agitation toward self or others.

▶ The patient eats well-balanced meals and gets adequate rest and sleep.

▶ The patient interacts appropriately.

▶ The patient maintains reality orientation.

▶ The patient discusses losses with staff and family or significant others.

▶ The patient sets realistic goals for him- or herself.

▶ The patient identifies aspects of self-control over his or her life situation.

▶ The patient can concentrate and make decisions.

Improvement outcomes for patients with suicidal (SI) or homicidal (HI) ideation or aggressive behaviors:

▶ The patient will seek help through the mental health system.

▶ The patient will state that he or she is no longer having SI, HI, or aggressive feelings.

▶ The patient will be able to recognize anger and seek staff to talk about feelings.

▶ The patient will exert internal control over anger.

▶ The patient will not cause harm to self or others.

▶ The patient will use problem-solving to seek solutions.

Anxiety Disorders

Pathogenesis: Anxiety

The anxiety disorders are characterized by fear and worry that can be polarizing. Polarization leads to dysfunction by interfering with the ability to make a decision. The neurobiology of fear is thought to involve brain circuits that are regulated by the amygdala—the small, almond-shaped brain structure that is responsible for detecting threat and initiating the stress response. Conditions of worrying may involve a different brain circuit that passes through the basal ganglia. The connection with the basal ganglia is especially important in obsessive-compulsive disorder (OCD), where we see overlap with other disorders linked to basal ganglia dysfunction, such as ADHD and tics.

Anxiety disorders and depression often share symptoms that are associated with a chronic stress response. Is anxiety a symptom, a syndrome, or a disorder? Symptoms associated with chronic stress include tension headaches, migraine headaches, and musculoskeletal pain. In addition, a chronic response to stress by way of the HPA axis (Chapter 2, Figure 2–1), with increased circulating levels of cortisol, has been linked to increased abdominal fat, impaired immune function, disrupted glucose metabolism, cardiovascular symptoms (e.g., hypertension), gastric ulcers, and hippocampal atrophy with learning and memory impairments.

As noted previously, sympathetic nervous system activation of the autonomic nervous system activates the fight-or-flight mechanism with its automation of increased heart and respiratory rates, dilation of pupils, and sweating responses due to noradrenergic norepinephrine release. HPA activation is elicited when anxious. Do anxiety disorders, therefore, suggest alteration of norepinephrine (NE), gamma-amino-butyric acid (GABA), epinephrine (E)?

The brain's GABA receptors can be modulated by central nervous system depressants such as alcohol and benzodiazepines. When people drink alcohol or take benzodiazepines, anxiety levels tend to subside. During withdrawal from those same substances, anxiety increases. These findings support the hypothesis that the neurotransmitter GABA and its receptors are important in the symptoms of anxiety, with too little GABA associated with symptoms of anxiety. On the other hand, too much arousal from NE or glutamate may also lead to symptoms of anxiety.

Anxiety can be a normal emotion in threatening circumstances. It is the emotional component of the "fight or flight" stress response and has important survival functions. Anxiety can also be part of a syndrome or symptom complex associated with certain medical or substance-related conditions. Examples include hyperthyroidism, attention-deficit hyperactivity disorder (ADHD), and alcohol or benzodiazepine withdrawal. Finally, anxiety can be the primary component of a disorder.

Anxiety is common at all ages. Children can develop all the anxiety disorders experienced by adults in addition to separation anxiety disorder. Separation anxiety is a normal stage of development at around 6 through 18 months of age. The infant or toddler with separation anxiety should exhibit some resistance to being passed to someone not as familiar as the primary caretaker. However, separation anxiety becomes a disorder when school-aged children continue to express fear of separation along with significant functional impairment. Anxiety states in children can manifest as enuresis (repeated voiding of urine in bed or clothing) or encopresis (voluntary or involuntary passage of stool in a child who has previously been toilet trained, typically over age 4). Although anxiety has a heritable component, anxiety disorders such as posttraumatic stress disorder (PTSD) and phobias occur after a threatening event. Evidence of self-mutilation (referred to as nonsuicidal self-injury disorder) may accompany many psychiatric presentations (e.g., psychosis, mood dysregulation, anxiety, substance use, feeding and eating disorders, gender dysphoria). Additional risk factors for the development of anxiety and anxiety disorders include:

- ▶ Genetics
- ▶ Biology
    - ▸ Temperament, physiologic abnormalities
- ▶ Medical conditions
    - ▸ For example, acute MI or hypoglycemia
- ▶ Psychoanalytic
    - ▸ Unconscious fear expressed symbolically
    - ▸ Lack of ego strength and coping resources
- ▶ Learning theory
    - ▸ Fears are learned and become conditioned responses
    - ▸ Lack of recovery environment (social supports)
- ▶ Cognitive theory
    - ▸ Faulty cognition or anxiety-inducing self-instructions

Common features of several anxiety disorders are reviewed below.

Panic Disorder

- ▶ Recurrent, unexpected panic attacks
- ▶ Can present before puberty; peak age 15 to 20 years
- ▶ At least one of the attacks has been followed by 1 month of:
    - ▸ Persistent concern about having additional attacks
    - ▸ Worry about implications (e.g., losing control, having a heart attack)

Generalized Anxiety Disorder (GAD)

▶ Excessive anxiety and worry; "worry warts" (worrying more days than not for at least 6 months, about a number of events or activities)

▶ Average age of onset is in 20s

▶ The anxiety and worry are associated with 3 or more of the following 6 symptoms:

  ▸ Restlessness

  ▸ Being easily fatigued

  ▸ Difficulty concentrating

  ▸ Irritability

  ▸ Muscle tension

  ▸ Sleep disturbance

Phobia: Specific, Social, or Agoraphobia

▶ Marked or persistent fear that is excessive or unreasonable, cued by the presence or anticipation of a specific object or situation

▶ Exposure to the phobic stimulus almost invariably provokes an immediate anxiety response, which may take the form of a panic attack.

▶ The person recognizes that the fear is excessive.

  ▸ The phobic stimulus is avoided.

Obsessive-Compulsive Disorder (OCD)

▶ Highly co-occurring with ADHD and tic disorders

▶ Can occur before age 9 (rule out PANDAS)

▶ Either obsessions or compulsions that cause marked distress, are time-consuming, and interfere with functioning

  ▸ Obsessions: recurrent and persistent thoughts, impulses, or images that are intrusive and inappropriate

  ▸ Compulsions: repetitive behaviors that the person feels driven to perform; aimed at anxiety reduction

Body Dysmorphic Disorder

▶ Physically normal appearance and body, but patient believes that parts of the body are abnormal, misshapen, or ugly

▶ Impairs function

Hoarding Disorder

▶ Tendency to collect and accumulate objects without apparent value, to the point of functional impairment; functional paralysis

Trichotillomania

▶ Hair-pulling disorder; hair may be pulled from various areas of body (head, eyelashes, pubic area, armpits)

▶ Pulling is accompanied by tension release.

  ▹ May result in development of a bezoar (hair ball in stomach) that may require surgical removal

Excoriation (Skin Picking) Disorder

▶ New to DSM5 (APA, 2013)

▶ Usually begins in adolescence; mostly focuses on face or head

  ▹ Picking at skin to the point of trauma, bleeding

Separation Anxiety Disorder

▶ Normal developmental achievement at around 6 to 18 months of age

▶ Suggests significant functional impairment if continues in toddlers and older children.

Trauma-Related Anxiety Disorders

Posttraumatic Stress Disorder (PTSD)

▶ Person has been exposed to a traumatic event

▶ Traumatic event is persistently re-experienced

▶ Persistent avoidance of stimuli associated with the trauma and numbing of general responsiveness

▶ Persistent symptoms of increased arousal

▶ Duration is longer than 1 month

  ▹ Can occur in children and adolescents

Acute Stress Disorder

▶ Similar to PTSD except that onset follows during or immediately after a stressful event

▶ Lasts a month or less

Adjustment Disorder

▶ Person feels overwhelmed by one or multiple stressors (e.g., marriage, relocation, witnessing parental discord)

▶ Can occur in children and adolescents

  ▹ Starts within 3 months of stressor; stops within 6 months of stressor's end

Rape Trauma Syndrome

▶ Similar to PTSD except that onset follows during or immediately after a rape or sexual assault

  ▹ Lasts a month or less

NANDA-I: Anxiety and Anxiety Disorders

▶ Panic anxiety: real or perceived threat

▶ Powerlessness related to anxiety

▶ Ineffective coping related to intrusive or inappropriate thoughts

▶ Ineffective role performance related to ritual performance

▶ Posttrauma syndrome related to war exposure

▶ Posttraumatic rape syndrome related to sexual abuse, assault, or molestation

▶ Dysfunctional grieving

▶ Fear

▶ Social isolation

Psychiatric–Mental Health Practice Standard 4: Planning

Improved outcomes for patients with anxiety and anxiety disorders:

▶ The patient will recognize signs of anxiety and utilize anxiety reduction skills.

▶ The patient will verbalize an understanding of the relationship between anxiety and maladaptive coping.

▶ The patient will deal with stress using coping strategies.

  ▹ Thought stopping

  ▹ Relaxation techniques

  ▹ Physical exercise

▶ The patient will attend to school or work.

PRIMARY FEEDING AND EATING DISORDERS

Pathogenesis: Theories for Obesity, Anorexia Nervosa, Bulimia Nervosa, and Binge-Eating Disorders

Obesity is defined as a condition of excess body fat in an amount large enough to have a negative effect on the person's health. The prevalence of childhood obesity has doubled since 1980 in the United States. Hormonal causes may include hypothyroidism, hypercortisolism, primary hyperinsulinism, pseudohypoparathyroidism, acquired hypothalamic problems (e.g., tumors, infections, traumatic syndromes). Psychological causes include complex self-perceptions, such as an unconscious wish to make oneself unattractive after experiencing sexual assault, abuse, or rape. Physical complications of obesity include a lower metabolic rate that results from a lack of exercise, and increased risk for other health problems including diabetes, hypertension, and premature heart disease.

Anorexia nervosa and bulimia nervosa are eating disorders found primarily in highly developed cultures such as in the United States, especially those with a focus on youth and beauty. They are serious conditions that can be fatal if not successfully treated. Both involve cognitive distortions concerning body shape and weight (a body dysmorphic disorder). General risk factors include:

- ▶ Biological
  - ▸ Illnesses that cause changes in appetite or weight
  - ▸ More common in females
- ▶ Sociocultural
  - ▸ Family dynamics.
  - ▸ Cultural focus on being thin
- ▶ Psychological
  - ▸ Difficulties with growing up
  - ▸ Poor sexual adjustment or sexual trauma or abuse history

Anorexia is characterized by refusal to maintain body weight at or above 85% of the expected based on age and height. Multiple physiological, psychological, and social factors are involved in the complex regulation of eating. The self-induced state of starvation seen in anorexia has serious physical consequences, including cardiac arrhythmias, bradycardia or tachycardia, hypotension, hypothermia, skin dryness with possible lanugo (a soft, fine, downy hair on the arms and other body parts that is normal in infancy), edema, and amenorrhea. Basically, all organ systems are affected by starvation. Hospitalization is indicated for patients who are 20% or more below the expected weight for their height.

Bulimia is characterized by recurrent episodes of binge eating followed by inappropriate compensatory mechanisms. Vomiting or laxative abuse can lead to metabolic disturbances and electrolyte abnormalities (e.g., hypokalemia, hypochloremic alkalosis, hypomagnesemia). Recurrent self-induced vomiting can result in the loss of dental enamel, scars on the hand, and esophageal tears. Nonpurging type of bulimia may include fasting or excessive exercise, but not laxatives, vomiting, or enemas.

TABLE 4-3.
PRIMARY FEEDING AND EATING DISORDERS

Anorexia Nervosa	▸ Refusal to maintain body weight at or above 85% of expected
	▸ Intense fear of gaining weight
	▸ Disturbance in self-perception
	▸ Amenorrhea for at least two consecutive cycles
	▸ Cachexia: loss of fat, muscle mass, reduced thyroid metabolism, cold intolerance, difficulty maintaining temperature
	▸ Cardiac: loss of muscle, arrhythmias, bradycardia, tachycardia
	▸ Dermatologic: lanugo; edema
	▸ Hematologic: leukopenia
	▸ Skeletal: osteoporosis
Bulimia Nervosa	▸ Recurrent episodes of binge eating
	▸ Eating greater amounts than most people
	▸ Sense of lack of control
	▸ Recurrent, inappropriate compensatory behavior
	▸ Compensatory behaviors at least two times a week for 3 months
	▸ Purging type or nonpurging type
Binge-Eating	▸ New to DSM5 (APA, 2013)
	▸ Recurring episodes of eating significantly more food in short period of time with feelings of lack of control
	▸ Eating quickly and uncontrollably despite feeling full
	▸ Feels guilt, shame, or disgust afterwards
	▸ Eats alone
	▸ Less common, more severe than simply overeating
	▸ Associated with significant physical and psychological problems

NANDA-I: Eating Disorders, Including Infantile Failure-to-Thrive and Geriatric Failure-to-Thrive

- ▶ Risk for electrolyte or fluid imbalance
- ▶ Nutrition, altered, and less or more than body requirements
- ▶ Readiness for enhanced nutrition
- ▶ Risk for self-injury
- ▶ Self-care deficit or feeding
- ▶ Body image disturbance
- ▶ Ineffective coping
- ▶ Risk for impaired attachment
- ▶ Dysfunctional family processes

Psychiatric–Mental Health Practice Standard 4: Planning

Improved outcomes for patients with feeding and eating disorders:

- ▶ The patient will regain healthy eating patterns.
- ▶ The patient will normalize BMI.
- ▶ The patient will accurately describe body dimensions.
- ▶ The family will demonstrate positive interactions.

SUBSTANCE USE DISORDERS

Substance use disorders are a problematic pattern of substance use leading to significant impairment with at least two criteria in a 12-month period (DSM5; APA, 2013). Biochemical and neuroanatomical brain alterations from chronic use may influence vulnerability and promote addiction. Abused substances derive their rewarding properties from altering dopamine levels in limbic system, triggering cravings. Dopamine in the brain mediates pleasure and motivation.

Substance use disorders and mental illnesses are linked and share both risk and protective factors CDC, 2014a). Up to half of persons with a serious mental illness will develop a substance use disorder at some time in their lives. Substance users are almost three times as likely to have a serious mental illness as those who do not have a substance use disorder. Three in four mental illnesses emerge early in life, and 1 in 5 children have had a serious mental illness. Stress increases alcohol and drug use and is associated with higher rates of relapse, and sociocultural factors point to social learning theories (e.g., cultural, ethnic, peer influences). The brain continues developing into young adulthood (age 25 or so). Risky behaviors and poor choices are characteristic of youth and young adults, reflective of the fact that the brain is still developing. Psychological factors that may increase risk are:

▶ Low self-esteem, frequent depression, or passivity

▶ Inability to relax or defer gratification

▶ Higher risk in impulsive groups (violent offenders, conduct disorder, intermittent explosive disorder)

BOX 4-4.
SUBSTANCE DISORDERS AND DEFINITIONS OF ABUSE, DEPENDENCE, INTOXICATION, AND WITHDRAWAL

Substance Disorders

▶ Alcohol-Related

▶ Stimulant-Related

▶ Inhalant-Related

▶ Opioid-Related

▶ Sedatives, Hypnotics, Anxiolytic–Related

▶ Cannabis-Related

▶ Hallucinogen-Related

▶ Tobacco-Related

Abuse

▶ Administration of any drug in a culturally disapproved manner that causes adverse consequences

▶ Recurrent use causing:

  ▶ Failure in role responsibilities

  ▶ Physically hazardous situations

  ▶ Legal problems

▶ Continued use despite social and interpersonal problems

Dependence

▶ Physical dependence:

  ▶ A physiologic state of neuro-adaptation produced by repeated administration of a drug, necessitating continued administration to prevent withdrawal syndrome

  ▶ Tolerance: need for increasing amounts for desired effect

▶ Psychological dependence:

  ▶ Repeats use to produce pleasure or avoid discomfort

  ▶ Cravings for the substance

▶ Substance is often taken in larger amounts or over a longer period than intended

▶ Time is spent in activities necessary to obtain the substance

▶ Social, occupational, recreational activities given up because of use

▶ Unsuccessful efforts to cut down use

Intoxication

▶ Reversible substance-specific syndrome caused by substance ingestion

▶ Maladaptive behaviors due to substances

▶ Symptoms not due to medical conditions or other mental disorder

Withdrawal

▶ Substance-specific syndrome caused by cessation of prolonged and heavy use

▶ Substance-specific syndrome causing impairment in social, occupational, and other areas of functioning

▶ Symptoms not due to medical condition or accounted for by other mental disorder

▶ Withdrawal symptoms are generally the opposite of intoxication symptoms

Genetic factors and environmentally induced alterations in brain neurochemistry appear to influence vulnerability for addiction. Addiction to drugs is a chronic, relapsing disease of the brain characterized by compulsive drug-seeking and use (Volkow, 2007). All drugs of abuse are thought to increase brain dopamine in the pathways that drive motivation and enhancements to reward systems. Chronic use of alcohol or other drugs may produce alterations in brain neurochemistry that help to maintain addictive behaviors. Higher rates of substance abuse are found in impulsive groups: violent offenders, and those with conduct disorder or intermittent explosive disorder. Stress increases alcohol and drug use, and is associated with higher rates of relapse. Substance use disorders are frequently comorbid with other mental disorders (dual diagnosis). New entries to DSM5 (APA, 2013) include cannabis withdrawal, caffeine withdrawal, and tobacco use disorder. Combined, addiction to substances is "a chronic, relapsing, disease of the brain that has imbedded behavioral and social context aspects" (Leshner, 1997; former head of NIDA. For further information about the effects of specific substances on brain neurophysiology, visit the website of the National Institute on Drug Abuse (http://www.nida.nih.gov).

Alcohol

Alcohol is a central nervous system depressant. It exerts desired effects by enhancing GABA. It is a legal substance that is usually ingested by swallowing but may be taken in via new routes (e.g., smoking vapors or rectal instillation by way of tampon-soaked insertion). These routes bypass the liver's cytochrome enzyme (CYP450) first-pass system, bringing the chemical directly into the bloodstream.

The nurse assesses current symptoms and history to determine intoxication or withdrawal state (evidenced by anxiety, tremor, seizure, delirium, alcohol poisoning which can lead to death). Screening, with the CAGE, Brief Drug Abuse Screening Test (B-DAST), or other tools is a standard of care. Structurally, with chronic use, affected brain structures such as the prefrontal cortex (executive functioning) and the hippocampus (memory) show evidence of less brain growth and more brain shrinkage (amount of shrinkage increases with age) as well as enlargement of the brain sulci, fissures, and ventricles from loss of gray and white matter. Chronic alcohol users may show evidence of

▶ Peripheral neuropathy, myopathy, or cardiomyopathy;

▶ Wernicke's encephalopathy, Korsakoff's psychosis;

▶ Esophagitis, pancreatitis, gastritis, hepatitis, cirrhosis;

▶ Serum or urine analysis: leukopenia, thrombocytopenia, increased liver enzymes (GGT, AST, ALT, ALP), mean corpuscular volume (MCV), ammonia, amylase, or triglycerides;

▶ Sexual dysfunction; and

▶ Jaundice.

Psychiatric–Mental Health Practice Standard 4: Planning

Improvement outcomes for patients in alcohol or benzodiazepine withdrawal may be facilitated by use of:

- ▶ Clinical Institute Withdrawal Assessment for Alcohol, revised version (CIWA-Ar): evidence-based tool

- ▶ Nurse-administered valid and reliable tool to monitor withdrawal and guide medication treatment while hospitalized

- ▶ 10 distinct symptom areas each scored between 0 and 7

    - ▸ Nausea and vomiting, tremor, paroxysmal sweats, anxiety, agitation, tactile disturbances, auditory disturbances, visual disturbances, headache, orientation and clouded sensorium

    - ▸ Score 10 or more: plan to administer tapered benzodiazepine withdrawal prevention protocol

- ▶ CIWA-B for benzodiazepine withdrawal also available

Amphetamine and Other Substances

Amphetamines, methamphetamines, bath salts, khat, cocaine, caffeine, nicotine (nonamphetamine stimulant) and some over-the-counter (OTC) medications, such as ephedrine, are CNS stimulants that increase both dopamine (DA) and norepinephrine (N). The initial euphoria may be followed by crashing; repeated use can lead to acute paranoid psychosis. Basal ganglia effects can cause increased stereotypic behaviors (pacing, scratching) and peripheral nervous system (PNS) effects may appear as tremors, emotional lability, or restlessness. Physical examination reveals cardiovascular effects (tachycardia, ventricular irritability), respiratory depression, constipation, and urinary retention.

Inhalants

Inhaling or "huffing" substances such as gasoline, varnish remover, lighter fluid, glue, or spray paint results in intoxication presentations of belligerence, assaultiveness, apathy, impaired judgment, psychosis, dizziness, nystagmus, incoordination, slurred speech, unsteady gait, depressed reflexes, tremor, blurred vision, euphoria, or anorexia. Withdrawal profiles are similar to those of alcohol.

Opioids

Narcotics and analgesics, such as morphine, codeine, hydromorphone (Dilaudid), methadone, meperidine (Demerol), hydrocodone (Vicodin), and oxycodone are the most commonly abused legal drugs, whereas heroin is the most commonly abused illegal drug. Prescription drug abuse is the most common problem today and has been for several years. Intoxication with opioids can lead to death because of severe respiratory depression. Effects of opioid use are pain relief, euphoria (rush), tranquility, drowsiness (nodding), mood swings, mental clouding, apathy, and constricted pupils. The PNS exhibits slowed motor movements. In states of withdrawal, patients look as though they have a bad case of the flu with drug craving, lacrimation, rhinorrhea, yawning, diaphoresis, and flu-like symptoms. The Clinical Opioid Withdrawal Scale (COWS) or another standardized measure may be used to monitor patients as they come down from the intoxicated (high) state.

Sedative-Hypnotics

Central nervous system (CNS) depressants that enhance GABA include the benzodiazepines (including midazolam [Versed]), barbiturates, alcohol, and propofol. They are often prescribed on an as-needed basis and have psychoactive properties that make them highly sought after and abused. Assessment of patients using medications of the sedative-hypnotic types is evidenced by cognitive slowing or memory problems, sedation and desire to sleep, decreased anxiety or decreased musculoskeletal tension, and sexual impairment. Benzodiazepines are used to treat alcohol and other substance withdrawal; they have anticonvulsant and antiseizure effects.

Cannabis

Various substances containing cannabis include marijuana (active ingredient is tetrahydrocannabinol [THC]), hashish, and K2 ("spice"), a synthetic marijuana. According to Nasrallal and Weiden (2014), "marijuana is the number one trigger for the development of schizophrenia" among genetically vulnerable persons. He purports that "marijuana is very bad for the brain." Marijuana has both stimulant and sedative effects on the CNS. It induces a state of well-being, relaxation, loss of temporal awareness, slowing of thought processes, shortened attention span, easy distractibility, impairment of short-term memory (hippocampal damage), apathy, panic, toxic delirium, and sometimes psychosis. Increased appetite and antinausea effects make it useful for oncology patients. Chronic use damages the hippocampus, with evidence of memory impairment. It has both physical and psychological dependence ramifications. Difficulty sleeping or irritability results when the drug is withdrawn.

Hallucinogens

Hallucinogens are psychedelic substances that interfere with glutamate functioning. They come in various forms, such as mescaline, psilocybin, LSD, STP, PCP (a veterinary anesthetic), "designer drugs" (ecstasy or Molly), or ketamine (Special K). Ecstasy or Molly is a synthetic psychoactive drug that is neurotoxic; it works by increasing serotonin, dopamine, and norepinephrine. The enhancement of serotonin triggers the release of oxytocin and vasopressin, which play important roles in love, trust, sexual arousal, and other prosocial experiences. A sense of emotional closeness and empathy results (NIDA, 2015). The surge of serotonin, however, depletes the brain of serotonin, causing negative after-effects on the CNS such as "trips" (changes in sensory experience, including illusions and hallucinations), impaired judgment, fear of losing one's mind, anxiety, and delirium. Intoxication is evidenced by heightened sensory awareness, staggering gait, slurred speech, tachycardia, increased blood pressure, hyperthermia, nausea. Dangerous flashbacks have been reported. A new plant-based substance known as ayahuasca promoted in the popular press as a therapy for PTSD, anxiety, and suicidal ideation is attracting tourism in Iquitos, Peru, promising spiritual catharsis.

Nicotine (Tobacco)

Nicotine is a CNS stimulant. The mild euphoria experienced from nicotine results from affecting acetylcholine (Ach), dopamine (DA), and gamma-amino-butyric acid (GABA), and endogenous opioid peptides. Approximately 60% to 90% of patients with schizophrenia use nicotine by way of cigarette smoking in an attempt to relieve the negative symptoms of schizophrenia. By inducing liver enzymes, nicotine lowers serum plasma levels of antipsychotics (Ciraulo et al., 2006). A chemical biomarker called cotinine can be measured in saliva to determine whether a person currently uses nicotine. Nicotine is highly addictive, and withdrawal uncomfortable. The half-life of nicotine is about 2 hours, meaning users will experience physiological discomfort if they go without it for several hours. The Fagerstrom Test for Nicotine Dependence (smoker and smokeless versions) is a clinical scale to measure withdrawal severity. Replacements for cigarettes today are the newly popular hookah bars, which sell flavored smokes, and electronic cigarettes (e-cigs) that deliver nicotine by way of "vaping" without burning tobacco.

NANDA-I: Substance Use Disorders

▶ Impaired judgment

▶ Imbalanced nutrition

▶ Ineffective coping

▶ Risk of injury

Psychiatric–Mental Health Practice Standard 4: Planning

Improvements for patients with substance use disorders:

▶ The patient has not experienced injury.

▶ The patient demonstrates good judgment.

▶ The patient acknowledges problems and personal responsibility.

▶ The patient learns adaptive coping mechanisms when stressed.

▶ The patient will engage in patient and family (if applicable) education.

▶ The patient eats well-balanced meals.

▶ The patient obtains adequate rest.

▶ The patient is willing to follow through on his or her treatment plan.

PERSONALITY DISORDERS

Personality is the enduring pattern of inner experience and behavior that is established in the late adolescence or early adulthood. Temperamental traits are present at birth. Personality forms during childhood and is influenced by attachment, parenting style, and other experiences. Personality traits are enduring characteristics that are present by late adolescence. Personality changes may occur because of conditions such as AIDS, dementia, or substance abuse, although the pathophysiology is not well understood.

Personality disorders have their onset in adolescence or early adulthood. They are long-standing and inflexible mental conditions, not usually the focus of clinical attention, especially in inpatient settings (Table 4–4). They are diagnosed when persons experience clinically significant distress or impairment related to long-standing, inflexible, and pervasive patterns of thought, emotion, and behavior. Problematic behaviors are manifested in two or more of the following:

▶ Cognition (ways of perceiving and interpreting self, other people, and events)

▶ Affectivity (the range, intensity, lability, and appropriateness of emotional response)

▶ Interpersonal functioning problems

▶ Impulse control problems

TABLE 4-4.
CLUSTER TYPES AND CHARACTERISTICS OF PERSONALITY DISORDERS

Cluster A Odd and Eccentric Types	▸ **Paranoid:** suspicious, mistrustful, appears defensive or resistant to control, very skeptical of most things, copes by projection, attributes shortcomings to others to justify actions
	▸ **Schizoid:** asocial pattern—aloof, introverted, seclusive, uninterested in social activities, apathetic, unengaged; thought to be schizophrenic prodrome; copes by intellectualizing
	▸ **Schizotypal:** odd, bizarre, strange, magical, eccentric, socially anxious, secretive and private; copes by undoing; easily overwhelmed by stimulation; many bizarre acts or thoughts reflect a retraction of previous acts or thoughts
Cluster B Dramatic and Emotional Types	▸ **Antisocial:** the psychopath; delinquent, criminal; lack of superego; impulsive, thrill-seeking, irresponsible; gets pleasure from swindling others; copes by acting out; highly manipulative
	▸ **Borderline:** unstable, intense affect, impulsivity with self-damaging acts, identity disturbance, chaotic relationships, manipulative, abandonment concerns, demanding, unpredictable, "black or white," "all or nothing;" copes by regression, projection, and denial
	▸ **Histrionic:** gregarious, seductive, dramatic, tendency to sexualize all relationships, extreme extraversion, attention-seeking, superficial, difficulty in maintaining deep relationships; copes by creating facades
	▸ **Narcissistic:** egotistical, preoccupied with power and prestige, sense of superiority, arrogant, entitled; copes by rationalizing, repressing, and using fantasy
Cluster C Anxious and Fearful Types	▸ **Avoidant:** withdrawn pattern, sensitive to rejection and humiliation, slow and constrained speech, shy and uncomfortable with others, sees self as inferior; copes by using fantasy and daydreams
	▸ **Dependent:** submissive pattern, need for social approval, clingy, feels inadequate, wants other to manage life, relates to others in an immature and childlike way, naïve; copes by using introjections—internalizing beliefs of others
	▸ **Obsessive–Compulsive:** conforming, meticulous, rigid, disciplined, concerned with order and conformity, stubborn, usually copes by using reaction-formation (doing the opposite of their feelings), isolation, and undoing

HUMAN SEXUALITY

Gender Dysphoria (GD)

Gender dysphoria describes a person's desire to be treated as a member of the opposite sex than what has been biologically assigned. GD manifests as personal convictions that one has typical feelings, thoughts, and behaviors of the other gender; these perceptions may begin as early as 3 or 4 years of age. A desire to transform sex characteristics often accompanies these self-perceptions. Gender reassignment surgeries are currently available in the United States. Prepubertal patients (age 11 or so) may begin the transformation with specific hormonal therapies that either boost or inhibit testosterone and estrogen or may receive hormonal suppression therapy to delay puberty.

Particular struggles experienced by transgender persons include nonacceptance and stigma, which are believed to be the cause of higher than average rates of suicide among transgender persons. Gender reassignment outcomes are described in several publications geared to children and adolescents. *Some Assembly Required: The Not So Secret Life of a Transgender Teen* (Andrews, 2014) was co-written by a transgender pair (female-to-male and male-to-female). *Rethinking Normal: A Memoir in Transition* (Hill, 2014) was written by a transwoman. The highly popular and Emmy award–winning Netflix show *Orange Is the New Black* includes a storyline of a transwoman, played by an actress who is also a transwoman and incidentally an identical twin to a male sibling in real life; her twin portrayed her in pretransition scenes on the show. Open discussions about transgender lifestyles targeted to youth are planned in the upcoming MTV documentary entitled *The "T" Word*.

These and other portrayals in popular media reflect paradigm shifts in our understanding and recognition of diverse sexual identity. Organizations and groups that serve this population often also serve persons with diverse sexual orientations, generally referred to under the rubric LGBTQI (lesbian, gay, bisexual, transgender, queer, questioning, and intersex). In light of still-widespread lack of understanding, discrimination, and stigma associated with gender role nonconformity experienced by transgender persons, it is the psychiatric–mental health nurse who addresses the needs and concerns of the patient with compassion and empathy, and without prejudice or judgment.

NANDA-I: Gender Dysphoria

- ▶ Disturbed body image
- ▶ Disturbed personal identity
- ▶ Risk for compromised human dignity
- ▶ Role confusion
- ▶ Depression
- ▶ Hopelessness

SLEEP DISORDERS

Many variations of sleep disorders are recognized in DSM5 (APA, 2013). On the whole, sleep disorders emanate from one of the two principle phases of sleep: (1) rapid eye movement (REM) sleep, during which most dreaming occurs, or (2) non-REM sleep. For our purposes, we will review insomnia, the most commonly reported sleep disorder. Insomnia is defined as sleep that is too brief or unrestful. It is a common disorder that can be acute or chronic and is more prevalent in older adults, affecting approximately 30% to 50%, and in young and middle-aged African Americans. On the whole, African Americans take longer to fall asleep, experience lighter sleep, don't sleep as well, take more naps, and have more sleep-related breathing problems than others (National Heart, Lung, and Blood Institute [NHLBI], 2011). Children generally need at least 9 hours of sleep each night, but adult needs may vary. Insomnia is diagnosed by patient report of the issue or observation of sleep architecture (quality and quantity) in children.

Sleep quality and quantity are important. Sleep is a crucial time for learning and the way that memories are first encoded, transferred, and downloaded to other regions of the brain where they are thought to be processed and stored (Smith, 2013). Adequate sleep plays an important role in regulating metabolism; in fact, sleep inadequacy has been linked to problems in the immune system, resulting in low-grade inflammation and an undermining of responses to vaccines. Inflammatory markers are associated with cardiometabolic problems and atherosclerosis (Dolgin, 2013). Many medical conditions, such as Parkinson's disease, cognitive disorders, sleep apnea, cardiovascular disorders, hyperthyroidism, diabetes, esophageal reflux, urinary frequency or infections, pain and discomfort, CNS stimulants, some antidepressants, anti-arrhythmic drugs, corticosteroids, thyroid medications, diuretics, overuse of sleeping pills (rebound insomnia), and stress factor into sleep insufficiency.

Altered sleep and circadian rhythm disturbances may occur as a result of travel, (especially to different time zones), shift work, sundowner syndrome, narcolepsy, sleep apnea, restless leg syndrome, and hospitalization (increased exposure to noise and light at night). Fatigue states that result from insomnia can precipitate falls and motor vehicle accidents. Linkages between sleep disruption and psychiatric disorders are well established. Poor sleepers are more likely to develop depression; in fact, insomnia is often the first symptom to appear and the last to go. Sleep disturbances may also be an early sign of neurodegenerative disease (Costandi, 2013). Similarly, sleep loss may precipitate episodes of mania or hypomania (DeWeerdt, 2013). Alterations in sleep can also result in hypervigilance, fear, or psychoses. What is unclear is whether sleep disorders trigger mood and anxiety disorders, or mood and anxiety disorders trigger sleep problems.

The psychiatric–mental health nurse recognizes that sleep is an opportune time to promote parasympathetic restoration and adapts the milieu to facilitate and closely monitors sleep hygiene. The hospital or home and social environment may generate obstacles to quality sleep. A polysomnogram (sleep study) that records brain activity, eye movements, heart rate, and blood pressure while a patient sleeps overnight may be ordered. It is important to accurately assess and document hours of sleep achieved to determine outcomes for improved sleep quality and quantity.

Dementia: Neurodegenerative Disorder

Dementia is a syndrome of acquired cognitive deficits that result from various levels of neurodegenerative and ischemic processes. Dementia manifests by a progressive, global deterioration of mental activity and self-care abilities, memory impairment, and cognitive deficits that are disabling and represents a decline from previous functioning. The progression is slow, insidious, and nonreversible. A score of 24/30 or less on the Mini Mental State Exam (MMSE) (Folstein et. al., 1975) is suggestive of cognitive difficulties and should be confirmed with more extensive neuropsychological testing. *Sundowning* is the term used for the disorientation that persons with dementia may experience when familiar environmental cues diminish at nighttime.

The most common cause of dementia is Alzheimer's disease (AD). Nearly 13% of adults over the age of 65 and 45% of those over the age of 85 are estimated to have AD (Liu, Kanekiyo, Xu, & Bu, 2013). Early changes in Alzheimer's disease and other dementias appear to be related to a decrease in the brain's levels of acetylcholine (ACh), a neurotransmitter essential to learning and memory (cholinergic deficit hypothesis). Support for this assumption comes from the observation that by boosting cholinergic functioning with cholinesterase inhibitors (therefore reducing the metabolism and increasing the availability of Ach), memory function is enhanced in early dementia. As AD progresses, an accumulation of aggregation-prone proteins called beta-amyloids are not removed from the body (Kingwell, 2012), and bundles of tangled proteins called neurofibrillary tangles begin to interfere with the functioning of neuronal cells. The process of excitotoxicity related to glutamate overactivity is also thought to be responsible for some of the neurodegeneration and atrophy of the brain seen on magnetic resonance imaging (MRI) scans. Another recently identified factor is hippocampal atrophy, leading to development of mild cognitive impairment and dementia (Kingwell, 2012). Numerous studies demonstrate a reduction in hippocampal size associated with various cardiovascular diseases, diabetes, obesity, obstructive sleep apnea, vitamin B12 deficiency, head trauma, specific genotype, and psychiatric disorders (Fotuhi, Do, & Jack, 2013). A definitive diagnosis is made at autopsy. Three stages of dysfunction are noted:

- ▶ Early or mild
  - ▹ Forgetfulness and short-term memory loss
  - ▹ Difficulty with activities of daily living

- ▹ Disturbed executive functioning

- ▹ Impairment in social or occupational functioning

▶ Middle or moderate

- ▹ Difficulty with activities of daily living and familiar tasks such as cooking or balancing a checkbook

- ▹ Changes in ability to communicate

- ▹ Agnosia

- ▹ Apraxia

- ▹ Aphasia

▶ Late or severe

- ▹ Inability to perform activities of daily living; complete dependence

- ▹ Becomes disoriented, incoherent, amnesic, or incontinent

Although two-thirds of all dementias are AD, there are other types and many secondary causes for neurodegeneration which include:

▶ Infection

▶ Vascular dementia: cognitive functioning declines in a stair-step fashion (rather than progressively) after cerebrovascular accidents, cerebrovascular disease, atherosclerosis

▶ Electrolyte (metabolic) imbalances

▶ Drug toxicity

▶ Sensory impairment or deprivation (visual or auditory)

▶ Emotional disturbances

▶ Nutritional disturbances

▶ Cerebral or head trauma: direct injury to brain tissue

▶ Pick's disease (frontotemporal impairment): characterized by atrophy in the frontotemporal brain regions due to neuronal loss, gliosis, Pick's bodies (masses of cytoskeletal elements), and protein build-up in areas of the brain

▶ Lewy body: more common in persons with Parkinson's disease and characterized by the deposition of Lewy bodies (protein) that accumulates in the neurons; persons with Lewy body dementia may have visual hallucinations, a characteristic that distinguishes it from other dementias

▶ Huntington's disease: autosomal-dominant degenerative disorder

▶ Tertiary syphilis (or neurosyphilis): occurs in persons who have untreated syphilis for many years; usually occurs about 10 to 20 years after a person is first infected with syphilis

▶ HIV/AIDS: dementia results from the direct effects of HIV infection in the brain, opportunistic infections, or the toxic effects of drug treatments; HIV may gain entrance to the central nervous system by infecting the macrophages and monocytes that cross the blood-brain barrier. Symptoms of the resulting AIDS dementia complex can be confused with clinical depression because of the presentation of apathy and cognitive and motor problems. HIV has an affinity for the brain.

Sexually Transmitted Infections

Among the many sexually transmitted infections, including syphilis, gonorrhea, chlamydia, trichomoniasis, human papillomavirus (HPV), herpes simplex virus, and human immunodeficiency virus (HIV), two are of particular interest to the psychiatric–mental health nurse because they can cause dementia: syphilis and HIV. Syphilis is caused by spirochete bacterium and, if not diagnosed and treated, can cause dementia in stage 3 by way of the slow, progressive infection of the brain.

Similarly, dementia can develop during the advanced stages of AIDS, the disease caused by HIV infection. The progression of AIDS dementia mimics depression in early stages (e.g., hopelessness, insomnia). Later, cognitive signs, such as forgetfulness, slowness, poor concentration, possible delirium, delusions, hallucinations, and difficulties with problem-solving; behavioral signs, such as apathy and social withdrawal; and neurological findings, such as tremors, impaired rapid repetitive movements, imbalance, ataxia, hypertonia, hyperreflexia, frontal release signs, or CD4 depression, appear.

NANDA-I: Dementia

▶ Risk for injury

▶ Impaired verbal communication

▶ Self-care deficits (in bathing, hygiene, dressing, and grooming) related to cognitive impairment

▶ Disturbed social interactions

▶ Disturbed thought processes as evidenced by memory loss

▶ Disturbed sleep pattern

▶ Caregiver role strain

Delirium

Delirium is a serious medical condition that can be caused by any number of disturbances. Unlike dementia, which is generally a slowly progressing condition, delirium is quite acute, comes on rapidly, and is characterized by a clouding of consciousness with disorientation. Cognition changes rapidly; acute confusion fluctuates; psychomotor agitation or depression may be present. The patient may display a reduced ability to maintain and shift attention.

This change in cognition cannot be better accounted for by a preexisting or evolving dementia. Whereas a patient with dementia may remain relatively oriented until the later stages of the illness, persons with delirium may shift between periods of orientation and disorientation. If delirium is suspected, it is important to alert the medical team so a complete physical assessment can be completed. Often, in older persons, an infection such as pneumonia or a urinary tract infection is the etiology. Delirium occurs frequently in medical and rehabilitation settings but is often unrecognized and can result in considerable morbidity and mortality. Many medical issues may precipitate the onset of delirium. The mnemonic "I WATCH DEATH" serves as a reminder to rule out all potential medical causes as shown in Box 4.4 below.

> **BOX 4–4. DELIRIUM MNEMONIC: "I WATCH DEATH"**
>
> **I**nfection
>
> **W**ithdrawal
>
> **A**cute metabolic disturbance
>
> **T**rauma
>
> **C**NS pathology
>
> **H**ypoxia
>
> **D**eficiencies
>
> **E**ndocrinopathies
>
> **A**cute vascular
>
> **T**oxins
>
> **H**eavy metals

Psychiatric–Mental Health Practice Standard 4: Planning

Improved outcomes for neurodegenerative and neurocognitive disorders:

▶ The patient will achieve optimal functioning across health systems or domains:

  ▸ Health perception and health management, value-belief patterns

  ▸ Nutritional-metabolic, elimination patterns

  ▸ Activity-exercise, sleep-rest patterns

  ▸ Cognitive-perceptual patterns

  ▸ Self-perception and self-concept patterns

  ▸ Role-relationship, sexuality-reproductive patterns

  ▸ Coping-stress-tolerance patterns

NANDA-I Diagnoses: Spiritual Distress, Pain, Falls

Spiritual Distress

- ▶ Questioning life, death, pain, suffering
- ▶ Losing hope
- ▶ Requesting clergy; spiritual assistance
- ▶ Abandoning usual religious or spiritual practices

Psychiatric–Mental Health Practice Standard 4: Planning

Improvements for patients with spiritual distress:

- ▶ The patient verbalizes a sense of purpose.
- ▶ The patient accepts the reality of death.

Pain

- ▶ Anxiety
- ▶ Hopelessness
- ▶ Depressed mood
- ▶ Fear
- ▶ Insomnia
- ▶ Mobility and physical status impaired
- ▶ Acute and chronic
- ▶ Self-care deficit
- ▶ Sexual dysfunction
- ▶ Sleep pattern disturbance
- ▶ Caregiver role strain

Psychiatric–Mental Health Practice Standard 4: Planning

Improved outcomes for pain:

- ▶ The patient will participate in developing an individualized care plan based on multimodal therapies to achieve pain relief.
- ▶ The patient age 3 years or older, or with developmental or language deficits, will use the Wong-Baker FACES scale (range of faces going from happy to neutral to painful) to communicate pain. "point to the face that shows how bad the pain feels to you"; 0 = no hurt (smiling, happy face) to 10 = hurts worst (sad, crying face).

▶ The patient will report pain at an acceptable level.

▶ The patient will maintain a daily log of pain, interventions, and responses.

▶ The patient will participate in pain management in preparation for discharge.

Psychiatric–Mental Health Practice Standard 4: Planning

Improvements for patients experiencing pain:

▶ The patient will achieve an acceptable level of pain.

▶ The patient will engage in alternative and complementary practices designed to manage pain experiences.

Falls

▶ Risk for self-harm related to postural imbalance

▶ Impaired physical mobility

  ▸ General: over age 60; history of falls; history of smoking, alcohol, or drug abuse

  ▸ Mental status: lethargy, confusion, disorientation, inability to understand directions, impaired memory or judgment

  ▸ Physical conditions: vertigo, unsteady gait, weight-bearing joint problems, weakness, paresis or paralysis, seizure disorder, impaired vision, impaired hearing, slow reaction times, diarrhea, urinary frequency, urgency, nocturia, insomnia

  ▸ Vital signs alterations

  ▸ Advanced age, which can lead to:

    ▷ Increased sensitivity to environmental temperature

    ▷ Increased risk for hypothermia

    ▷ Increased blood pressure, especially systolic due to decreased vessel elasticity

    ▷ Decreased efficiency of respiratory muscles with increased breathlessness

▶ Medications: diuretics, psychotropics, hypotensive, or CNS depressants and medications that increase GI motility (e.g., laxatives); side effects can lead to:

  ▸ Orthostatic hypotension

  ▸ Systolic falls to 90mmHg or below

  ▸ Measure BP supine, sitting, and standing before initiating medications

▶ Ambulatory or other devices used: cane, crutches, walker, wheelchair, Geri chair, braces

Psychiatric–Mental Health Practice Standard 4: Planning

Improvements for patients at risk for falls:

▶ The patient will recognize the importance of dangling at the bedside and rising slowly before ambulation.

▶ The patient will accept the need for assistive devices that provide stability and support during ambulation.

PROBLEM IDENTIFICATION ACROSS THE LIFE SPAN (CHILD AND ADOLESCENT FOCUS)

DSM5 (APA, 2013) reestablishes disorders usually first evident in infancy, childhood, or adolescence to focus on the patient's development during the formative years when the nervous system is still developing. Hence, some of the most common psychiatric disorders and criteria are referenced under the heading neurodevelopmental disorders. The most common problems (psychiatric diagnoses) that compromise optimal functioning seen in child and adolescent populations are presented below for review.

Child and adolescent psychiatric–mental health diagnoses can be atypical, constantly changing, and unusually comorbid with other disorders. Accurate diagnoses must be made with consideration of the rapid and complex physical, emotional, and psychological changes co-occurring as a process of growth and development. Additionally, accurate diagnosis is important to avoid misdiagnosing and overmedicating young persons. ADHD, for example, is frequently comorbid with anxiety, depression, conduct disorder, oppositional behavior, substance abuse, and tics (Stahl, 2008). Children and adolescents may also experience disorders found in adult populations such as anorexia nervosa, bulimia nervosa, binge-eating disorder, obesity, schizophrenia, bipolar disorder, PTSD, acute stress disorder, adjustment disorder, and gender dysphoria. The sequelae of symptoms and treatments are similar; however, considerations may be different insofar as pharmacologic agents and dosing, and recommended therapies.

Pediatric autoimmune neuropsychiatric disorder associated with streptococcal infections (PANDAS) is associated with group A β-hemolytic streptococcus bacterial infection (GABHS), because it leads to a neural autoimmune response resulting in obsessive-compulsive disorder–like (OCD) behaviors and CNS symptoms (e.g., eye-blinking, hyperactivity, uncontrollable movements). PANDAS-induced OCD-type presentations typically are self-limiting after several weeks, and a clear association between the two events has not been satisfactorily established (Morrison, 2014).

TABLE 4-4.
NEURODEVELOPMENTAL DISORDERS

Intellectual Disability	▸ Usually begins in infancy
	▸ Low intelligence requires special help in coping with life
	▸ Communication, social interaction, and practical living skill impairments
	▸ Mild: IQ from 50–55 to approximately 70; this group is usually educable to the second to fifth grade functional level
	▸ Moderate: IQ from 35 to 55, trainable to live semi-independently
	▸ Severe: IQ from 20 to 40; cannot develop independent living skills; usually due to genetic causes
	▸ Profound: less than 20 to 25; dependent on others for self-care— institutionalized; genetic causes
Borderline Intellectual Functioning	▸ IQ range 71–84
Language Disorder	▸ Lag in spoken and written language compared to age group
	▸ Small vocabulary, impaired use of words to form sentences, reduced ability to use sentences to express ideas
Social (Pragmatic) Communication Disorder	▸ Difficulty with language usage, including ability to adapt communication to fit context, follow rules of conversation, and understand implied communication
Speech Sound Disorder	▸ Problems with producing sounds of speech, or errors in order of sounds
Childhood-Onset Fluency Disorder (Stuttering)	▸ Stuttering with consonant sounds; sounds drawn out or repeated
Selective Mutism	▸ Ability to speak normally, but doesn't speak in certain situations
Learning Disorders (Reading [Dyslexia], Mathematics [Dyscalculia], Written Expression [agraphia or dysgraphia], Drawing [Constructional Apraxia], Learning Disorder Not Otherwise Specified [NOS])	▸ Standardized test scores markedly less than expected for age:
	▸ Reading (dyslexia)
	▸ 60%–80% with reading disorder are male
	▸ Mathematics (dyscalculia)
	▸ Seldom diagnosed before second grade and may not become apparent until fifth grade or later
	▸ Written expression (agraphia or dysgraphia)
	▸ Difficulty copying simple drawings (constructional apraxia)
	▸ Approximately 5% of U.S. public school students are diagnosed with learning disorders; prevalence is 10%–25%
	▸ Co-occur with conduct disorders, oppositional defiant disorder, ADHD, major depressive disorder, or dysthymia
	▸ School dropout rate almost 40%
Stereotypic Movement Disorder	▸ Repetitive movements without goal attainment that begins in early childhood
	▸ Sometimes associated with congenital blindness, deafness, temporal lobe epilepsy, Wilson's disease, Lesch-Nyhan syndrome

(continued)

TABLE 4-4.
CONTINUED

Autism Spectrum Disorders (Autism, Rett's Syndrome, Asperger's Syndrome, Childhood Disintegrative Disorder)	▶ Affect 1 in 68 children (CDC, 2014b)
	▶ Social relationship difficulties vary from mild to almost complete lack of interaction since early childhood
	▶ Reduced use of eye contact, hand gestures, smiles, nods
	▶ Difficulty adapting to different social situations
	▶ Engages in repetitive and narrowly focused activities and interests
	▶ Needs routine; difficulty with changes in routine
	▶ Fascination with spinning or small parts of objects
	▶ Feeble or excessive reactions to stimuli
	▶ Stereotypic behaviors such as hand flapping, body rocking, or echolalia
	▶ Males 2 to 4 times more likely to be affected
	▶ Asperger's syndrome: cognitive and linguistic development intact; difficulties with social interaction and nonverbal communication
	▶ Rett syndrome only affects girls (genetic mutation on X chromosome; some live until middle age, then growth and development regression seen
	▶ Childhood disintegrative disorder: apparently normal growth and development until age 3, then regression noted
Tourette's Syndrome	▶ Tics that begin by age 6 and affect various parts of the body; often beginning with eye blinks
	▶ Vocal tics that involve coprolalia (vocalizing obscenities)
	▶ More common in males
	▶ Strong family history present
Persistent (Chronic) Motor or Vocal Tic Disorder; Provisional Tic Disorder	▶ Involuntary, sudden vocalization or body movement that is repeated, rapid, nonrhythmic
	▶ May be complex: several simple tics in rapid succession
	▶ May be occasional twitch
	▶ Usually involves upper part of face (grimaces and twitching eye muscles)
	▶ Vocal can be barks, grunts, coughs, throat clearings, sniffs, single syllables
	▶ May disappear as child matures
	▶ More common in males

(continued)

TABLE 4–4.
CONTINUED

Attention-Deficit Hyperactivity Disorder	▶ Onset before age 7, although diagnosis can be made at any age
	▶ Impaired work or educational, social, personal function
	▶ Inattentive, hyperactive, impulsive predominance may occur, or combined presentation
	▶ Patient always in motion; disruptive because of restlessness, fidgeting, talking; difficulty paying attention and focusing; easily distracted, neglects details, makes careless mistakes
	▶ Nigrostriatal and prefrontal pathway implications of norepinephrine or dopamine to and from basal ganglia
Disruptive, Impulse-Control, and Conduct Disorders	
Oppositional Defiant Disorder	▶ Onset at age 3–4 years; diagnosis few years later (by age 8)
	▶ Negativism and defiance beyond quest for normal independence-seeking, lasting longer than 6 months
	▶ Hostile towards others
	▶ Blames others
	▶ Behavior must occur with persons other than siblings
Conduct Disorder	▶ Onset at age 5–6
	▶ Consistently violates basic right of others
	▶ Breaks rules, sets fires, shows cruelty to others or animals, lies, and steals
Intermittent Explosive Disorder	▶ Frequent, repeated, spontaneous outbursts of aggression towards people, property, or animals
Kleptomania	▶ Irresistible urge to steal things they really don't need
	▶ Provides tension release
Pyromania	▶ Fire-setters feel tension and release it by setting fires
Disruptive Mood Dysregulation Disorder	▶ Persistently negative mood with frequent, severe temper explosions
	▶ Minor provocations can provoke to extremes; bullying, threatening, fighting
	▶ Outbursts occur every few days on average for at least a year
	▶ Nonsuicidal self-injury (NSSI) or self-mutilation, cutting, or burning self-behaviors may co-occur; one hypothesis: do tattoos represent a socially acceptable way to engage in NSSI?
Trichotillomania	▶ Engages in chronic hair, eyelash, eyebrow, or pubic hair pulling to the point of baldness
	▶ Highly comorbid with OCD and Tourette's syndrome
	▶ Causes significant embarrassment and shame
	▶ Provides tension release

(continued)

TABLE 4–4.
CONTINUED

Feeding and Eating Disorders	
Pica	▶ Commonly found in young children and pregnant women, children with autism spectrum disorder, intellectual disability
	▶ Persistent eating of dirt or other nonfood items
	▶ May be related to mineral deficiency (iron, zinc)
Rumination Disorder	▶ Regurgitation and reswallowing of food for at least 1 month
	▶ Can be associated with bulimia nervosa, intellectual disability
	▶ Males more likely to be affected
Elimination Disorders	
Encopresis	▶ Age 4 or older, moves bowels in inappropriate places
	▶ More common in males
Enuresis	▶ Age 5 or older, day and nighttime wetting
	▶ May have primary (never been dry) or secondary (toilet training initially successful)
	▶ May accompany non-REM sleep problems, especially during first 3 hours of sleep
Anxiety Disorders	
Separation anxiety disorder	▶ Resistance and severe anxiety with being alone because of fear that something might happen to significant other; or fear they may become lost.
	▶ Can be diagnosed in all ages (children, adolescents, adults, older adults).
Trauma and Stress-Related Disorders	
Reactive Attachment Disorder	▶ Poor attachment; poor bonding to primary caregivers during early childhood
	▶ Child fails to seek comfort from parents or surrogates
	▶ Child extremely withdrawn
Disinhibited Social Engagement Disorder	▶ Child fails to show normal reticence in the company of strangers
	▶ Child pathologically outgoing; no social reserves evident

NANDA-I: Childhood Disorders in General

- ▶ Risk for self-directed violence
- ▶ Risk for other-directed violence
- ▶ Ineffective coping
- ▶ Enuresis or encopresis
- ▶ Problems with social skills, problem-solving, school performance
- ▶ Disturbed thought processes
- ▶ Disturbed sleep patterns
- ▶ Anxiety
- ▶ Chronic or situational low self-esteem
- ▶ Risk for caregiver role strain
- ▶ Readiness for enhanced family processes among family members

NANDA-I: Family-Related Nursing Diagnoses

- ▶ Ineffective therapeutic regime management
- ▶ Ineffective family coping
- ▶ Ineffective parenting
- ▶ Knowledge deficit
- ▶ Caregiver role strain
- ▶ Ineffective denial
- ▶ Complicated grieving

NANDA-I: Suicide, Abuse, and Violence (Intrapersonal, Interpersonal)

Ineffective (Maladaptive) Coping: Suicide

Suicide is the 10th leading cause of death in the United States and according to Puntil, et. al. (2013), there are approximately 90,000 psychiatric–mental health nurse generalists working on inpatient psychiatric units where the most acutely suicidal patients are cared for. Psychiatric–mental health nurses are particularly called upon to provide leadership in developing, implementing, and evaluating competency-based education and training in suicide prevention. The National Suicide Prevention Lifeline is a confidential, free network (800.273.TALK/800-273-8255) to educate and intervene with persons with suicidal ideation and with persons who are concerned about someone.

Ineffective (Maladaptive) Family Coping: Features of Domestic or Intimate Abuse, Sexual Abuse, Assault, and Violence and Neglect

Domestic or intimate partner violence refers to an escalating, and usually persistent, pattern of abuse in which a person in an intimate relationship controls a vulnerable person or persons through force, intimidation, threat of violence, control of finances, or any combination thereof. The three most common categories of violence associated with domestic violence involve child abuse, intimate partner abuse, and elder abuse. As nurses, we recognize family violence patterns that can originate early in life such as failure to thrive (manifestation of infantile depression; poor parent-child bonding?), shaken baby syndrome (maladaptive parenting or discipline?), domestic violence (personal boundary violations; rape, incest), and elder abuse and neglect. Does caregiver role strain play a role in our sandwich generation households (parents raising and caring for own children as well as their own parents)?

Vulnerable population groups include children, women ages 15 to 44 (reproductive age), frail older adults, persons with mental illnesses, cognitive impairments, and children and adults with mental delays and physical disabilities. Women are more at risk of suffering abusive behavior, particularly during pregnancy and the period immediately after a separation (Stuart, 2009). Intimate partner abuse in heterosexual relationships tends to be gender-related, with more women being victimized; the majority of spousal or intimate partner perpetrators are men. However, intimate partner abuse also occurs in gay relationships where it is not gender-related: both abuser and victim are of the same sex. Domestic violence is a serious event in which the victim can be physically injured, psychologically traumatized, or neglected. More pregnant women die as victims of domestic violence than from any other cause.

Perpetrators of abuse and violence come from all walks of life, socioeconomic strata, educational levels, races, ethnicities, and occupations. They are more likely to have grown up in an abusive household or been exposed to community or peer group violence. Most perpetrators have low self-esteem and dependent personalities. They tend to lack impulse control and frequently view their victims as their property. Poverty, stress, and cultural values supportive of violence as a way of controlling behavior contribute to the development of abusive behaviors. Alcohol and other substance abuse is frequently a precipitating factor, although not the cause of domestic violence. Perpetrators can be paid caregivers or long-term-care personnel as well as family members or persons with legal authority to make healthcare or financial decisions for a victim.

Abuse should be suspected when injuries are not explainable, family members provide different explanations, or the explanation does not fit the observed injuries. A history of similar injuries, multiple visits to the Emergency Department, and a delay between the onset of injury and seeking medical care should raise suspicion. Although no single injury informs the nurse that physical abuse has occurred, the nurse should look for patterns of injury or more than one indicator related to the possibility of physical and other forms of abuse. Always believe a patient who reports abuse.

There is a predictable cycle to spousal or intimate partner abuse. Without treatment, it always repeats.

▶ Tension-building (escalation or buildup) phase: Tension rises with minor abuses; the victim tries to appease the perpetrator.

▶ Explosion (acute battering) phase: Abuse in the form of physical injury, psychological harm, or both occurs.

▶ Honeymoon phase: The abuser is remorseful and apologetic, promising that the abuse will not happen again. Undoing, a common defense mechanism, may be observed.

▶ Later, the tension-building phase reappears and the cycle repeats (Dugan & Hock, 2006).

Domestic abuse, assault, and violence can take many forms:

▶ Emotional: systematic degradation of a person's self-worth through verbal attacks, controlling or limiting the victim's rights, isolating the victim from social contacts, and destroying the victim's personal property or pets.

▶ Physical: intentional infliction of bodily harm through punching, beating, kicking, burning, shoving, twisting hair or body limb, withholding food, or forcing compliance through actual or threatened physical force. Physical abuse also includes denying the victim food, fluids, or sleep. Indicators can include dislocations, fractures, burns, abrasions on limbs or torso consistent with strap or rope marks, bruising (particularly bilateral bruising to the arms or inner thighs), evidence of repeated bruising without medical cause, or traumatic loss of teeth or hair.

▶ Psychological indicators: requires further exploration with children when school performance suddenly changes; presenting as overly compliant, passive, withdrawn, or demanding without reason; running away or doesn't want to go home; descriptions of the relationship with parent or caregiver as negative; inability to concentrate that cannot be attributed to a physical or psychological cause; reports physical or sexual abuse by a parent or caregiver; refuses to change clothes for gym periods.

▶ Sexual: forcing sex on an unwilling person, unsolicited sexual intimacy (fondling breasts or buttocks, or genital contact with no penetration), indecent exposure, or forced exposure to sexually explicit material or unusual sex practices. It also includes sexual behaviors with a person who is unable to give valid consent (e.g., a minor, a person with cognitive impairments, an unconscious person). Use of a child for pornography or other sexually exploitive activities is sexual abuse. Sexual abuse can consist of not revealing a sexually transmitted disease and failing to take precautions to safeguard the other person. Women with disabilities may be at greater risk.

▶ The most common form of sexual abuse of children is incest —sex with a family member. Possible indicators requiring further exploration with children include

  ▸ Unusual incidence of urinary tract infections,

  ▸ Bruises, itching, rawness in the perineal area or inner thighs,

  ▸ Nightmares, fear of going to bed,

  ▸ Changes in behavior, extreme mood swings, or withdrawal,

  ▸ Unusual interest or highly developed knowledge in sexual matters,

  ▸ Enuresis; encopresis, and

  ▸ Presence of a sexually transmitted disease.

▶ Neglect: the most common form of child and elder abuse; can be active or passive. Active neglect refers to the intentional disregard by caregivers and others for the physical, emotional, or financial needs and welfare of a child, disabled or cognitively impaired adult, or frail older adult. It can include withholding of care or finances, or failure to provide adequate supervision needed by the victim. Passive neglect is not intentional; the caregiver may not be able to provide appropriate care or supervision because of his or her own disability, lack of resources, lack of maturity, or ignorance. Possible indicators of child or frail older adult neglect include

  ▸ Consistently dirty or has a distinct body odor,

  ▸ Lacks appropriate clothing for the weather,

  ▸ Doesn't have lunch or lunch money,

  ▸ Lacks adequate medical or dental care, medications, or eyeglasses,

  ▸ Appears apathetic, or afraid something is happening to her or him,

  ▸ Lack or inappropriate supervision of a child's leisure and adolescent sexual activities,

  ▸ Abuses alcohol or other drugs,

  ▸ Child frequently absent from school,

  ▸ Not in approved age-appropriate car seat, and

  ▸ Left alone; unattended.

Referral to have a rape kit collected by a Sexual Assault Nurse Examiner (SANE), if available, is prudent. SANEs are experts in history-taking, physical and emotional assessment, recognition, and documentation of trauma response and injury—experts at collecting and managing forensic evidence. SANEs also provide emotional and social support during the courtroom testimony if required by the judicial system (see www.iafn.org for more information).

Nurses must follow state laws that mandate reporting of child or elder abuse. In most states, healthcare professionals are protected from breach of confidentiality in reporting suspected child or elder abuse and neglect. Specific reporting guidelines are incorporated into state laws. In a court of law, the judgment about reporting of child or elder abuse or neglect will be made on the basis of these published guidelines, and what a reasonable and prudent nurse would do in a similar situation.

Treatment of the victim begins with the assessment. Interview the alleged victim alone. Believe the abuse claim. Validate the person's feelings. Document signs of abuse and encourage treatment; children entering treatment for depression, anxiety, or eating disorders often have underlying abuse issues, requiring assessment.

Children in abusive situations may need to be removed from the home or placed temporarily with a relative to prevent further episodes of abuse. Educate the abused child about self-protective strategies and remind the child that the abuse was not his or her fault. Treatment approaches for children should reflect their developmental level.

For adult victims of abuse, help to identify and explore a safe environment in which the person has safe alternatives should she or he need them (e.g., a shelter, staying with a friend or relative). Develop a safety plan that details the steps the adult victim should take in case of abuse, including collecting of important papers, money, and phone numbers. Educate adult victims about the cycle of abuse, and explore and correct misperceptions that the victim provokes the perpetrator to become abusive.

Patient Injuries in Healthcare Facilities

The Joint Commission mandates that any unexpected occurrence involving death or serious physical or psychological injury in a healthcare facility be reported. The purpose of identifying unexpected occurrences, referred to as sentinel events, is to reduce their frequency. A sentinel event is defined as any unanticipated event in a healthcare setting not related to the natural course of the patient's illness that results in serious physical or psychological injury to, or death of, a person or persons. *Root cause analyses* are enacted to identify lapses or oversights in processes for the purpose of constructing safety nets to close those gaps. The aviation industry boasts of thousands of flights worldwide on a daily basis with very few casualties. Many healthcare facilities have adopted the check–check–recheck with a partner strategy similar to that used by the aviation industry to eliminate errors, sentinel events, near-misses, and injuries and fatalities. Examples of sentinel events relevant to mental health settings include medication error, restraint resulting in injury or death, suicide or suicide attempt, patient elopement, delayed treatment, and fall resulting in injury or death.

Psychiatric–Mental Health Practice Standard 4: Planning

Improved Outcomes for Children and Adolescents in General

▶ Teach proactive interventions systematically.

▶ Respond warmly to positive behaviors.

▶ Ignore negative behavior when appropriate.

▶ Refrain from giving unnecessary commands (demonstrating control when unnecessary).

▶ Avoid unrealistic demands.

▶ Use therapeutic play with children.

▶ Involve family, school, and other supports.

▶ Believe reports of bullying, reports of sexual abuse.

Improved Outcomes for Children and Adolescents: Tools

▶ Therapeutic play

▶ Pharmacotherapy

▶ Expressive therapies

▶ Bibliotherapy

▶ Children's games

▶ Storytelling

▶ Cognitive behavioral therapy (CBT)

▶ Milieu management

▶ Special education

▶ Computer-based treatment

▶ Speech and language therapies

▶ Social skills training

▶ Sensory integration training

▶ Music therapy

Improved Outcomes for Autism Spectrum Disorders

▶ The patient will maintain safety (self and others).

▶ The patient will use socially appropriate behaviors.

▶ The patient will use coping skills.

▶ The patient will gain restorative sleep.

Improved Outcomes for ADHD

▶ Targeted symptoms:

  ▹ Problems with social skills

  ▹ Problem-solving

  ▹ School performance

  ▹ Behavioral inhibition

  ▹ Communication

CRISIS AND CRISIS INTERVENTION

Gerald Caplan (1964), a pioneer in crisis intervention, described crisis as a psychological state that occurs when a person is faced with insurmountable situations or problems and their usual ways of coping are inadequate to deal with the stress. Every crisis presents an opportunity for personal growth. Caplan believed that the crisis state resolves itself in 4 to 6 weeks. Crises are typically self-limiting, with resolution occurring within 72 hours without intervention. There are three general types of crises:

▶ Situational: specific external event upsets equilibrium, occurring at a personal or family level (e.g., cancer diagnosis, job loss)

▶ Maturational: occurs at transition points in life (e.g., menopause, puberty, childbirth)

▶ Adventitious or global: accidental, unexpected, usually occurring to larger segments of the population (e.g., natural disaster)

The *crisis state* is conceptualized as a normal response or reaction to an overwhelming, traumatic event. Flannery (2002) reviews this crisis response as one in which a person's psychological homeostasis is disrupted, usual coping strategies are unable to reestablish homeostasis, and the level of stress associated with the crisis has resulted in functional impairment. When people are unable to resolve significant problems in their lives, they can begin to experience tension and anxiety, a decline in their overall functioning, inability to organize and regulate behavior, and increased defensiveness. What can result are somatic complaints, perceptual changes, intense feelings (e.g., sense of urgency, "going crazy" hallucinations), impaired impulse control, and limited capacity to express feelings or draw support from their usual sources of help (support system). A person in a crisis state may even experience survivor guilt.

Of course, preventing crises from occurring in the first place is ideal. The psychiatric–mental health nurse, in adopting tenets proposed by Hildegard Peplau (1988) invoking the "therapeutic use of self" (Chapter 7), can go a long way, in some cases, toward averting patient decompensation before it happens. First-line implementations focus on the therapeutic alliance, patient triggers, feelings, and environmental monitoring. It behooves nurses to take time to implement basic strategies to strengthen alliances with patients who already are presenting with a myriad of psychosocial stressors, psychiatric impairments, and substance-induced intoxication or withdrawal that compromise good judgment and *best behaviors*. Behaviors are attempts to get needs met; these behaviors may be healthy, straightforward, and adaptive ways; or unhealthy, subversive, destructive, and maladaptive ways for the patient to meet his or her needs. Prevention strategies compel nursing staff to pay attention to, and addresses:

▶ Basic physical needs

  ▶ Offer water, food; plan to sit with patient and patient groups at varying times without intention to focus solely on their problems; identify supports and strengths.

  ▶ Attend to emergencies and complaints of pain.

▶ Basic psychological needs

  ▶ Listen, give support, support adaptive defenses, provide structure, encourage constructive activity.

  ▶ Encourage preferred coping mechanisms.

  ▶ Teach simple techniques for reducing stress (journaling, adequate sleep or rest, diet and exercise, sublimation through safe outlets for strong energy, deep breathing, meditation and prayer).

  ▶ Support previous successes and beliefs in self-efficacy.

  ▶ Assist in setting up new supports or activating those already available.

  ▶ Refer or link to social services for assistance with basic living needs.

Crisis intervention is an acute, short-term therapeutic intervention. The goal is to return persons in crisis to their precrisis adaptive level of functioning and to prevent or reduce the negative effects of the stressors creating the stress. Constructive resolution of a crisis can provide a person with stronger coping ability, whereas an inability to resolve a crisis can lead to psychiatric symptoms or personal breakdown. A generalized model of crisis intervention is built on a four-phase strategy:

1. Develop an alliance with patients.

   ▸ Build trust and use empathy.

   ▸ Begin where the person wants.

   ▸ Acknowledge helplessness.

2. Gather information about triggers and events.

   ▸ Focus on precipitating event.

      ▷ It may not be therapeutic to describe a traumatic event in detail.

      ▷ Gather timeline and precipitating events.

   ▸ Determine precrisis level of functioning.

      ▷ Review similar past symptoms.

   ▸ Determine acute and long-term needs, threats, and challenges.

   ▸ Review past successful coping mechanisms.

   ▸ Identify usual resources.

3. Problem-solve with patients; give them some credit for input.

   ▸ Begin basic problem-solving.

   ▸ Set realistic goals.

   ▸ Focus on termination from the beginning.

   ▸ Support patient strengths.

   ▸ Suggest additional coping strategies.

4. Evaluate.

   ▸ Have identified outcomes been achieved?

   ▸ Are adequate support systems in place?

   ▸ What does the patient need?

Nursing Model of Crisis Intervention

According to Aguilera's (1998) nursing model, a person, family, or group can experience a biological or psychosocial event that creates a state of disequilibrium and anxiety. If balancing factors are present in the form of realistic perception of the event, adequate situational support, and adequate coping mechanisms, the person will be able to resolve the problem, regain a sense of equilibrium, and avert the crisis state. On the other hand, if one or more balancing factors are absent, then the problem remains unresolved, the disequilibrium and anxiety continue or escalate, and the person experiences the crisis state. Crisis intervention treatment focuses on helping patients to create or restore these essential balancing factors to achieve the precrisis level of functional coping. Three phases are described; stabilization, problem-solving, and resolution.

Aguilera's First Phase of Crisis Intervention

The *first* priorities in treating a person in a crisis state are to *stabilize* the patient and to ensure the safety of the patient, family, and others in the immediate environment. This requires the nurse to remain calm and in control of the situation, setting limits when needed. Depending on the nature and severity of the crisis state, short-term medication may be indicated. When a patient is threatening the safety of the milieu, nursing interventions focus on reducing the likelihood of harm. Interventions are focused on an immediate crisis situation or problem that is perceived as overwhelming and traumatic to the patient. Because immediate relief is called for, it is essential to determine the services and resources needed to return the patient to his or her precrisis level of functioning. Support networks can help persons in crisis begin to function independently.

▶ Reduce stimulation in the milieu.

▶ Remove lethal material.

▶ Separate the person from other patients.

▶ Establish a contract for safety.

▶ Provide constant one-on-one monitoring.

▶ Maintain safety: observe for escalation.

▶ Remain calm: defuse with least restrictive means.

Use deescalating communication strategies:

▶ Speak in a calm, low voice.

▶ Respect the need for personal space.

▶ Avoid intense eye contact.

▶ Acknowledge the patient's feelings and reassure that staff is there to help.

▶ Avoid power struggles.

▶ Communicate expected behavior.

▶ Communicate consequences of unacceptable behavior.

▶ Give an opportunity for time out.

Use seclusion or restraints only if necessary, as last resort. In high-risk, potentially violent, or life-threatening situations where preventive and deescalating strategies have failed, seclusion or restraints might be required. It is always understood that all patients have a basic right to treatment in the least restrictive setting. State regulations vary on rules about seclusion and restraint; however, the psychiatric–mental health nurse must always adhere to the strictest standard, whether defined by state regulatory agencies, The Joint Commission, or the Centers for Medicaid and Medicare Services (CMS). Families must be notified when a patient has been in restraints and the patient must be checked for injuries or bruising that may have occurred because of the restraint.

▶ Seclusion and restraint require a team response with a designated team leader.

▶ Notify security if necessary.

▶ Remove all other patients from the area.

▶ The leader should expresses concern for the patient's safety and behavior.

▶ At given signal, the team secures the patient's limbs.

▶ The patient is escorted to an appropriate room and informed of the intervention.

▶ If necessary, administer restraints or medications.

Aguilera's Second Phase of Crisis Intervention

In the second phase of intervention, it is important that nurses take an active role with patients and families to engage in problem-solving strategies. Once the patient is stabilized medically and is safe, the focus turns to collecting comprehensive assessment data. This is accomplished by gathering specific information about the crisis—that is, concentrating on recent events, what led up to the present state of disequilibrium, the duration of the crisis state, and its impact on others. This is also the time to explore information about support systems, previous coping strategies, and the meaning of the crisis to the patient. These strategies include:

▶ Developing a working alliance with the patient and his or her family. Appeal to the fact that you are the nurse (most trusted healthcare providers) and are there to help. Suggest the need to obtain blood pressure (as a distraction). Offer the patient water and a seat at the table with you.

▶ Identify and encourage patient strengths and abilities.

▶ Identify coping mechanisms used successfully in the past.

▶ Give the patient an opportunity to express emotions; acknowledge fear, anger, helplessness, or resentment.

▶ Help the patient externalize the events of the crisis in a realistic manner.

▶ Set realistic goals. Help the patient explore other options when strong feelings recur.

▶ Mutually identify possible solutions, and encourage self-responsibility.

▶ Help the patient to identify and mobilize social supports and develop new ones.

▶ Assist the patient, when needed, to make appropriate community support contacts.

Aguilera's Third Phase of Crisis Intervention

In the *resolution phase* of crisis intervention, the nurse assists crisis patients to restabilize their lives and to achieve precrisis adaptive functioning. This involves helping crisis victims understand the negative impact of the crisis on their lives, and active assistance with use of available resources and support networks to achieve independent functioning. This potentially is a teachable moment.

Successful resolution is evidenced by a decrease in the original presenting symptoms to manageable proportions, satisfaction with the outcome of the crisis intervention, and articulated plans for future action. During this phase, the nurse helps the patient summarize goal achievement and identify healthy ways of coping to prevent further problems. If the patient needs further assistance, or the problems for which the person sought crisis intervention are not resolved to the patient's and nurse's satisfaction, referrals for psychotherapy or additional support can be made.

PSYCHIATRIC–MENTAL HEALTH PRACTICE STANDARD 5F: MILIEU THERAPY

Milieu therapy is a form of spatial interaction that uses the social environment of the unit or facility as a primary therapeutic agent. People are in constant interaction and transaction with their environments. The psychiatric–mental health registered nurse has responsibility for providing the socio-cultural-environmental structure and for maintaining a safe and therapeutic (purposeful) environment. Essential components of a therapeutic milieu includes safety, structure, norms, limit-setting, and balance. These components, discussed in this chapter, include consideration of treatment in the least restrictive environment. Milieu therapy components that pertain to patient basic rights, and education needs that are obtained through individual, group, family, and community modalities, are presented in Chapter 7.

Safety in the Milieu

Safety is the priority goal in patient care. Every healthcare provider avows to a basic tenet to do no harm. This compels healthcare providers to know how to promote safety, how to evaluate sentinel events and near misses, and how to avoid and prevent compromises to safety. Safety standards are articulated by The Joint Commission (TJC) through annual published standards referred to as National Patient Safety Goals (2015), one of which is to identify safety risks among patients; find out which patients are most likely to try to commit suicide.

Of late, the healthcare industry is taking note of the highly rated safety margin found within the aviation industry. Among all the thousands of flights that occur all over the earth, flight mishaps are few. Some of the check-recheck policies and practices occurring in operating room suites and in personal protective equipment dressing and undressing practices noted today stem from application of aviation safety-check modeling. In psychiatric care settings, prevention of suicide and homicide, assaults, aggression, and violence are top priority. Crisis states, theories, and interventions are discussed here to facilitate nurses' understanding of this level of patient decompensation.

Seclusion and Restraint Safety: Regulatory Guidelines

Restraint-free environments are the ultimate goal. The Joint Commission (2009) invokes federal guidelines for the use of seclusion or restraints to manage violent or self-destructive behaviors of reduce the risk of harming patients. Anyone restrained must be evaluated by a physician or licensed independent practitioner within 1 hour. The patient must be monitored continuously and the procedure must be terminated as soon as the patient meets the criteria for release. The nurse must document the behaviors, the attempts to use less restrictive interventions, nursing care provided, the patient's response to the treatments, and rationale for terminating the intervention. TJC (2009) also provides very specific guidelines for implementing restraints. Types of available restraints are:

▶ Physical: any device, garment, or hold that restricts a person's voluntary movement and cannot be easily removed by the person

▶ Chemical: psychotropic medication given for the specific purpose of controlling behavior; its therapeutic value lies in decreasing a patient's escalating anxiety and potential to harm self or others. When restrictive measures are necessary, nurses should document which less restrictive measures were tried unsuccessfully, and specifically why the particular restrictive measure is necessary.

Patients can be restrained temporarily for serious medical or behavioral symptoms. Examples of medical reasons for restraints include the patient's inability to cooperate with an essential physical treatment or device such as an IV, in-dwelling catheter, respirator, or dressing; or because of confusion or irrational thinking. Behavioral health reasons consist of severe behaviors that potentially could cause injury to self or others because of violent, aggressive, or acute agitation related to an emotional or behavioral disorder, or symptoms associated with acute drug use. Restraining a patient, either physically or chemically with medication, is an emergency form of treatment reserved for situations in which the patient's behavioral symptoms justify temporary restraint or seclusion to protect the patient from harming him- or herself or others. Nurses and staff who restrain patients must be trained in cardiopulmonary resuscitation (CPR) techniques.

Regardless of the reason for the restraint or seclusion, TJC standards apply. The CMS outlines require written and time-frame guidelines when implementing restraint or seclusion. Only the minimal amount of restraint necessary to ensure the safety of the patient and others, while promoting the patient's personal autonomy to the highest level possible, can be used. The initial evaluation of the person must be made within 1 hour by a licensed independent practitioner (LIP) and length-of-time maximums are based on age:

▶ Adults: 4 hours

▶ Adolescents (ages 9–17): 2 hours

▶ Children (ages younger than 9): 1 hour

During the entire time of emergency treatment, physical assessment of the patient in seclusion or restraints must be documented in the chart at designated intervals. Remember, the legal assumption is that if it's not documented, it wasn't done! Required documentation of the care offered to the person in restraints or seclusion and evidence of staff debriefing includes

▶ Document that risk was assessed

▶ Least restrictive options tried without success

▶ Description of the event (triggers?); rationale for use

▶ Rationale for the restraint or seclusion, including the patient's condition or symptoms

▶ Evidence of at least hourly face-to-face medical and behavioral evaluation, including a description of the behavior and interventions attempted

▶ Patient's physical condition

▶ Adequate nutrition and hydration offered regularly

▶ Circulation and range of motion in extremities checked frequently

▶ Vital signs, especially respiratory functioning monitored

▶ Hygiene and elimination offered

▶ Physical and psychosocial status and comfort provided

▶ Medications administered

▶ Notification of family of need for intervention

▶ Discontinuation of restraints as soon as feasible

▶ Signs of injury associated with the application of restraint or seclusion, if any

▶ Rationale for terminating the intervention

▶ Debriefing with patient, patient's family, and staff to identify triggers precipitating loss of control, options for alternatives that can be used in the future, barriers to providing least restrictive interventions

▶ The patient's response to treatment interventions, and rationale for continued use of restraint or seclusion, if warranted

Structure in the Milieu

The structure and process environment of milieu therapy is particularly helpful with disorganized patients or those who require close supervision and guidance. Milieu therapy is used in inpatient, partial hospitalization, community, and rehabilitation settings. This planned treatment environment acts as a therapeutic agent, where patients must be willing to actively participate in group and decision-making activities. Communication is open and direct between staff and patients, and reality testing and problem-solving exercises are the goal of implementations. When the nurse opens curtains to bring in sunshine during the day, throws scrunched tissues in the trash, empties the urinal, arranges tables and chairs for a group, or is involved in developing unit rules or patient orientation handbooks, or weighs in on the new color suggested for renovation, this represents engagement in the tenets of milieu therapy. Structure and environmental modification focuses on the following:

▶ Comfort during treatment

▶ Confidentiality of sensitive information

▶ Organization of healthful activities

▶ Structuring time and monitoring fatigue in both patients and staff

▶ Cleanliness of environment

▶ Access to communication (mail, visitors)

▶ Provision of space for privacy

▶ Provision of space when needed

Norms in the Milieu

Clear communication is vital to enhance effectiveness and promote recovery for all. Norms, or expectation should be clearly spelled out in patient handbooks and posted as reminders. They include elements such as being respectful to all others, speaking in turn, calling others by given name not derogatory names, using respectful language, attending groups and classes on time, remaining for groups and classes until the end, allowance to go to room if anxious or too acutely ill for interaction (give attention to the number of days that patient has been in hospital; presentations expectedly are variant depending on whether it is day one or day 5. The longer a patient has been in the hospital, the higher your expectations, given the patient is responsive to medications, is used to the milieu, and has gained increased comfort and confidence). Other areas for setting norms include

- ▶ Community rules posted or accessible,

- ▶ Consequences discussed before actions occur,

- ▶ Violence, aggression, abuse prohibited,

- ▶ Independence encouraged,

- ▶ Communication safeguarded within group, milieu,

- ▶ Cultural differences accepted,

- ▶ Feedback promoted if positive, and

- ▶ Visitors and visitation monitored.

Limit-Setting in the Milieu

Another clearly effective way to promote a therapeutic milieu is to be consistent in engagements with patients and other staff. Each patient, despite his or her particular presentation or nuances, deserves the understanding by the nurse that it is the patient who is sick and in need, not the nurse. It behooves the psychiatric–mental health nurse to remember that patients, because of their illness, may not be engaging in their best behaviors. Testing staff and manipulating others are tactics that many patients, even nonpatients, have learned to get personal needs met in their socioeconomic, family, and community environments. At the end of the day, this is exactly what we all engage in—getting personal needs met, perhaps in more prosocial ways.

Modification of the therapeutic milieu results from continual evaluation of effectiveness of the interventions and recognition of the need for improvements. Rules can change in accordance to the patient mix. At times there may be grey areas. This is the time for team decisions and conflict resolution (Chapter 7). Behavior modification strategies assist with limit-setting in the environment. These elements address several of the following concerns:

▶ Limits are set appropriately; no power plays.

▶ Staff enforces rules consistently.

▶ Individual uniqueness and needs considered.

▶ Time-out opportunities offered.

▶ Crisis intervention implemented.

▶ Advocacy promoted.

▶ One-on-one observation available.

▶ Seclusion and restraints are last resort.

▶ Medications taken as prescribed.

▶ Token economy implemented:

  ▸ Interpersonal skills and self-care behaviors rewarded

  ▸ Positive and negative reinforcement used

Balance, the desired outcome, "is the process of gradually allowing independent behaviors in a dependent situation" (Keltner, Schwecke, & Bostrom, 2003, pp. 280–281). Independence needs to be gained in increments and staff monitors to ensure that one's need does not overpower another's need, both in and between patients.

REFERENCES

Agency for Healthcare Research and Quality. (2012). *Five major steps to intervention (the "5 A's")*. Retrieved from http://www.ahrq.gov/professionals/clinicians-providers/guidelines-recommendations/tobacco/5steps.html.

Aguilera, D. (1998). *Crisis intervention: Theory and methodology*. Philadelphia: Mosby.

American Psychiatric Association. (2013). *Diagnostic and statistical manual of mental disorders, 5th ed.* Arlington, VA: American Psychiatric Publishing.

Andrews, A. (2014). *Some assembly required. The not so secret life of a transgender teen*. New York: Simon & Schuster.

The Associated Press. (2012, May 11). FDA panel backs Truvada, first pill to block HIV infection. Retrieved from http://www.nydailynews.com/life-style/health/fda-panel-backs-truvada-pill-block-hiv-infection-article-1.1076327.

Caplan, G. (1964). *Principles of preventive psychiatry*. New York: Basic Books.

Centers for Disease Control and Prevention. (2014a). *Substance use and mental disorders: Early detection, prevention and treatment*. Retrieved from http://www.cdc.gov/nchs/ppt/hp2020/hp2020_MH_MD_and_SA_progress_review_presentation.pdf.

Centers for Disease Control and Prevention. (2014b). *Facts about ASD.* Retrieved from http://www.cdc.gov/ncbddd/autism/facts.html.

Ciraulo, D. A., Shader, R. I., Greenblatt, D..J., & Creelman, W. (2006). *Drug interactions in psychiatry, 3rd ed.* Philadelphia: Lippincott Williams & Wilkins.

Costandi, M. (2013). Neurodegeneration: Amyloid awakenings. *Nature Outlook: Sleep, 497*(7450); S19–S20.

DeHert, M., Correll, C. U., Bobes, J., Cetkovich-Bakmas, M., Cohen, D. Asai, I. & Leucht, S. (2011). Physical illness in healthcare consumers with severe mental disorders. I. Prevalence, impact of medications and disparities in health care. *World Psychiatry, 10*(1), 52–77.

Deratnay, P., & Sidani, S. (2013). The effect of insomnia on functional status of community-dwelling older adults. *Journal of Gerontological Nursing, 39*(10); 22–30.

DeWeerdt, S. (2013). Mood disorders: The dark night. *Nature Outlook: Sleep, 497*(7450); S14–S15.

Dolgin, E. (2013). Deprivation: A wake-up call. *Nature Outlook: Sleep, 497*(7450); S6–S7.

Dolgin, E. (April 2014). Negative feedback. *Nature, 508*; S10–S11.

Dugan, M. K., & Hock, R. (2006). *It's my life now: Starting over after an abusive relationship or domestic violence, 2nd ed.* New York: Brunner-Routledge.

Farrington, E. *Relationship of vitamin D deficiency to depression in older adults: An integrative review for 2008–2013.* Faculty Advisor: Mary Moller, Yale School of Nursing. Poster presented at 27th Annual APNA Conference 2013, San Antonio, TX.

Flannery, R. & Everly, G. (2002). Crisis intervention. A review. *International Journal of Emergency Mental Health, 2*(2), 119–125.

Folstein, M., Folstein, S., & McHugh, P. (1975). Mini-Mental State: A practical method for grading the cognitive state of patients for the clinician. *Journal of Psychiatric Research, 12*, 189–198.

Fotuhi, M., Do, D., & Jack, C. (2013). Modifiable factors that alter the size of the hippocampus with ageing. *Nature Reviews: Neurology, 8*, 189–202. Retrieved from http://www.nature.com/nrneurol/journal/v8/n4/full/nrneurol.2012.27.html.

Hanrahan, N., Lee, M., Longmire, W., Olamijulo, G., Blair, L., & Seng, L.,(2014). *PTSD toolkit for nurses.* University of Pennsylvania School of Nursing, Little Bird Games, & American Nurses Foundation. Retrieved from http://www.nurseptsdtoolkit.org/index.php.

Hearn, K. (March 2013). The dark side of Ayahuasca. *Men's Journal.* Retrieved from http://www.mensjournal.com/magazine/the-dark-side-of-ayahuasca-20130215.

Hill, K. R. (2014). *Rethinking normal: A memoir in transition.* New York: Simon & Schuster.

The Joint Commission. (2009). Restraint/Seclusion for hospitals that use The Joint Commission for deemed status purposes: Author. Retrieved from http://www.jointcommission.org/mobile/standards_information/jcfaqdetails.aspx?StandardsFAQId=260&StandardsFAQChapterId=78.

The Joint Commission. (2015). National Patient Safety Goals. Retrieved from http://www.jointcommission.org/assets/1/6/2015_BHC_NPSG_ER.pdf.

Keltner, N. L., Schwecke, L. H., & Bostrom, C. E. (2003). *Psychiatric nursing, 4th ed.,* pp. 280–281.

Kingwell, K. (2012). Neurodegenerative disease: Modelling connectivity networks of the brain: Can neurodegeneration and dementia progression be predicted? *Nature Reviews: Neurology;* 8, 237–237 1.

Lee, J. (2010). Adolescent brain development and implications for drug abuse prevention. Retrieved from http://www.drugabuse.gov/international/abstracts/adolescent-brain-development-implications-drug-abuse-prevention.

Leshner, A. (1997). Addiction is a brain disease, and it matters. *Science, 3*; 278(5335). 45–47. Retrieved from http://www.sciencemag.org/content/278/5335/45.abstract.

Liu, C. C., Kanekiyo, T., Xu, H., & Bu, G. (2013). Apolipoprotein E and Alzheimer's disease: Risk, mechanisms and therapy. *Nature Reviews: Neurology, 2*(9), 106–118.

Morrison, J. (2014). *DSM-5 made easy: The clinician's guide to diagnosis.* The Guilford Press; New York.

NANDA International. (n.d. a) *The complete list of NANDA nursing diagnosis for 2012–2014, with 16 new diagnoses.* Retrieved from http://faculty.mu.edu.sa/public/uploads/1380604673.6151NANDA%202012.pdf.

NANDA International. (n.d. b) List of diagnosis. Retrieved from http://www.nclex.ucoz.net/_ld/0/30_NANDALISTOFDIAG.pdf.

Nasrallal, H. A., & Weiden, P. J. (2014). Paradigm shifts in the biology, diagnosis, and treatment of schizophrenia. *Medscape Education webinar;* released October 15, 2014. Retrieved from http://www.medscape.org/viewarticle/830903.

National Heart, Lung, and Blood Institute. (2011). *Who is at risk for insomnia?* Retrieved from http://www.nhlbi.nih.gov/health/health-topics/topics/inso/atrisk.html.

National Institutes of Health. (2012). *Intravenous immunoglobin for PANDAS (pediatric autoimmune neuropsychiatric disorders associated with streptococcal infections).* Retrieved from clinicaltrials.gov/ct2/show/NCT01281969.

National Institute of Mental Health. (2015). *Schizophrenia.* Retrieved from http://www.nimh.nih.gov/health/topics/schizophrenia/index.shtml.

National Institute of Neurological Disorders and Stroke. (2014). *Rett syndrome fact sheet.* Retrieved from http://www.ninds.nih.gov/disorders/rett/detail_rett.htm.

National Institute on Drug Abuse. (2015). *MDMA (Ecstasy/Molly).* Retrieved from http://www.drugabuse.gov/drugs-abuse/mdma-ecstasymolly.

Owen, D. C., Armstrong, M. L., Koch, J. R., & Roberts, A. E. (2013). College students with body art. *Journal of Psychosocial Nursing, 51*(10), 20–28.

Owens, B. (2013). Obesity: Heavy sleepers. *Nature Outlook: Sleep, 497*(7450); S8–S9.

Peplau, H. (1988). *Interpersonal relations in nursing.* London: Macmillan.

Puntil, C., York, J., Limandri, B., Greene, P., Arauz, E., & Hobbs, D. (2013). Competency-based training for nurse-generalists: Inpatient intervention and prevention of suicide. *Journal of the American Psychiatric Nurses Association, 19* (4); 205–210.

Rank, O. (1957). *The trauma of birth.* New York: Brunner.

Rosedale, M., Ecklesdafer, D., Kormos, T., Freedland, M., & Knapp, M. (October 9, 2013). *The significant promise of therapeutic neuromodulation: Implications for psychiatric mental health nurses.* Paper presented at the 27th Annual APNA Conference 2013, San Antonio, TX.

Schizophrenia: What's in my head? Directed by Charlotte Stoddart. Nature, 508(7494). Retrieved from http://www.nature.com/nature/outlook/schizophrenia/#video.

Selye, H. (1956). *The stress of life.* New York: McGraw-Hill.

Smith, K. (2013). Off to night school. *Nature Outlook: Sleep, 497*(7450); S4–S5.

Stahl, S. (2008). *Stahl's essential psychopharmacology. Neuroscientific basis and practical applications,* 3rd ed. New York: Cambridge University Press.

Stuart, G. W. (2009). *Principles and practice of psychiatric nursing, 9th ed.* Philadelphia: Mosby.

Swanson, K. M., & Wojnar, D. M. (2004). Optimal healing environments in nursing. *The Journal of Alternative and Complementary Medicine, 10*(1); S43–S48.

Volkow, N. (2007). Director's message to medical and health professionals. National Institute on Drug Abuse. Retrieved from http://www.drugabuse.gov/about-nida/directors-page/messages-director/2007/02/medical-health-professionals.

Walter, C., Edwards, N. E., Griggs, R., & Yehle, K. (2014). Differentiating Alzheimer's disease, Lewy body, and Parkinson's dementia using DSM-5. *The Journal for Nurse Practitioners, 10*(4); 262–270.

World Health Organization. (2014). *Mental disorders: Fact sheet.* Retrieved from http://www.who.int/mediacentre/factsheets/fs396/en/.

CATEGORY II

IMPLEMENTATION AND EVALUATION

IMPLEMENTATION AND EVALUATION OF THE COMPREHENSIVE CARE PLAN ACROSS THE LIFE SPAN

By this point in the nursing process, the psychiatric–mental health nurse can synthesize an understanding of presenting symptoms and etiologies, has defined patient problems in nursing diagnostic terms, can develop short- and long-term mutually agreeable goals with the patient, and can better engage in critical thinking as he or she implements and evaluates treatment options. Nursing actions (Standard 5: Implementations; what the nurse does) is followed by nursing evaluation (Standard 6: Evaluation; effectiveness of the actions and implementations). The American Nurses Association's (2014) *Scope and Standards of Practice: Psychiatric–Mental Health Nursing* states that the nurse works with the interprofessional team to implement the comprehensive plan of care that incorporates pharmacological, biological, and integrative therapies. The nurse assures safe and timely implementation of the care plan; documents the plan and any modifications; uses evidence-based interventions; uses care strategies that are both age-appropriate and culturally and ethnically sensitive; incorporates available community resources; collaborates with the interprofessional team regarding care plan implementation; and manages psychiatric or behavioral emergencies through determination of risk level and coordination of effective emergency care interventions.

Specifically, this chapter reviews psychopharmacology; pain management; somatic therapies; and complementary, alternative, and integrative therapies. The standards compel the nurse to evaluate the efficacy of the implementations and interventions. Joint Commission Standards for 2015 compel the nurse to improve the safety of using medications. Evaluation begins with forming of measurable outcome goals (derived from the assessment, nursing diagnosis, and planning process steps). Evaluation is the last step of the evidence-based nursing process and is systematic and ongoing. As the nurse evaluates outcomes, care plans are revised as necessary until treatment goals are met. The following information sources may be used to evaluate individual response to treatment:

▶ Scores on rating scales (e.g., AIMS, CIWA-Ar, BPRS) that are used to evaluate the response to nursing care or medications

▶ Physical exam findings (e.g., weight changes, muscle strength and endurance, vital signs)

▶ Mental status changes (e.g., evaluating thought process and listening to content, reviewing psychological test results)

▶ Laboratory test results (e.g., drug levels, blood glucose levels)

▶ Results of screening tools (e.g., APGAR, CAGE)

▶ Observation and documentation of medication response)

PSYCHIATRIC–MENTAL HEALTH PRACTICE STANDARD 5E: PHARMACOLOGICAL, BIOLOGICAL, AND INTEGRATIVE THERAPIES

Principles for Safe and Effective Medication Administration and Management

Nursing interventions support physiological functioning. Many nursing interventions are physician-initiated, such as medications ordered by the physician in charge of caring for the patient. Generally speaking, management of patient symptoms is the target for treatments. When symptoms are managed, the patient is more amenable to other interventions that further support or complement a return to optimal functioning.

Biological treatments may include interventions that involve self-care activities, exercise or other physical activities, sleep, nutrition and hydration, pain management, relaxation training, and medication management. Having a good understanding of neurotransmitter and brain receptor functions (reviewed in Chapter 2) is helpful for learning and understanding indications for pharmacologic treatments and how pharmacokinetic and pharmacodynamic properties affect individual biological responses. With the first physical map of the human genome completed in 1995, the fields of pharmacogenomics and ethnopharmacology are rapidly advancing. Genetic testing capabilities permit the identification of pharmacodynamic factors that elucidate the advent of personalized medicine. Personalized medicine uses genes involved in the cytochrome P450 (CYP450) to identify individual and ethnic differences in medication efficacy.

Think back to biochemistry classes when you would mix one compound with another in a fluid medium and observed for a reaction. A person's body is like a chemical flask, and any compound that enters has potential to evoke a reaction. The nurse needs to know what medications or substances (food, fluids, etc.) the patient has recently taken, understand the dosing of what currently is intended to be given, then stay alert to observe patient response after administration. The psychiatric–mental health nurse applies current research findings to guide actions that

- ▶ Assesses patient responses to expected benefits, drug-drug interaction effects, expected side effects, potential untoward effects, and therapeutic doses of pharmacological agents;

- ▶ Communicates observations of patient responses to biological interventions to other health clinicians;

- ▶ Intervenes in alleviating untoward effects of biological interventions; and

- ▶ Provides health teaching about mechanisms of action, proper management and administration, ways to cope with transitional side effects, and other treatment options.

Safe Medication Management and Just Culture

The Institute of Medicine (IOM) published a summary of research findings on the unacceptable level of medication errors in hospitals (2000) and followed up with *Preventing Medication Errors* (2007). These seminal reports, in combination with The Joint Commission's 2015 (TJC) National Patient Safety Goals (NPSG), provide evidence-based strategies for preventing medication errors across the healthcare spectrum. Holloway & Kusy (2014) references a 2011 report in the *American Journal of Medical Quality*, of research findings that point to a strong association between disruptive behaviors in the workforce and 70% of sentinel events reported by TJC that could be traced to communication errors; 71% occurrence of medical errors; 67% of adverse events; 51% of patient safety compromises; and 27% of patient mortality. Recommendations center on providing patient-centered care with a goal of improved provider-patient communication about medication benefits and risks and organizing a culture of safety around medications. To this end, organizations are expected to engage in electronic prescribing and to take actions to prevent errors from "look-alike, sound-alike" medications, avoid use of confusing abbreviations and symbols, and label all medications and containers. The official "Do Not Use" list for confusing abbreviations can be found on the Joint Commission's (2005) website http://www.jointcommission.org/assets/1/18/Do_Not_Use_List.pdf

The *Just Culture* model (Wise, 2014) is a set of management tools and skills that aligns the behaviors, duties, and skills of healthcare providers in identifying, understanding, and categorizing choices in patient care performances to improve patient outcomes.

Medication Reconciliation Across All Settings

The Joint Commission presents annual national patient safety goals for behavioral health patients. To achieve and retain accreditation, behavioral health organizations must reconcile medications at all points of care and whenever medications are updated or changed. Reconciliation is intended to identify and resolve discrepancies by comparing medications a patient is and should be taking with newly ordered medications. The comparison addresses duplications, omissions, interactions, and the need to continue current medications. To reconcile medications, the nurse identifies the medication name, dose, frequency (routine times and as needed), route, and purpose. The nurse is also responsible for ensuring that the patient knows which medicines to take when he or she is at home; reviewing dosing and special instructions (Black Box Warnings), and telling patients to bring their up-to-date list of medicines every time they visit a physician or healthcare provider.

The word *psychotropic* is an umbrella term that refers to a chemical substance that can readily cross the blood-brain barrier and that affects brain functioning and the central nervous system, resulting in alterations in mood, cognition, behavior, consciousness, or perceptual states. Further, because of psychotropic medications' powerful effects on multiple organs and neurotransmitter systems, it is crucial that psychiatric–mental health nurses have a clear understanding of *what* and *why* they are administering these medications. The nurse also must consider medication mechanisms of action, as well as expected effects, side effects, and perhaps untoward or adverse effects that might arise at any point in the medication treatment schedule. This is a most important responsibility and should be thought of with a sense of high ethics, morals, knowledge, and accountabilities. Important terminology related to mechanistic actions and properties of psychotropic medications follows.

Potency: The relative dose required to achieve certain effects. This term is generally applied to the first-generation antipsychotics to describe the relationship between therapeutic dose and side effects. The more potent the drug, the lower the dosage, and the higher the risk of extrapyramidal side effects (EPS). Antipsychotics with low potency tend to be more sedating and have more anticholinergic side effects than the high-potency antipsychotics. *Example:* Haloperidol (Haldol) 5mg is more potent than chlorpromazine (Thorazine) 300–800mg because less is needed to achieve the same therapeutic effect. Haloperidol has a much higher risk for EPS. Chlorpromazine is more sedating.

Therapeutic Index: The relative measure of the toxicity or safety of a drug, defined as the ratio of the median toxic dose to the median effective dose. *Example:* The therapeutic index of lithium is quite low and requires careful monitoring of serum levels.

Tolerance: The need for an increased amount of drug to achieve the same effect. It is the process of becoming less responsive to a particular drug as it is administered over time.

Pharmacokinetics: How the body moves a drug throughout the body by way of four processes: (1) absorption, (2) distribution, (3) metabolism, and (4) elimination. For most psychiatric drugs, the principal route of administration is oral. Oral drugs are absorbed through the small bowel, passing into the portal (liver or hepatic) circulation. Most of the psychotropic drugs are partially metabolized by the cytochrome P450 (CYP450) enzymes as the drugs pass through the liver. This process, called "first-pass metabolism," is avoided by drugs that are given intravenously (IV) or intramuscularly (IM). After the first pass through the liver, the drug metabolites enter the systemic circulation, where they are distributed to organs in direct proportion to their fat and protein content. Most psychotropic drugs are highly lipophilic ("love fat") and highly protein-bound (attach to proteins). The unbound (free) concentration of the drug then readily passes the blood-brain barrier. These drugs also have rapid and extensive distribution in other tissues.

Many factors affect pharmacokinetics, including alterations in hepatic CYP450 enzyme concentrations, kidney functioning, the amount of bound protein in the circulation, the half-life of the drug, and the time to onset of action. Therefore, consider conditions of malnutrition or hepatic or renal disease on drug effectiveness.

▶ **Hepatic CYP450 enzyme** interactions can induce or inhibit the metabolism of certain drugs, changing the desired concentration levels. For example, nicotine is an inducer of CYP450 enzymes. Heavy nicotine users, therefore, may require a lower dose of a drug after they have quit smoking. Hepatic disease will affect liver enzyme activity and first-pass metabolism. For drugs that have high first-pass effects, hepatic disease can result in elevated or toxic plasma drug levels.

▶ **Renal disease or drugs that reduce renal clearance** (e.g., NSAIDs) may increase serum concentration of these drugs (e.g., lithium). Some drugs rely more on excretion by way of the kidneys than metabolism by the liver.

▶ **Malnutrition, wasting, and aging** affect the amount of free-circulating drug that is bound to proteins in the bloodstream. If a highly protein-bound drug is displaced from its protein by another, more strongly protein-bound drug, it can result in increased circulating levels of the first drug. Any condition that shifts the ratio of bound to free drug can change the concentration of the drug.

▶ **Half-life** is the time needed to clear 50% of a drug from the plasma. Half-life is the determinant of the duration of action of a drug. It also determines the length of time necessary to reach steady state and how frequently drugs must be taken to maintain the desired effect.

▶ **Steady state** is reached when the amount administered per unit of time equals the amount eliminated per unit of time. It takes five half-lives for concentration to build to steady state. Likewise, it takes five half-lives to wash out a drug.

▶ **Onset of action** is the length of time that it takes for a medicine to start to work. Drugs within a category may be chosen based upon their onset of action. For example, sedatives with rapid onset of action will be useful for persons with sleep-onset insomnia.

▶ **Cardiovascular disease and reduced cardiac output** can affect both renal and hepatic drug clearance. Cardiovascular disease especially increases the risks of using drugs with potential cardiac effects (e.g., tricyclics). A common side effect of many of the psychotropic drugs, orthostatic hypotension, greatly increases the risk for falls in older adults. Gastrointestinal disease and decreased gastric acid secretion may slow absorption. Brain changes and reduced acetylcholine (ACh) output increase the risk for anticholinergic toxicity. In general, older adults are more susceptible to adverse drug effects and interactions (particularly cardiac).

▶ **Age and gender** differences affect how the body processes drugs.

  ▸ **Children** may have greater hepatic capacity, more glomerular filtration, and less fatty tissue, and may be less able to store drugs in their fat, resulting in quicker elimination and shorter half-lives. These differences in children and adolescents may result in recommended dosages that approach those of adults despite smaller body size.

  ▸ **Older adults** may have less efficient livers and kidneys (in fact lower levels of functioning in most organ systems compared to younger persons), resulting in slower metabolism and excretion of drugs. Most psychotropic drugs are lipid-soluble, so when lean body mass is lost and body fat concentration increases, the lipid-soluble psychotropic drugs distribute widely in fat tissue, resulting in unexpectedly prolonging drug actions.

  ▸ **Women** may have certain pharmacological risks during pregnancy. Most fetal malformations (teratogenic effects) occur during the embryonic period (weeks 3 to 8 of gestation) and positive pregnancy tests are possible at weeks 4 to 7. Overall, recommendations to women of childbearing age are to prevent first-trimester exposure to psychotropic medications by using birth control. However, untreated maternal mental illness during pregnancy and postpartum periods can result in the infant having lower Apgar scores, lower serotonin levels, difficulty being consoled, sleep problems, and behavior problems even into school age. If pregnancy occurs and psychotropic drugs must be used during pregnancy, the risk–benefit ratio must be clearly established. Antidepressant prophylaxis during the third trimester may be used to prevent postpartum depression in women with a history of depression. Again the risk–benefit ratio must be assessed because there is risk to the baby of having withdrawal symptoms from the antidepressant. Because of lipid solubility, psychotropic drugs pass readily into breast milk, so mothers should be advised of alternatives.

Pharmacodynamics refers to what a drug does to the body at four specific target sites: receptors, ion channels, enzymes, and transport pumps. Think of these actions as chemical reactions within the laboratory flasks (our bodies).

▶ **Receptors:** Psychotherapeutic drugs produce a wide range of effects on neurotransmitter receptors. Each neurotransmitter has several receptor types, and each given receptor type may have multiple subtypes with different actions. Thus, one drug can have multiple actions in different areas of the brain and spinal cord, depending on the distribution of neurotransmitter pathways and receptors. Newer drugs are developed with greater selectivity and specificity in the hope that they will have fewer side effects.

    ▸ **Agonist:** Naturally occurring neurotransmitters stimulate receptors and are thus agonists. Drugs that mimic the actions of the neurotransmitters are also agonists.

    ▸ **Antagonist:** Substances that block the actions of agonists *in the presence of the agonist.* In the absence of the agonist, the antagonist has no effects. For example, naloxone (Narcan) is an opioid antagonist. It precipitates withdrawal in the presence of opioids, but otherwise has no effect.

    ▸ **Inverse agonist:** Drugs that have the opposite actions of their agonists.

    ▸ **Partial agonist:** Drugs that stimulate receptors to a lesser degree than the natural neurotransmitter.

In general, the most concerning side effects and their causes are summarized below:

    ▸ **Anticholinergic effects:** acetylcholine (muscarinic) receptor blockage (antagonism)

    ▸ **Extrapyramidal side effects (EPS):** dopamine receptor blockage (antagonism)

    ▸ **Sedation:** histamine receptor blockage (antagonism)

    ▸ **Orthostatic hypotension:** adrenergic receptor blockage (antagonism)

    ▸ **Sexual dysfunction, anxiety, akathisia, insomnia, gastrointestinal upset, and diarrhea effects:** serotonergic receptor excessive activation (agonism)

▶ **Ion channels** exist for many ions, including sodium, potassium, chloride, and calcium. Drugs such as calcium channel blockers act by blocking the movement of calcium through the channel. Unlike ions, neurotransmitters do not actually pass from one neuron into another. Instead the neurotransmitter interacts with the receptor, causing it to change configuration. The effects of this "gating" action depend upon whether the neurotransmitter has an excitatory or inhibitory action at the receptor. For example, glutamate is an excitatory neurotransmitter. One of the glutamate receptors (N-nitrosodimethylamine or NMDA) gates a calcium channel. When glutamate interacts with the NMDA receptor, calcium is allowed in, depolarizing the postsynaptic cell.

▶ **Enzymes** are proteins important for drug metabolism. For example, monoamine oxidase (MAO) is an enzyme that metabolizes the monoamine neurotransmitters (5HT, D, and NE). MAO is located inside the terminals of catecholamine neurons. After the neurotransmitter is released into the synaptic cleft and reacts with the receptor, it is pumped back into the terminal where MAO can destroy it. Antidepressant drugs that block MAO (such as MAO inhibitors) decrease the metabolism of monoamines in the cytosol (i.e., once they have been pumped back into the terminal), and thus increase the availability of the neurotransmitter for recycling and rerelease from the neuron.

▶ **Transport pumps** are proteins that actively carry neurotransmitter molecules out of the synapse and back into the presynaptic neuron. When reuptake pumps are inhibited, the concentration of certain neurotransmitters or ions builds up in the synapse or extracellular space. For example, selective serotonin reuptake inhibitors (SSRIs) block re-uptake of serotonin, increasing the synaptic availability.

PSYCHOPHARMACOLOGY: GENERAL PRINCIPLES

The psychiatric–mental health nurse understands that baseline assessment information about the patient's overall health, well-being, and illness states are elucidated before the administration of any pharmacological agent. The physical review of systems, allergy lists, documentation of past and present health alterations, clinical laboratory and radiological study results, and current medication regimen are important foundations before initiating any new therapies. Because biotransformation (or metabolism) of psychopharmaceutical agents is so integral to the absorption–distribution–metabolism–elimination process, baseline electrocardiograms (ECG), liver function tests (LFT), thyroid function studies (TFS), renal clearance studies, serum chemistry analyses (electrolytes and blood components), as well as measures of weight and height, waist circumference, vital signs, blood glucose, and fasting lipid profiles, assist with recognizing psychopharmaceutical tolerability and effect factors. When a person is healthy, an assumption is made that medication interventions may be effective; paradoxically, medication interventions may have deleterious effects on body systems, perhaps over time. It is useful to understand that, for most disorders, medication treatment dosing targets one of three phases in the illness continuum:

1. **Acute phase:** Prevent harm, manage aggressive behaviors, reduce positive symptoms, return patient to baseline functioning, form an alliance with patient to develop treatment goals, and begin referrals to community resources. In this phase, new medications may be started or current medications adjusted. The psychiatric–mental health nurse intervenes by implementing continuous monitoring of responses, as well as providing ongoing education about the medication's expected benefits (or response) and expected side effects to the patient, as well as the family.

2. **Stabilization phase:** Minimize stress and enhance adaptation, with continued reduction in symptoms and recovery of functioning. Medication may need to be adjusted. The nurse continues to monitor response and side effects, providing information as necessary to patient and family. During this phase, the nurse can help the patient learn self-management skills.

3. **Maintenance phase:** Ensure that symptom remission or control is sustained. The patient is asked to report increases in symptoms or relapses, and any adverse effects from medications. The nurse will monitor weight, BMI, blood glucose, lipids, and other factors depending upon medication side effects. During this phase, the goal is recovery: to maintain or improve level of functioning and quality of life with the expectation that the patient is in recovery, understands how to maintain this state, and is aware of signs and symptoms of either medication side effects or break-through symptoms that require possible intervention by a healthcare provider.

It is helpful to classify medications according to the broad categories of neurotransmitters (hence, symptoms) they affect. In practice, however, because of overlapping pathophysiological mechanisms, medications are often offered across the different categorizations to affect varying symptoms simultaneously because more than one neurotransmitter is affected by the newer psychopharmaceuticals. For example, antidepressants may be used to treat anxiety disorders, pain, and eating disorders, in addition to major depression. The major classes of medications reviewed in this chapter include the following:

- ▶ **Anticholinergics:** side effects that develop with most psychotropic medications
- ▶ **Antipsychotics, neuroleptics, major tranquilizers** for psychosis, bipolar disorder, aggression, tic disorders
- ▶ **Antidepressants** for depression, pain, anxiety
- ▶ **Mood stabilizers** for bipolar disorder, aggression, mood disorders
- ▶ **Anxiolytics, sedative-hypnotics** for anxiety, sleep disorders, substance withdrawal
- ▶ **Psychostimulants** for attention-deficit hyperactivity disorder, narcolepsy
- ▶ **Cognitive enhancers** for dementia

Anticholinergic and Gastrointestinal Side Effects

Commonly occurring side effects experienced by patients receiving psychotropic medications include anticholinergic and gastrointestinal symptoms. Both types are relatively easily managed or may be transient in nature. The nurse observes for both expected and unexpected patient responses to medication interventions.

Anticholinergic side effects: One of the major complaints from patients about typical antipsychotic medications is side effects. Educating patients about potential side effects and possible treatments might help with medication compliance. Side effects that can be ameliorated are the anticholinergic effects that cause drying of mucus membranes. Anticholinergic effects result in constipation, dry mouth, nasal congestion, blurred vision, and urinary retention. Nurses should check with the patient daily about bowel movements because constipation can be particularly uncomfortable. If the patient reports constipation, a diet high in fiber should be encouraged, water intake should be increased, and sometimes it is helpful to give a laxative. Dry mouth is helped by small sips of water, sugarless hard candies or gum, and mouth rinses. Nasal congestion can be improved with saline spray or over-the-counter nasal decongestants (which must be used carefully to reduce risk of developing tolerance). Blurred vision during acute phases of treatment implementation is self-limiting. The nurse should reassure patients that their normal vision should return in approximately three weeks and until it does they should avoid any potentially dangerous tasks. If the blurred vision becomes uncomfortable, pilocarpine eye drops can be used for a limited time. Urinary retention might require bethanechol.

Anticholinergic toxicity: Anticholinergic side effects are manageable and usually do not require switching or reducing antipsychotic medications. However, if symptoms worsen and the patient becomes toxic, this can be life-threatening. A useful mnemonic for remembering the symptoms is "Dry as a bone, red as a beet, hot as a hare, blind as a bat, and mad as a hatter." Patients may become agitated. Because ACh is so important to cognitive functioning, the lack of it creates severe cognitive symptoms including possible disorientation to time, person, and place, as well as hallucinations. Seizures, stupor, and coma may ensue. Older adults are especially vulnerable. Regular monitoring of anticholinergic symptoms will help prevent toxicity. If symptoms of toxicity do arise, discontinue the causative agents, provide close medical supervision, and give medication (physostigmine) to reverse symptoms.

Gastrointestinal discomfort, hypotension or orthostatic hypotension, and weight gain: Complaints of feeling overly sedated and having difficulty getting up and attending to required tasks may be helped by asking the prescriber to administer at bedtime rather than in the morning or during the midday or afternoon. Gastrointestinal distress may lessen if the medication is given at mealtime as long as there is no contraindication to taking food. For dizziness or loss of balance complaints, the nurse should recommend that the patient first get into a sitting position and then slowly stand. Blood pressure should be measured before giving the dose. Because some of the medications can cause weight gain, patients should be advised about this and encouraged to exercise regularly and maintain a healthy diet. Education about nutrition is essential for this population, who might have knowledge deficits regarding diet.

TYPICAL (OLDER OR CONVENTIONAL) ANTIPSYCHOTICS

Dopamine Receptor Antagonists: Implementations and Evaluations

The terms *antipsychotics, neuroleptics*, and *major tranquilizers* may be used interchangeably. Typical antipsychotics were the first generation of antipsychotics available in the 1950s, but are no longer considered first-line treatments because of their side effect profiles. Chlorpromazine (Thorazine) was first used in 1952 (incidentally, the same year that Hildegard Peplau penned her nurse-patient relationship tome and the first DSM was published). These events revolutionized psychiatric and mental health care at that time. Trust-building, patient and family education, symptom management, support services, case management, milieu therapy, reality-oriented group therapy, and psychopharmacology are key intervention strategies for patients with psychotic disorders.

There are over 20 different typical antipsychotics, each generally efficacious, but with very different side effect profiles. Typical antipsychotics work by blocking dopamine (dopamine antagonists) in the brain, generally reducing or eliminating positive symptoms (hallucinations and delusions) of psychosis. The nurse assures that baseline measures, such as weight, waist circumference, blood pressure, fasting blood glucose, fasting lipid profiles, serum blood analyses, and family history of obesity, dyslipidemia, hypertension, and cardiac disease are noted. Neuroleptic side effects related to all these analyses may result and are discussed later. The psychiatric–mental health nurse observes for efficacy when administering medications, and advocates when the patient reports or is observed to experience side effects. High-potency typical antipsychotic use lends itself to a greater concern for EPS risk and less sedation, cardiotoxicity, seizures, and anticholinergic effects than the low-potency typical antipsychotics. The low-potency typical neuroleptics have greater sedation and anticholinergic effects, with lower risk for EPS than the high-potency neuroleptics. Potency comparatives refer to dosing amounts between the high and low and are outlined here. Box 5–1 lists some of the common typical or conventional antipsychotics.

▶ **High-potency:** haloperidol (Haldol), 6–20mg a day, and fluphenazine (Prolixin), 1–20mg a day

▶ **Low-potency:** chlorpromazine (Thorazine), 300–800mg a day

---

BOX 5–1.
TYPICAL (OLDER OR CONVENTIONAL) ANTIPSYCHOTICS

Generic Name	Trade Name
chlorpromazine	Thorazine
fluphenazine	Prolixin
haloperidol	Haldol
loxapine	Loxitane
mesoridazine	Serentil
molindone	Moban
perphenazine	Trilafon
pimozide	Orap
thioridazine	Mellaril
thiothixene	Navane
trifluoperazine	Stelazine

Indications: Positive symptoms of schizophrenia and other psychotic disorders; mood instability, severe agitation; assaultive behaviors; Tourette symptoms; in children or adolescents, severe aggressive behaviors

Mechanism of action: Widespread antagonism of dopamine receptors, especially the D2 receptor. The intended target for blocking dopamine is in the limbic system; however, these drugs tend to block dopamine in dopamine pathways that serve other brain areas as well, resulting in Parkinsonism (effects on the basal ganglia, nigrostriatal pathway), increased negative symptoms (effects on the prefrontal cortex, mesolimbic pathway), and hyperprolactinemia (effects on the pituitary gland, tuberoinfundibular pathway).

Evaluation: Efficacy, Side Effects, and Adverse Effects of Typical (Older or Conventional) Antipsychotics (Neuroleptics or Major Tranquilizers)

Expected benefits (clinical response, efficacy): Clinical effects of medications can occur in 30 to 60 minutes; therefore, some aggressive behaviors may improve in that time frame. Antipsychotic action takes approximately 7 to 10 days; full therapeutic effect occurs in 4 to 6 weeks. These medications do not seem to influence the negative symptoms of schizophrenia, so additional medications may be necessary to treat those behaviors. Conventional antipsychotics have long half-lives and are eliminated slowly.

Untoward or Adverse Effects and Treatments

Gynecomastia and galactorrhea: Antipsychotics antagonize the D2 receptor sites resulting in increased levels of prolactin leading to gynecomastia (enlarged breast tissue) and galactorrhea (expression of milk from mammary glands in the breast). This can be especially difficult for male adolescents. Patients need reassurance and support about what is occurring. Because these side effects can be quite distressing and result in nonadherence, the patient might be switched to another medication without this side effect profile.

Photosensitivity, or sensitivity to sunlight, may place the patient at increased risk for sunburn while outdoors. A wide-brimmed hat and sunglasses are recommended to shield the patient from harm incurred from the sun.

Extrapyramidal side effects (EPS): Because no antipsychotic medication can directly target the positive symptoms without influencing other pathways, the patient must be advised of possible short-term and long-term movement disorders that may result from decreased dopamine in the nigrostriatal pathways, which results in extra pyramidal side effects (EPS). Specific reversible movement disorders, such as a medication-induced Parkinsonism (pseudoparkinsonism), dystonias, and akathisia can be assessed by way of regular ratings using the AIMS or other abnormal movement tool and direct observations by the nurse.

▶ *Akathisia* presents as motor restlessness or an inner, subjective feeling of restlessness: "I feel like my bones are on fire."

▶ *Pseudoparkinsonism* presents with muscle stiffness, cogwheel rigidity, shuffling gait, stooped posture, drooling, or slow resting tremor.

▶ *Dystonic reactions* result in abnormal muscle tonicity and spasms such as of eyes (oculogyric crisis), face (glossopharyngeal spasms), head, neck (wry neck or torticollis), and back (spasms). The above movement dysphorias can be readily identified and reversed with as-needed administration of select medications (below). If antipsychotic medications are otherwise promoting expected benefits, there may be no need to discontinue them. Medications used to treat extrapyramidal side effects work by releasing the neuromuscular dystonia and includes compounds across several categories:

  ▸ Anticholinergics: benztropine (Cogentin) and trihexyphenidyl (Artane)

  ▸ Antihistamines: diphenhydramine (Benadryl)

  ▸ Dopamine agonists: amantadine (Symmetrel)

  ▸ Alpha-adrenergic agonists: clonidine (Catapres) and guanfacine (Tenex)

  ▸ Beta-adrenergic antagonists: propranolol (Inderal)

  ▸ Benzodiazepines: clonazepam (Klonopin) and lorazepam (Ativan).

▶ *Tardive dyskinesia (TD):* This *irreversible* side effect can occur in 10% to 20% of the population on typical or conventional antipsychotic medications, especially for those on high-dose, high-potency medications. TD does not present until after a patient has been on the medication for at least 6 months. TD affects the muscles of the face, mouth, tongue (periorbital areas), fingers, and toes with a presentation of lip-smacking, grimacing, tongue movements, and writhing movements of the fingers and toes. Regular monitoring with the AIMS scale will aid early symptom detection and the dosing may be decreased or the patient may be switched to an atypical antipsychotic medication. The use of vitamin E has shown some benefits but is not a standard therapy.

Neuroleptic malignant syndrome (NMS): A rare, life-threatening complication that can occur anytime during treatment with neuroleptics. Motor and behavioral symptoms include muscular rigidity or dystonia, akinesia, mutism, obtundation (mental dullness as a result of a medical condition), and agitation. Autonomic symptoms include hyperpyrexia, sweating, and increased pulse and blood pressure. An order for the immediate discontinuation of the dopamine receptor antagonist drug is warranted with medical support to cool the patient, and vital signs, electrolytes, fluid balance, and renal output must be monitored. Symptomatic treatment of elevated body temperature is necessary to reverse this syndrome.

Because of these serious side effects, the typical neuroleptics are no longer considered first-line psychopharmaceutical treatment for psychosis and psychotic features. Additionally, the typical neuroleptics didn't seem to do much for reducing or eliminating negative symptoms (alogia, amotivation, poor judgment and insight) of psychosis. They have been supplanted by the advent of the atypical (newer or novel) antipsychotics, which are reputed to be efficacious for both positive and negative symptoms of psychosis and with reduced evidence of EPS. They are discussed in the next section.

ATYPICAL (NEWER OR NOVEL) ANTIPSYCHOTICS: SEROTONIN-DOPAMINE ANTAGONISTS (SDAS)

The atypical antipsychotic medications have now become the first-line treatments for psychotic disorders. The atypicals have two major distinctions from the older, conventional antipsychotic medications. The atypical medications are considered to have fewer extra pyramidal side effects and have shown better efficacy for reducing the negative symptoms of schizophrenia. There are 10 different atypical antipsychotics; efficacy of all 10 is similar but they have distinct side effect profiles. Some medications in this category are approved for Bipolar I and Bipolar II disorder. Some been approved for treatment of schizophrenia in children and adolescents and for use with autism spectrum disorders. Psychotic symptoms can improve within 1 week, but it may take several weeks for the full effect on behavior; therefore, full efficacy cannot be determined for 4 to 6 weeks.

Indications: Atypical antipsychotics show efficacy in the treatment of psychotic disorders, acute bipolar mania, maintenance phase and bipolar depression, severe agitation, behavioral disturbances, impulse control disorders, autistic behaviors, Tourette symptoms, dementia-related psychosis (see black box warning on package inserts), and as an adjunct in treatment-resistant depression.

Atypical Antipsychotics and Specific Nursing Considerations

Clozapine (Clozaril, Leponex): The first atypical antipsychotic medication. The usual dosage range is 300 to 450mg a day (may go as high as 900mg). It may reduce positive symptoms in patients who do not respond to other antipsychotics and may reduce tardive dyskinesia (TD). It is no longer considered a first-line treatment because of some of its life-threatening side effects such as agranulocytosis, dose-related increased risk for seizures, hyperglycemia with ketoacidosis, dyslipidemia, increased salivation, sweating, pulmonary embolism, myocarditis, and neuroleptic malignant syndrome (NMS). Patients receiving this medication must have white blood counts (WBC) monitored as well as weight, blood pressure, fasting plasma glucose, lipids, and ECG.

Risperidone (Risperdal): Adults 2 to 8mg a day; children and older adults 0.5 to 2mg a day; long-acting (Consta) 25 to 50mg depot IM every 2 weeks. Increased risk of EPS and hyperprolactinemia at dosages greater than 6mg a day.

Olanzapine (Zyprexa): Adults 10 to 20mg a day; not officially recommended for children, but used at 2.5 to 10mg a day; long-acting Zyprexa Relprevv is administered every 2 to 4 weeks. Risk of metabolic syndrome and significant weight gain.

Quetiapine (Seroquel): Adults 150 to 750mg a day; not officially recommended for children, but used at 25 to 500mg a day. Used as an adjuvant for treatment-resistant depression. Sedation and weight gain can be problematic. If patient stops medication for longer than one week, medication must be retitrated.

Ziprasidone (Geodon): Adults 40 to 200mg a day; not officially recommended for children. May have activating effects at low doses. Risk of QTc prolongation; need to monitor ECG. Weight gain is uncommon. Medication should be taken with 500-calorie meal.

Aripiprazole (Abilify): Adults 10 to 15mg twice a day; children 2 to 15mg a day; Abilify Maintena 200 to 400mg IM monthly depot injection. Used as an adjuvant for treatment-resistant depression. Risk of akathisia, agitation, insomnia, headache, and weight gain.

Paliperidone (Invega): Adults 6 to 12mg a day; safety and efficacy not established for children. Risk of akathisia and hyperprolactinemia. Extended-release product: paliperidone palmitate (Invega Sustenna), adult doses 234mg initially in deltoid muscle IM to 156mg 1 week later, then monthly maintenance of 117mg; maximum 12mg a day.

Asenapine (Saphris): Adults 5 to 10mg sublingual; safety and efficacy not established for children. Risk of somnolence, oral hypoesthesia, and possible anaphylactic reaction. Maximum 10mg twice a day.

Iloperidone (Fanapt): Adults 6 to 12mg twice a day; safety and efficacy not established for children. Risk of dizziness, somnolence, and orthostatic hypotension. Titrated to maximum of 12mg a day.

Lurasidone (Latuda): Adults 40 to 80mg a day; take with at least 350 calories; safety and efficacy not established for children. Risk of somnolence, akathisia, agitation, nausea, and pseudoparkinsonism. Maximum 80mg a day.

Regarding efficacy profiles, the evidence (Clinical Antipsychotic Trials of Intervention Effectiveness—CATIE Trial) supports that either the typical (conventional) or atypical medications will have similar results in controlling the positive symptoms of schizophrenia (National Institute of Mental Health, 2005).

High-potency antipsychotics can be used as depot (decanoate) injections. Decanoate formulations are administered intramuscularly (IM) and are useful when patients are noncompliant with oral preparations or prefer less frequent dosing. The available depot formulations are:

▶ Haloperidol (Haldol): every 4 weeks IM injection

▶ Fluphenazine (Prolixin): every 2 weeks IM injection

▶ Risperidone (Risperdal Consta): every 2 weeks IM injection

▶ Paliperidone palmitate (Invega Sustenna): every month IM injection

▶ Aripiprazole (Abilify Maintena): every month IM injection

Mechanism of action: Dopamine antagonism is not as robust at the D2 receptors; therefore, there is a much lower risk for EPS, negative symptoms, and hyperprolactinemia than seen with the typical antipsychotics.

Evaluation: Efficacy, Side Effects, and Adverse Effects of Atypical (Newer or Novel) Antipsychotics (Neuroleptics or Major Tranquilizers)

Untoward or Adverse Effects and Treatments

Metabolic syndrome: The most notable adverse effect is metabolic changes. Before starting atypical antipsychotics, baseline values of weight, waist circumference, BP, fasting plasma glucose, and fasting lipid profile must be obtained. Additionally, obtain personal and family history of obesity, dyslipidemia, hypertension, and cardiovascular disease. Consider that patients may be switched to another atypical antipsychotic if excessive weight gain occurs (overweight, obese), or if insulin resistance (prediabetes or diabetes), hypertension, or dyslipidemia develops. Implementations for dealing with the various metabolic changes include:

▶ Weight gain: Monitor weight and BMI, start exercise programs, and recommend dietary management.

▶ Hyperglycemia with ketoacidosis: Monitor fasting plasma glucose.

▶ Hyperlipidemia: Monitor cholesterol and lipid levels.

Agranulocytosis: With the use of clozapine, a patient can develop flu-like symptoms, sore throat, or signs of infection. Suspend treatment if white blood cell count (WBC) falls below 2,000/mm3. Patients receiving clozapine need their WBC monitored weekly, which may be reduced to biweekly after 6 months.

EPS: Although some EPS may be evident with the atypical antipsychotic medications, they present significantly less overall. Anticholinergics may be necessary to reduce motor symptoms. There is evidence that African-American men have higher rates of developing EPS than other group members.

Hypersomnia: This common side effect of the atypical antipsychotic medications is due to histaminic receptor blockage. If patient becomes highly sedated during the daytime, the nurse can recommend switching to night-time dosing.

Black box warning: Older adults with dementia-related psychosis should be administered atypical antipsychotics with caution because these create an increased risk of cardiovascular complications.

Some antipsychotics are approved for children and adolescents with psychoses or agitated and self-injurious behaviors that may accompany neurodevelopmental disorders, conduct disorder, and Tourette's syndrome. Expected benefits, side effects, and adverse effect profiles are similar to what may be seen among adults.

ANTIDEPRESSANTS: IMPLEMENTATIONS AND EVALUATIONS

Clinical depression is so common that it is referred to as the "common cold of mental illnesses." Antidepressants are the first line of treatment for depression as well as for pain and chronic anxiety disorders. All antidepressants are generally equally efficacious in treating symptoms of depression, so they are chosen based upon individual treatment response and side effect profiles. For example, more sedating antidepressants would be chosen for depressed persons with sleep disorders. Treatment with antidepressants may be an option for a patient with mild depression; however, they are highly recommended for patients with moderate to severe symptoms. For persons with psychotic symptoms, an antipsychotic could be added.

Treatment in the acute phase centers on establishing a therapeutic alliance, providing safety for the patient and the milieu, and promoting support and education. During the stabilization phase, antidepressant medication and psychotherapy are continued with a goal of preventing relapse of symptoms. This may take 16 to 20 weeks of consecutive medication therapy. Electroconvulsive therapy (ECT) may be added if the patient's depression is treatment-resistant. During the maintenance phase of medication treatment, the goal is to prevent recurrence of symptoms. Antidepressants may be tapered over several weeks if recurrence risk is low.

Because suicidal ideation commonly accompanies depressed states and mood instability, a high-priority role for the psychiatric–mental health nurse is to establish trust and rapport; determine suicide and homicide risk; identify patient's plan, means, lethality (remove lethal items), and if risk is high, recommend hospitalization and place on constant 1:1 monitoring. As part of hospitalization care, plan for psychopharmacology, discuss current crisis, develop an individualized crisis and safety plan, and identify supports and suicide hotline numbers. Psychoeducation is given to patient, family, and friends. Antidepressant medications are effective.

Indications: Antidepressant medications are recommended in the treatment of major depressive disorders to reduce or alleviate symptoms. Patients with a mood-congruent depression with psychosis, and with no personal or family history of a bipolar disorder, may benefit from an antidepressant along with administration of an antipsychotic agent. Antidepressants are also useful to treat chronic generalized anxiety disorder (GAD), obsessive compulsive disorder (OCD), panic disorder, social anxiety disorder, posttraumatic stress disorder (PTSD), eating disorders, and depressive symptoms that present in many of the personality disorders.

Mechanisms of action: Deficits in the monoamine system (serotonin, norepinephrine, dopamine) result in symptoms of depression. The evidence supporting this hypothesis is that all antidepressants increase one or more of the monoamines with resultant reduction or elimination of symptoms. Evidence suggests that medication in combination with brief psychotherapy, such as cognitive behavioral therapy or interpersonal therapy, produces quicker results. Medication alone is not adequate treatment for children and adolescents. The patient (and family and significant others) should be taught that antidepressant medications can take 3 to 6 weeks for some of the depression symptoms to improve. When depression symptoms begin to lift, patients are at increased risk for having the energy to act impulsively on suicidal ideation.

Potency in select population groups: Studies on children and adolescents regarding antidepressant use have been limited, although children may not respond to tricyclic antidepressants (TCAs). Fluoxetine (Prozac) is the most studied medication in this population, which studies have shown responds best to and has fewer adverse effects from the selective serotonin reuptake inhibitors (SSRIs). However, the Food and Drug Administration (FDA) warns of a 2% to 3% greater risk of suicidal thought in children taking antidepressants (see the black box warning on package inserts) but reports that the risk is ameliorated if the medication is given in combination with cognitive behavioral therapy.

Concerns with older adults exist. The standard edict to "start low and go slow" should be considered. Women are especially concerning during pregnancy, the postpartum period, and postmenopausal period. Because most malformations and teratogenic effects occur during the 3rd to 8th week of embryonic gestation, the risk-versus-benefits ratio must be carefully weighed. If a woman has experienced depression, or develops postpartum depression, this is another high-risk time for both mother and infant. Without antidepressants, a mother may relapse during or after pregnancy and negatively affect maternal-infant bonding and attachment.

> **BOX 5-2.**
> **ANTIDEPRESSANT CLASSIFICATIONS**
>
> ▸ Tricyclic antidepressants (TCAs)
> ▸ Monoamine oxidase inhibitors (MAOIs)
> ▸ Selective serotonin reuptake inhibitors (SSRIs)
> ▸ Dual serotonin and norepinephrine reuptake inhibitors (SNRIs)
> ▸ Norepinephrine dopamine reuptake inhibitors (NDRIs)
> ▸ Serotonin 2 antagonist/reuptake inhibitors (SARIs)
> ▸ Alpha 2 antagonist/noradenaline and specific serotonergic agents (NaSSAs)

Untreated postpartum depression may be a factor in infanticide. During the postmenopausal period, women on estrogen replacement therapy may be effectively treated with antidepressants. Knowledge of all medications that the patient is taking is paramount, because there are many drug-drug interactions with the SSRIs and increased risk of cardiac complications with the tricyclic antidepressants (TCAs; Box 5–2).

Tricyclic Antidepressants (TCAs)

This category of antidepressants has a strong history of efficacy for the treatment of depression. However, TCAs are used less frequently because of their high toxicity in overdoses (fatality potential). They block the reuptake (reabsorption) of both serotonin and norepinephrine but also block acetylcholine, histamine, alpha-adrenergic, and sodium channels, thus causing multiple expected side effects. Before any treatment with TCAs, the patient must obtain a baseline ECG, liver function tests, complete blood cell count, and thyroid function studies, which must be repeated annually as long as the patient continues on TCAs.

Indications: Depression, anxiety disorders, obsessive-compulsive disorder (clomipramine [Anafranil]), chronic pain (e.g., neurogenic pain, trigeminal neuralgia, diabetic neuropathy, sciatica, fibromyalgia), sleep disorders, insomnia, and cataplexy.

Tricyclic Antidepressants and Specific Nursing Considerations

▸ **Imipramine (Tofranil):** 150 to 300mg; effective for treatment of both depression and panic disorders; sometimes used in children for ADHD treatment or enuresis

▸ **Desipramine (Norpramin; Pertofrane):** 150 to 300mg; fewer anticholinergic and antihistaminic adverse effects than other TCAs

▸ **Trimipramine (Surmontil):** 150 to 300mg; strong anticholinergic effects

▸ **Amitriptyline (Elavil, Endep, Tryptizol, Laroxyl):** 150 to 300mg; strong efficacy in management of pain

▶ **Nortriptyline (Pamelor; Aventyl):** 5 to 150mg; useful in treatment of migraine headaches

▶ **Protriptyline (Vivactil):** 15 to 60mg

▶ **Amoxapine (Asendin):** 150 to 400mg

▶ **Doxepin (Adapin; Sinequan):** 150 to 300mg

▶ **Maprotiline (Ludiomil):** I 150 to 230mg

▶ **Clomipramine (Anafranil):** 130 to 250mg (adults), 50 to 200mg (children and adolescents); useful for treating OCD in children and adults

Mechanism of action: Tricyclics block the reuptake of serotonin, norepinephrine, or both, increasing their availability for neurotransmission. These are desired actions of the drugs. Unfortunately, they also block many other receptors (ACh, histamine, alpha-adrenergic, and sodium channels), causing numerous unwanted side effects.

Evaluation: Efficacy, Side Effects, and Adverse Effects

▶ **Expected benefits (clinical response):** Improvements in energy and sleep may occur within the first 1 to 2 weeks; full effects may take 3 to 4 weeks.

▶ **Expected side effects:** Blockade of ACh receptors results in anticholinergic symptoms. Blockade of histamine receptors results in sedation and weight gain. Blockage of alpha-adrenergic receptors causes orthostatic hypotension and dizziness. Blockade of sodium channels can result in cardiac arrhythmias with possible cardiac arrest and resultant death, as well as CNS symptoms, vertigo, and possible seizures.

Untoward or Adverse Effects: Special Considerations

▶ TCAs are contraindicated for older adults because of the potential cardiac effects.

▶ TCAs are relatively contraindicated in older adults, children, pregnant women, and suicidal persons because of the potential for severe side effects and even death. Prescribers may consider providing smaller amounts to decrease or prevent suicidal overdosing.

Monoamine Oxidase Inhibitors (MAOIs)

Indications: MAOIs show significant efficacy in the treatment of depression with anxiety or phobic symptoms. They came on the market after the TCAs because of the high fatality rates associated with the TCA type of antidepressants.

Mechanisms of action: Inhibiting the MAO enzyme from metabolizing (or breaking down) the monamines (serotonin, norepinephrine and dopamine) and, thereby, allowing for more availability of these monoamines in the synapses when depolarization happens.

TABLE 5-1.
MONOAMINE OXIDASE INHIBITORS (MAOIS) AND USUAL DOSES

GENERIC	TRADE	DOSE
Phenelzine	Nardil	30–60mg
Tranylcypromine	Parnate	20–60mg
Isocarboxazid	Marplan	10–40mg
Selegiline*	Zelapar, Eldepryl, Emsam	6–12mg

*Long-acting topical patch; no dietary restrictions due to bypassing GI system

Evaluation: Efficacy, Side Effects, and Adverse Effects

Expected side effects: The most frequent side effects are orthostatic hypotension, insomnia, weight gain, edema, sexual dysfunction, and potential for severe drug-drug interactions. They may require 3 to 6 weeks before efficacy is noted.

Untoward or adverse effects: There is a risk of tyramine-induced hypertensive crisis (rare). Symptoms of hypertensive crisis include sudden elevation of blood pressure, severe occipital headache, tachycardia, sweating, fever, and vomiting. Patients are advised to be on a low-tyramine diet. Foods to be avoided (because they contain high levels of tyramine) are preserved or aged foods (e.g., pickled beets, aged cheese, cured or smoked meats or fish, red wine, alcoholic beverages). Patients also need to avoid over-the-counter decongestants, St. John's wort, and all herbal weight-loss products because these drugs and others that have sympathomimetic properties increase the patient's risk for a hypertensive crisis. Anticholinergic side effects can also appear. Because of these dietary restrictions, the MAOIs were supplanted with the selective serotonin reuptake inhibitors discussed below.

Selective Serotonin Reuptake Inhibitors (SSRIs)

The SSRIs have a broad range of clinical indications: major depression, obsessive-compulsive disorder (OCD), panic disorder, social anxiety, posttraumatic stress disorder (PTSD), eating disorders, and borderline personality disorder.

Indications: If treating depression, it can take 3 to 6 weeks to see efficacy. If treating OCD, it can take at least 12 to 16 weeks for a decrease in obsessional thoughts or compulsive behaviors. When the patient starts treatment, educate on the need to be aware of the activation of an undiagnosed bipolar disorder or a presence or increase of suicidal ideation. For children and adolescents, this risk factor must be emphasized with parents or guardians. Children and adolescents respond well to SSRIs and these are considered first-line treatments. However, the FDA warns of a 2%

to 3% greater risk of suicidal behavior in children taking antidepressants, thought to be because of the delay between early energizing effects of the drugs and improvement in depressed mood. Adolescents can be titrated to adult dosing but will start with lower doses than adults. Children will start and maintain lower doses. It can be helpful for a child to use a liquid form so they can be titrated by drops. Commonly prescribed SSRIs include:

▶ **Fluoxetine (Prozac, Sarafem):** 20 to 80mg a day for depression and anxiety disorders; 60 to 80mg a day for bulimia; Prozac weekly: 90mg

▶ **Fluvoxamine (Luvox):** 100 to 300mg a day for OCD; 100 to 200mg a day for depression

▶ **Paroxetine (Paxil):** 20 to 50mg a day

▶ **Sertraline (Zoloft):** 50 to 200mg a day

▶ **Citalopram (Celexa):** 20 to 60mg a day

▶ **Escitalopram (Lexapro):** 10 to 20mg a day

▶ **Vilazodone (Viibryd):** 10 to 40mg a day

Evaluation: Efficacy, Side Effects, and Adverse Effects

Expected side effects: Anxiety, agitation, akathisia, insomnia, nausea, diarrhea, and sexual dysfunction are common side effects of SSRIs. The nurse needs to discuss these potential side effects with patients and reassure them that many of these are transient and will resolve. It is also necessary to discuss the potential for sexual dysfunction, because this is a frequent reason for nonadherence. Sometimes adding bupropion (Wellbutrin, Zyban) to the SSRI is helpful for sexual dysfunction; if it is not, switching to another medication is necessary.

Untoward or Adverse Effects

Serotonin syndrome results from excess serotonin in the brain. Signs of serotonin syndrome include diarrhea, restlessness, extreme agitation, hyperreflexia and autonomic instability, myoclonus, seizures, hyperthermia, rigidity, delirium, coma, and possible death. Serotonin syndrome causes "HARM" (hyperthermia, autonomic instability, rigidity, myoclonus).

Serotonin discontinuation syndrome is caused by a rapid or sudden discontinuation of a serotonin medication. Educate patients to not suddenly stop a medication, but to work with the provider to taper off it gradually. Adverse effects of rapid discontinuation include agitation, nausea, disequilibrium, and dysphoria. SSRIs need to be tapered to discontinuation to avoid these symptoms.

Serotonin 2 Antagonist/Reuptake Inhibitor (SARI)

▶ **Trazodone (Desyrel):** 150 to 600mg a day; there is also a once-daily sustained release product (Oleptro). Trazodone is generally used in lower doses for treatment of insomnia because one of its properties is sedation. It should be used cautiously in children and adolescents. Men must be advised of the risk for priapism and generally patients should be aware of the risk for orthostatic hypotension.

▶ **Nefazodone (Serzone):** 300 to 600mg a day. The risk for hepatotoxicity is a major concern so this is not a first-line medication choice.

Dual Serotonin and Norepinephrine Reuptake Inhibitors (SNRIs)

Mechanisms of action: These antidepressants increase the availability of both serotonin and norepinephrine by inhibiting the reuptake of both. They are frequently used in patients with pain and fatigue as part of the depressive symptoms.

▶ **Venlafaxine (Effexor):** 75 to 225mg a day. There is some risk for hypertension so BP should be monitored. It is indicated in treatment of depression and concomitant anxiety; it is occasionally used to treat children with ADHD.

▶ **Desvenlafaxine (Pristiq):** Adults 50 to 100mg a day; safety and efficacy not established in children. It is an active metabolite of venlafaxine, indicated in treatment of major depressive disorder.

▶ **Duloxetine (Cymbalta):** 40 to 60mg a day. It has shown positive results in patients with neuropathic pain.

Alpha 2 Antagonist/Noradrenaline and Specific Serotonergic Agent (NaSSA)

Mirtazapine (Remeron) makes serotonin and norepinephrine more available. Dosing is 15 to 45mg at bedtime. It is indicated for patients whose depression presents with insomnia and anxiety. The nurse must advise patients of its highly sedating effects and subsequent risk for falls. It can cause significant weight gain, but has fewer sexual side effects than other medications with serotonin.

Norepinephrine Dopamine Reuptake Inhibitors (NDRIs)

Bupropion (Wellbutrin) is dosed at 225 to 450mg a day with slow titration. It is available in SR (slow release) and XL (extended release) forms. Wellbutrin inhibits reuptake of both dopamine and norepinephrine and is used in the treatment of depression and as an augmenting agent with other antidepressants. It has been used with children in the treatment of ADHD and has shown efficacy as a smoking cessation agent (Zyban). Bupropion (Zyban) is avoided as a nicotine replacement therapy in patients younger than age 18, and as with all antidepressant therapy, the psychiatric–mental health nurse observes and monitors for worsening or emergence of neuropsychiatric reactions that may result from use of bupropion (Zyban) as a smoking cessation aid. Evidence shows that, when used with patients with bipolar II disorder, there is less risk of becoming manic than with other antidepressants. Wellbutrin does not cause any sexual side effects and also seems to reduce sexual side effects when used with an SSRI. An adverse effect is that it can lower the seizure threshold in persons with a history of a seizure disorder or bulimia.

ANTIMANICS AND MOOD STABILIZERS: IMPLEMENTATIONS AND EVALUATIONS

Lithium

Lithium is a well-absorbed salt that is not bound to protein and is excreted by the proximal tubules of the kidneys. Once in the circulation, peak levels occur in 2 to 4 hours. Acute bipolar episodes are generally treated with lithium or valproate, or an atypical antipsychotic. If symptoms are inadequately managed after 10 to 14 days, another first-line medication may be added. The initial goals are to manage any unsafe behavior; decrease symptoms of agitation, irritability, and impulsivity; and return the person to usual levels of psychosocial functioning. Theoretical mechanisms explain concepts of sensitization and rekindling. The theory supposes that with recurring stressors and episodes of bipolar exacerbation, a person becomes predisposed to increased vulnerability for future recurrences that may last longer than previous episodes. The kindling idea hypothesizes that with repeated and intermittent subthreshold stimulation of a given region of the brain, a full-blown amygdala seizure ensues, resulting in the expressive affective instability so characteristic of bipolar disorders. Once stability is achieved with medications, the goal for maintenance is recovery with prevention of relapse and recurrence.

Because of the nature of the illness and the side effects of the medications, it is especially important to obtain usual baseline patient information, with particular focus on the functioning of the kidneys because of lithium metabolite excretion by way of the urinary system, and to determine the most effective drug with the fewest side effects for each patient. Damage to the thyroid and kidneys occur from lithium use over decades. Before initiating therapy, baseline renal function (including BUN and creatinine clearance) and liver function should be assessed, and then reassessed every 6 months. The nurse should assess for family history of kidney disease, diabetes, and hypertension and obtain baseline ECG, electrolyte, and thyroid levels. Pregnancy should be ruled out before lithium therapy initiation because of potential teratogenic effects. Patients need to be taught to avoid NSAIDs (nonsteroidal anti-inflammatory drugs) because of reduced renal clearance (Carlat Psychiatry Report, 2013) because increased thirst and polyuria can develop when taking lithium, sodium levels should be monitored; the patient should avoid excessive salt intake. Also, the potential for negative outcomes from known drug-drug interactions should be avoided. NSAIDs, hydrochlorothiazide, and ACE inhibitors can cause lithium levels to be high, whereas caffeine increases the glomerular filtration rate (GFR), resulting in increased urination and lowered lithium levels.

Indications: Acute mania and mood stabilization

Mechanism of action: Lithium's mechanism of action is not well understood. Clinical response in acute mania may take 7 to 14 days. The usual adult dosage is 900 to 1,800mg a day in divided doses. Lithium has a long half-life, yet narrow therapeutic window. This contributes to a risk for lithium toxicity (levels above 2.0mEq/L). The narrow therapeutic index requires frequent physical exams and labs. Serum blood levels for an acute episode are 0.8 to 1.4mEq/L for acute episodes and 0.4 to 1.0mEq/L for maintenance level.

Lithium toxicity: The psychiatric–mental health nurse is responsible for being alert to signs of lithium toxicity. Lithium toxicity is a medical emergency. Arrhythmias, coma, seizures, vascular collapse, hypotension, and stupor may result with lithium levels over 3.0mEq/L. If it occurs, discontinue lithium immediately. Obtain lithium blood level, electrolytes, BUN, creatinine, urinalysis, CBC, and electrocardiograph. Rehydration, emesis, lavage, dialysis, or a combination of these may be required.

Evaluation: Efficacy, Side Effects, and Adverse Effects

Expected side effects: Thirst, nausea, increased urination, fine hand tremor, and gastrointestinal (GI) upset are common side effects. Teach patients to avoid dehydration and excessive salt or fluid intake. Administration of propranolol (Inderal) and reduced caffeine intake may reduce tremor. Take with meals to reduce GI upset. Avoid NSAIDs because of decreased renal clearance. Other potentially distressing side effects include hair loss, acne, sedation, decreased cognition, and lack of coordination.

Untoward or adverse effects: Lithium toxicity is prevented by keeping the lithium blood level within the narrow therapeutic window. Polypharmacy with lithium and other mood stabilizers keeps the dosage of lithium lower and reduces the risk for toxicity. Instruct patients to avoid dehydration or excessive salt intake. Patients on lithium need to be educated to seek medical attention at first signs of diarrhea, nausea, vomiting, drowsiness, tremor, muscle weakness, or nystagmus. Signs of early toxicity include tremors; later signs include fever, decreased urine output, decreased blood pressure, irregular pulse, ECG changes, and impaired consciousness. This is considered a medical emergency; hold the next dose of lithium, plan to obtain labs, and support physiology (i.e., fluids, by mouth or intravenously). Long-term risk for metabolic abnormalities requires monitoring BMI, fasting triglycerides, and other factors (see metabolic syndrome related to atypical antipsychotic use).

ANTICONVULSANTS AND MOOD STABILIZATION: IMPLEMENTATIONS AND EVALUATIONS

The anticonvulsant medication category is a safer alternative to lithium therapy for mood stabilization. Therapeutic effects begin after days; mood stabilization may take weeks to months. They should never be discontinued abruptly or rebound effects may result. Weight gain is of particular concern with these medications, as well as thrombocytopenia and agranulocytosis. Specific interventions include protecting the patient from self-harm or injury because of hyperactivity, protecting patient from harm from others, monitoring responses to medications, helping to restore nutritional status and adequate sleep or parasympathetic restoration, helping to improve interactions, confronting anger that may be turned inward or outward, and enhancing self-esteem and personal hygiene. Patient and family education can help the patient maintain stability post-hospitalization. Other concerns that are linked to particular medications are cited below.

Indications: For acute mania and mood stabilization

Mechanisms of action: Exact mechanisms are not yet known. However, it is believed that anticonvulsants reduce the flow of ions through ion channels, increases inhibitory (GABA), or decreases excitatory (glutamate) neurotransmission.

Evaluation: Efficacy, Side Effects, and Adverse Effects

Expected benefits (clinical response): Therapeutic effects on mania begin after days but mood stabilization may take weeks to months.

Expected Side Effects and Treatments

- ▶ **GI system:** Nausea, diarrhea, and weight gain. GI effects can be reduced by using the extended-release formulations. Monitor weight and BMI; diet and exercise (lamotrigine [Lamictal] and topiramate [Topamax] have lowest risk).

- ▶ **Hematopoietic system:** Increased risk for thrombocytopenia; monitor prothrombin time. Risk for agranulocytosis (especially with carbamazepine); monitor WBCs.

- ▶ **Neurological system:** Tremor; consider low-dose beta blocker.

- ▶ **Cardiovascular system:** Sedation

- ▶ **Endocrine system:** Hair loss

Untoward or adverse effects on thyroid and liver: Obtain baseline and regular measures of hepatic and hematological levels; bleeding abnormalities may occur from reduced thrombocytes (platelets) or from the development of other blood dyscrasias. Check for pregnancy at least every six months.

Anticonvulsant Mood Stabilizers And Specific Nursing Considerations

▶ **Valproic acid (Depakote):** 1,200 to 1,500mg a day. Available as once-daily dosing; extended-release formulations (Divalproex CR, Depakote ER) are useful for reducing risk of GI side effects, and possibly sedation and hair loss. Valproic acid is most commonly used for the acute manic phase and is less effective for maintenance and treatment of bipolar depression. Therapeutic serum level is 40 to 100 mcg/mL.

▶ **Carbamazepine (Tegretol):** 400 to 1,200mg a day. Second-line augmenting agent for acute mania; because of risk for agranulocytosis, monitor WBC every 2 weeks for 2 months, then once every 3 months. Therapeutic serum level is 4 to 12mg/L.

▶ **Gabapentin (Neurontin):** 900 to 1,800mg a day; well tolerated but questionably effective for treating mania; good anti-anxiety and pain control effects.

▶ **Lamotrigine (Lamictal):** 100 to 200mg a day; indicated for bipolar maintenance. Useful for bipolar depression. Risk of rare toxic necrolysis (called Stevens-Johnson syndrome [SJS])—a life-threatening skin condition in which cell death causes the epidermis to separate from the dermis; usually begins with fever, sore throat, and fatigue, which is misdiagnosed and usually treated with antibiotics. Ulcers and other lesions begin to appear in the mucous membranes, almost always in the mouth and lips, but also in the genital and anal regions. A rash of round lesions about an inch across arises on the face, trunk, arms, legs, and soles of the feet, but usually not the scalp. Children and adolescents have higher incidence than adults of developing this life-threatening rash. Start very low and go slow.

▶ **Topiramate (Topamax):** 50 to 300mg a day; may be a useful adjunct in bipolar disorder. Not considered a first-line treatment. May cause weight loss.

COMBINATION BIOLOGICAL THERAPIES FOR MOOD STABILIZATION

Antipsychotics such as olanzapine (Zyprexa), quetiapine (Seroquel), and risperidone (Risperdal) have been approved for treatment of acute mania. Olanzapine (Zyprexa) and aripiprazole (Abilify) are FDA-approved for bipolar maintenance. Symbyax, a combination of olanzapine (Zyprexa) and fluoxetine (Prozac), is FDA-approved for bipolar depression.

ANTIANXIETY, ANXIOLYTICS: IMPLEMENTATIONS AND EVALUATIONS

Benzodiazepines

Because medications in this category are often prescribed in inpatient settings on an "as-needed" basis, the psychiatric–mental health nurse exercises critical thinking and clinical judgment before administering. "As-needed" benzodiazepines are administered by the nurse with the understanding of clinical indications for this medication. They are not given for the purpose of quelling annoyance of the nurse. Benzodiazepines potentiate the effects of gamma-amino-butyric acid (GABA) in the brain to exert its calming effects. The antianxiety effects are achieved in 30 to 60 minutes if taken by mouth.

Patient and family education are warranted to teach the nature and symptoms of the anxiety state, as well as strategies to manage the experience. Important strategies are learning skills associated with stress management, such as relaxation, cognitive and behavioral coping skills, individual counseling, group therapy, and systematic desensitization.

Psychopharmacology helps ameliorate symptoms so the patient can engage in adjunctive supports. Psychiatric nurses can use these medications to calm an acutely agitated, restless, or anxious patient, or can introduce an integrative or complementary approach for symptom management. Several of these alternative approaches, such as guided imagery, yoga, and exercise will be discussed later.

Indications: Used to treat anxiety symptoms and some anxiety disorders. Other indications include insomnia, seizures, muscle spasticity, alcohol withdrawal, and induction of anesthesia. Treatment recommendations say to use the lowest possible effective dose for the shortest possible period of time; avoid the desire to increase dose because needing a higher dosage is a sign of developing tolerance. As a general approach with children and adolescents, begin with a broad-spectrum agent such as an SSRI. Benzodiazepines can be used for acute anxiety and agitation. If ADHD symptoms are present, adjunctive use of a stimulant or bupropion should be considered and alpha-agonists such as clonidine (Catapres) and guanfacine (Tenex; Intuniv) should be considered if insomnia, hyperstartle, or hyperarousal symptoms are problematic.

Mechanism of action: Potentiation of the effect of GABA, inhibiting neurotransmission in the limbic system and cortex. All benzodiazepines have essentially equivalent pharmacologic actions. Selection is based on time course (onset and duration of effect). Onset of anxiolytic effects by route of administration are:

- ▸ PO: 30 to 60 min.
- ▸ IM: 15 to 30 min.
- ▸ IV: 1 to 5 min.

IM and IV preparations are available for lorazepam (Ativan), chlordiazepoxide (Librium), diazepam (Valium), and midazolam (Versed) used for preoperative sedation and amnesia. Faster onset is indicated for episodic burst of anxiety, need to fall asleep rapidly, and alcohol withdrawal. Onset of action is fastest for diazepam (Valium), lorazepam (Ativan), alprazolam (Xanax), triazolam (Halcion), and estazolam (ProSom).

Duration of action is a function of the half-life of the drug.

- ▶ Advantages of longer half-lives include less frequent dosing, less variation in plasma concentration, and less severe withdrawal.

- ▶ Advantages of shorter half-lives include no drug accumulation and less daytime sedation.

- ▶ Disadvantages of longer half-lives include drug accumulation, daytime sedation, and daytime psychomotor impairment.

- ▶ Disadvantages of shorter half-lives include more frequent dosing, earlier and more severe withdrawal syndromes, and rebound insomnia.

Long-acting benzodiazepines treat more chronic anxiety disorders, seizures, and alcohol and benzodiazepine withdrawal.

- ▶ Clonazepam (Klonopin): 18 to 50 hrs.
- ▶ Diazepam (Valium): 20 to 80 hrs.

Intermediate-acting benzodiazepines commonly treat more acute anxiety symptoms.

- ▶ Alprazolam (Xanax): 6 to 27 hrs.
- ▶ Lorazepam (Ativan): 10 to 20 hrs.

Short-acting benzodiazepines treat sleep onset insomnia, and may be used for preoperative anesthesia.

- ▶ Triazolam (Halcion): 1.5 to 3 hrs.

The "LOT" Benzodiazepines are considered safe in the patient with liver failure: **L**orazepam (Ativan), **O**xazepam (Serax), and **T**emazepam (Restoril).

Evaluation: Efficacy, Side Effects, and Adverse Effects

Expected side effects: Drowsiness, fatigue, depression, dizziness, ataxia, slurred speech, weakness, and forgetfulness are commonly seen. Teach patients to avoid driving or operating potentially dangerous machines; stand slowly to reduce dizziness. Patients may be able to adjust the time of the dosage to reduce daytime symptoms. Because of the risk of psychological and physical dependence, long-term use should be carefully monitored and the drugs should be tapered at discontinuation. Instruct patients not to increase the dosage of the drug unless ordered.

Generally, it takes approximately 12 to 18 weeks to initiate and stabilize anxiety states. Discontinuation syndromes depend on the length of time on drug, dosage taken, rate of taper, and half-life. The higher the dose and the shorter the half-life, the more severe the withdrawal symptoms. Withdrawal symptoms include anxiety, nervousness, diaphoresis, restlessness, irritability, fatigue, light-headedness, tremor, insomnia, weakness, risk for seizures and death. Benzodiazepines are cross-tolerant with alcohol, so the withdrawal is similar and very dangerous.

OTHER ANXIOLYTICS

Serotonin partial agonists such as buspirone (BuSpar) are alternative anxiolytics. Buspirone, given in 20 to 30mg a day doses, has no risk for physiological dependence. The therapeutic effects may take up to 4 weeks, limiting its use for severe acute anxiety. Beta blockers such as propranolol (Inderal) can be useful for reducing peripheral symptoms of anxiety and tremor. These are sometimes used by performers to reduce tremors and by persons with social anxiety to reduce peripheral symptoms. Propranolol can be used for non-anxiety–related tremors such as those resulting from the use of lithium.

PSYCHOSTIMULANTS AND NONPSYCHOSTIMULANTS: IMPLEMENTATIONS AND EVALUATIONS

Psychostimulants and nonpsychostimulants have utility in the management of attention-deficit hyperactivity disorder and narcolepsy, a sleep disorder. Before initiating stimulant and nonstimulant therapies, the nurse monitors the baseline ECG, BP, weight and height, serum analyses (CBC, platelets), and liver function. With children and adolescents, diagnoses can be atypical, constantly change, and be comorbid with other psychiatric disorders. The nurse needs to be aware of psychosocial aspects related to drug taking; some may feel sensitive and not want to be seen as "sick," whereas others may glorify the use of medications, especially some of the psychostimulants, which have high misuse and abuse potential. Because children have greater hepatic capacity, more glomerular filtration, and less fatty tissue, they likely have a lowered ability to store medications in fat, resulting in quicker elimination and shorter half-lives.

The stimulants are considered first-line treatments for ADHD. First-line stimulants make more dopamine (in the nigrostriatal and mesocortical pathways) or norepinephrine (in the prefrontal pathway), or both, available. The dose release is tailored to individual needs and response. Of the methylphenidate drugs, the immediate-release compounds last 2 to 4 hours (Ritalin, Focalin, Methylin, Dexedrine); the older sustained-release formulations last approximately 4 to 6 hours (Ritalin SR, Methylin ER, and Metadate ER), and the newer sustained-release formulations offer 8 to 12 hours of benefit (Metadate CD, Concerta, Focalin XR, Ritalin LA) and can be taken once daily. Second-line nonstimulant medications, such as atomoxetine (Strattera), a norepinephrine reuptake inhibitor (SNRI), and antihypertensives clonidine (Catapres) or guanfacine (Tenex; Intuniv) are considered third-line nonstimulant treatments. Second-line antidepressants are used to make more 5HT, DA, and NE available. Side effects may include sedation, headaches, depression, and potentially rebound hypertension. Blood pressure needs to be monitored by the nurse.

Indications: Inattentiveness, impulsivity, and motor hyperactivity

Mechanisms of action: Two pathways (norepinephrine prefrontal, and the dopaminergic nigrostriatal and mesocortical pathways) mediate attention, arousal, concentration, and other related cognitive functions. If they fail, inattentiveness and attention deficit may result. Motor hyperactivity and impulsivity are mediated by dopamine activity in the nigrostriatal pathway. In persons without ADHD, increasing dopamine in the nigrostriatal pathway with stimulants increases motor behavior and impulsivity, whereas patients with ADHD exhibit what may be a paradoxical reduction. Attention deficit disorder (ADD) and attention-deficit hyperactivity disorder (ADHD) are treated by increasing the levels of norepinephrine, dopamine, or both with psychostimulants.

Evaluation: Efficacy, Side Effects, and Adverse Effects

Expected side effects: The most common side effects include headaches, stomachaches, nausea, and insomnia. Psychostimulants may suppress normal growth so the nurse should monitor weight and height. So-called "drug holidays" may be initiated during summer months to allow catch-up from growth suppression. Advise to avoid taking stimulants in the late afternoon because of potential effects of impairing sleep states. Tolerance, dependence, or abuse may develop over time. Periodic monitoring of blood pressure, pulse, CBC, platelets, and liver function is recommended.

COGNITIVE ENHANCERS: IMPLEMENTATIONS AND EVALUATIONS

General considerations when initiating pharmaceuticals in older adults is to "start low and go slow;" use psychopharmaceuticals (all pharmaceuticals for that matter) with care. The nurse is alert to the potential for greater sensitivity to medication side effects and the effect of general medical conditions. Co-occurring medical problems with additional medications increase potential drug interactions. Medications are metabolized more slowly; therefore, lower doses may be beneficial. Lean body mass decreases, body fat increases, and lipid-soluble drugs are distributed more widely in fat tissue, so drug action may be prolonged. GI disease and decreased gastric acid secretion may slow absorption.

The initiation of medication for enhancing cognitive functioning is based on severity of symptoms. Treat psychosis and agitation pharmacologically when such behavior is dangerous or upsetting; treat co-occurring depression. There is some evidence for adding vitamin E 2000 IU a day (some evidence of increased risk of prostate cancer with use), and the Smith (2013) is conducting a clinical trial to evaluate the efficacy of coconut oil as a treatment for dementia. Alzheimer's dementia is progressive, so needs must continually be reassessed.

The main safety strategy in older adults is to prevent falls by reducing or eliminating hazards: have protective flooring installed, eliminate restraints and restraint hazards, increase staffing, place on close observation, and monitor vital signs and orthostatic blood pressure any time a medication is changed or added. Increased attention should be provided if the patient is on diuretics, a smoker, confused, or disoriented. Environmental safeguards, such as video monitoring and bed alarms, should be enlisted and safety hazards removed.

The nurse will address basic biological needs, such as adequate nutrition and hydration, and assists with hygiene, bathing, and activities of daily living (ADLs). Provide reality orientation, structure and consistency, and decrease stimulation. Offer opportunities to participate and make choices when possible. The nurse will communicate clearly and in simplistic form, keeping in mind memory problems, and explain procedures, help with reality testing, reorient, and decrease stimulation.

The nurse will monitor behavioral changes and mental symptoms and supervise medications, administering neuroleptic medications if the patient is psychotic. Restraints are used only if necessary for safety, and as a last resort. Dependency is a source of increased anxiety and stress, and hospitalization itself may be confusing and disorienting. One of the most important roles is to help caregivers cope with the strain of caring for a loved one with dementia and provide help with care planning, education, and grief or loss.

When communicating with a patient who has communication or language deficits, the nurse will identify barriers to compliance (e.g., hearing, visual, cognitive, or developmental deficits). Perhaps corrective lenses or hearing aids are needed. The nurse will use the same sequence and repeat phrases; speak slowly and clearly; use simple sentences. In addition, it is important to encourage the interaction by listening, smiling, using pictures and gestures; allow time for translation and processing; help the patient develop realistic, culturally relevant goals, and incorporate culturally specific teaching formats.

Older adults may have increased susceptibility to adverse effects (especially cardiac, GI, and mental status effects), and may have co-occurring cardiovascular disease (CVD); reduced cardiac output can affect renal and hepatic drug clearance. CVD risk increases cognitive enhancers are used with drugs that already affect the heart (e.g., tricyclic antidepressants). This fact places older adults at increased risk of orthostatic hypotension and falls as well as anticholinergic toxicity due to lower cholinergic output.

Indications: Cognitive enhancers are prescribed to slow the decline of cognitive function; they are not curative. Early in the course of the illness, acetylcholine (Ach) inhibitors are thought to enhance memory by slowing down the destruction of ACh. Tacrine (Cognex), donepezil (Aricept), rivastigmine (Exelon), and galantamine (Razadyne) are generally prescribed in mild to moderate levels of dementia. They are considered cholinesterase inhibitors that work by decreasing the destruction of acetylcholine, thereby improving acetylcholine levels in the synapse with resulting improvements in learning and memory abilities. The cholinesterase inhibitors also work to reduce behavioral symptoms, such as anxiety, depression, hallucinations, and agitation.

- **Donepezil (Aricept):** 5 to 10mg a day at night with slow titration

- **Rivastigmine (Exelon):** 12mg patch a day

- **Galantamine** (Razadyne; Razadyne ER): 4 to 24mg a day

- **Memantine (Namenda)** 10mg twice a day for severe dementia. It is a glutamate antagonist (N-methyl-D-aspartic = NMDA) that appears to have its therapeutic effect by blocking excessive glutamate (which may trigger an excitotoxic process leading to neurodegeneration) at one of the glutamate receptors (the NMDA receptor) and stabilizing neurodegenerative processes. It is therefore considered neuro-protective and helps slow the progression of AD when used in combination with one of the cholinesterase inhibitors. Memantine (Namenda) is well-tolerated with few side effects or drug interactions.

Side effects of the ACh inhibitors include nausea, diarrhea, vomiting, appetite loss, and increased gastric acid secretion.

MEDICATIONS, IMPLEMENTATIONS, AND EVALUATIONS TO TREAT AGGRESSIVE BEHAVIORS

Medications from all the classes of psychopharmacological agents are used to treat aggressive behaviors. Initially it is important to try to determine the cause of the aggression and attempt nonpharmacological interventions. If aggression continues and presents a risk to the patient or others, treatments are individualized and can involve the use of antipsychotics, anticonvulsants, antidepressants, lithium, benzodiazepines, or antihypertensive agents. Specific techniques when dealing with aggression in the milieu include:

- Maintain safety: Observe for escalation.

- Remain calm: Defuse with least restrictive means.

- De-escalation techniques and communication strategies

  - Speak in a calm, low voice. Use "I" language, don't take patient behavior personally, and avoid intense eye contact.

  - Respect patient's need for personal space.

  - Acknowledge patient's feelings; reassure that staff are there to help.

  - Clearly communicate patient behavior and expected behavior. Ask "What do you need?" Focus on disruptive behavior, not "bad patient."

- Environmental strategies

  - Structure the milieu with opportunities for less stimulation.

  - Offer opportunity for time out.

  - Always use least restrictive interventions.

  - Seclusion and restraints as a last resort.

MEDICATIONS, IMPLEMENTATIONS, AND EVALUATIONS TO PROMOTE SLEEP

Before resorting to sedative-hypnotics or benzodiazepines to facilitate parasympathetic restoration, the nurse will assist the patient with simple strategies that promote sleep hygiene: Remove or treat underlying causes. Assessment may include polysomnography.

- Rise at same time each day; avoid daytime napping.

- Maintain comfortable sleeping conditions; spend no longer than 20 minutes awake in bed; adjust sleep hours and routine to optimize daily schedule and living situation.

- Engage in calming activities at night (e.g., bath, relaxation).

- ▸ Avoid evening stimulation (e.g., TV); establish physical fitness habits earlier in day.

- ▸ Eat on regular schedule; light at night.

- ▸ Discontinue use of drugs that act on CNS.

Sedative-hypnotics or benzodiazepines may be used for short periods (less than 7 to 10 days up to 2 months) to promote sleep and may be continued 2 to 3 nights per week for refractory insomnia. A major concern is that they have physical and psychological dependence potential. Several benzodiazepine types are listed below:

- ▸ **Zolpidem tartrate (Intermezzo [sublingual], Ambien):** 5 to 10mg at bedtime

- ▸ **Triazolam (Halcion):** 0.125 to 0.25mg at bedtime

- ▸ **Temazepam (Restoril):** 15 to 30mg at bedtime

- ▸ **Eszopiclone (Lunesta):** 1 to 3mg at bedtime

MEDICATION TREATMENTS FOR SUBSTANCE USE DISORDERS: IMPLEMENTATIONS AND EVALUATIONS

Hospital detoxification is initially recommended, especially for alcohol, benzodiazepine, and sedative-hypnotic withdrawal in a safe and supportive environment. With close monitoring and supervision, the nurse can monitor lab tests and vital signs, and document status on an evidence-based clinical measure, such as the CIWA, Ar, CINA, or COWS. Rehabilitation, peer support groups (AA, NA, Al-Anon, Alateen), relapse prevention strategies, and harm reduction strategies can be introduced to the patient while in a detoxification setting. Pharmacological support is tailored to the specific problem identified:

- ▸ **Buprenorphine (Subutex):** Semisynthetic opioid used to treat opioid dependence; ceiling effect reduces risk of overdose; is less likely to cause respiratory depression.

- ▸ **Buprenorphine and naloxone (Suboxone):** Semisynthetic opioid used to treat opioid dependence.

- ▸ **Naloxone (Narcan):** Opioid antagonist; reverses the effects of opioids.

  - ▸ Now carried by first responders; possibility of allowing public access to this medication to reverse opioid overdosing currently under review.

- ▸ **Naltrexone (Revia):** Opioid antagonist; reverses the effects of opioids and alcohol.

- ▸ **Bupropion (Wellbutrin; Zyban):** Smoking cessation aid

- ▸ **Benzodiazepines:** Alcohol and benzodiazepine withdrawal

- ▸ **Methadone:** Maintenance therapy

EATING DISORDERS: IMPLEMENTATIONS AND EVALUATIONS

Hospitalization may be indicated as well as nutritional stabilization with dietary consultation. The nurse helps the patient become aware of cues that trigger problem eating responses; thoughts, feelings, and assumptions associated with cues; and connections. The nurse supports individual and family counseling. Referral to specialized eating disorders inpatient services is expensive and few are available.

GENDER DYSPHORIA: IMPLEMENTATIONS AND EVALUATIONS

The psychiatric–mental health nurse is in a pivotal position for advocating for antistigma and antidiscrimination behaviors and policies for transgender and questioning patients as well as those who are lesbian, gay, bisexual, queer, and intersex. Patients from these groups who come for psychiatric services are most likely coping with depression and anxiety associated with bullying and nonacceptance of these identities and lifestyles among more traditional family constructs. Those who engage in social and biological sex reassignment transitioning, including cross-sex hormonal therapy (estrogens, testosterones), are particularly likely to face extreme social, psychological, and emotional difficulties such as anxiety states related to impending surgeries, and health insurance policy omissions and inequities. Current ethical issues (such as whether mammograms are covered when performed on males transgendered to females) create new and additional barriers to holistic care that need to be addressed. It is estimated that African-American transgender women have the highest rates of suicide within this population.

PAIN MANAGEMENT: IMPLEMENTATIONS AND EVALUATIONS

The treatment goals for managing pain are to reduce acute and chronic pain to its lowest possible level, restore physical functioning by increasing activity levels, and to decrease the psychological impact of pain on the person. Comprehensive pain management that incorporates psychological and rehabilitative interventions, with or without pain medication, is the treatment of choice for patients with chronic pain. Therapies found to be of particular use in treating patients with chronic pain include cognitive therapy restructuring strategies and imagery.

If it is determined that a patient's pain level warrants medication, other decisions come into play. For mild to moderate pain, the patient may be started on a nonopioid analgesic given orally every 4 to 6 hours. Sometimes, an analgesic combined with behavioral interventions is sufficient to control lower levels of pain. If this intervention is not sufficient to control the pain, a low dose of a short-acting opioid may be started.

The use of opioids is often essential for moderate to severe pain management. The key to successful pain control with opioids is to "start low and go slow." If the pain is not controlled with lower doses, it may be necessary to titrate the dose upward with small increments until appropriate pain relief is achieved. Persons with chronic pain can also experience "breakthrough" pain, which occurs episodically as more severe pain. These pain spikes can occur with or without triggers, such as too much activity or added stress. When breakthrough pain occurs, rescue medications, which are faster-acting, can be used episodically.

Nurses need to become familiar with all drugs used for pain management, including duration of action, immediacy of effect, appropriate dosage, dosing intervals, and side effects. Other relevant information relates to the patient's previous response to pain medication, and the use of psychoactive drugs in the past.

Pain Management and Substance Use Comorbidity

The management of pain in patients with a history of substance abuse or with a comorbid psychiatric disorder such as depression, anxiety disorders, somatization disorders, or PTSD may require extra care in dosing and monitoring. Chronic pain and psychiatric disorders can be reciprocally interactive; the chronic pain can deepen psychological symptoms, and the heightened emotional reactivity of the mental disorder can intensify the level of pain.

Although physical dependence and tolerance are expected physiological correlates of extended opioid therapy for pain, their emergence should not be considered addiction. Physical dependence on a prescribed controlled substance represents a physiologic neuro-adaptation to the drug. It is not addiction per se but if the opioid is stopped abruptly, the person is likely to experience a withdrawal syndrome.

Patients with co-occurring substance dependence present a difficult problem. Patients with substance use disorders, even if in recovery, may need larger doses of opioid medications for pain relief than the general population because of cross-tolerance. Substance use problems in patients who need opioid analgesics for pain relief are not always self-evident. There are often few physical markers to identify patients who may be substance abusers or at risk before initiating opioid therapy. Yet these patients are entitled legally and ethically to receive pain management comparable to that for persons without this co-occurring disorder. Patients with co-occurring substance use disorders need to be carefully monitored and counseled before and during treatment to prevent abuse of drugs they may legitimately need for effective pain management. Consultation with an expert, or team management of such patients, may be warranted.

Use of screening instruments, a careful medication and substance use history, and monitoring medication compliance can alert the nurse to consider the possibility of addiction to pain medications in patients with comorbid substance use disorders. Clues to the possibility of addiction in patients seeking opioid medications include

- Seeking medication from more than one provider or resource (e.g., dentists, emergency departments, multiple pain clinics or providers),

- Not taking the medication as prescribed (e.g., taking multiple doses or at irregular times),

- Requesting prescriptions earlier than scheduled, or frequent reporting of prescription loss,

- Resisting recommended changes in drug choice or dosage despite clear evidence of adverse side effects,

- Routinely using alcohol or illegal drugs, and

- Routinely using prescribed benzodiazepines.

NONPHARMACOLOGICAL PAIN MANAGEMENT INTERVENTIONS AND EVALUATION

Nonpharmacological interventions can be used in combination with pharmacologic interventions to help patients self-manage their pain. Including family members in the individualized decision-making process regarding the types of treatment to be used empowers patients and helps ensure compliance. Cognitive models have proven quite useful in helping patients cope with chronic pain (Lebovits, 2007). Nonpharmacological interventions are based upon nursing assessment of human responses to actual or potential health problems.

Guided imagery in which a person is taught to shift attention from his or her pain to an imagined pleasant scene (such as watching the sun set or being with a special friend or at the beach) can be relaxing and decrease the perception of pain. There is both a relaxing and a distracting component to this therapeutic strategy.

Self-hypnosis, biofeedback, and relaxation strategies are also used to alter perceptions of pain. These techniques are active strategies that help patients to focus their mind in ways that can calm them and ease pain. Biofeedback is a methodology that allows patients to learn to control muscle tension, heart rate, breathing, and temperature as a way of reducing anxiety and stress. Patients are able to reduce autonomic arousal and consequently alter pain levels.

Pain Management With Children

In the small child, pain can manifest in the pitch, frequency, and duration of crying; changes in color; and body movements. The young child may be more emotional or irritable than usual. Changes in activity (e.g., listlessness or not playing) also can signify pain. Sometimes the child provides clues to pain location, or will respond with nodding or saying yes when asked specifically about pain in a body part. Once children are able to comprehend language, they can be shown pictures of faces indicating intensity of pain and asked which facial expression most closely matches their pain level. The Wong-Baker FACES (1988) scale can give the nurse an indication of the level of pain that a child is experiencing.

Anxiety and distress exacerbate discomfort and pain. Children can become sensitized over time to repeated procedures, causing anticipatory anxiety, which, in turn, can increase the perception of pain. It is difficult for parents to see their children in pain, and children respond to their parent's concern. Intervention to help parents feel more comfortable and confident in coping with a child's pain is essential. Suggestions for parents to help their young children who require pain management include:

▸ Let children know what to expect in simple terms; for example, the order of events for invasive or painful procedures (this should be done in a matter-of-fact but compassionate way, close to the time of the procedure).

▸ Adolescents may need more in-depth teaching and time to ask questions than younger children.

▸ Assure the child that you will be with him or her.

▸ Don't tell the child it won't hurt if it will.

▸ Touch and being held are comforting to the child.

▸ Light massage, back rubs, and hand-holding help reduce a child's tension.

For older children, guided imagery, relaxation exercises, meditation, Reiki, acupuncture, and the cognitive therapy interventions described above can be helpful.

Pain Management in Adults With Cognitive Impairments

Adults with cognitive impairments often cannot articulate their pain. Instead, they may demonstrate pain nonverbally through facial grimacing or wincing, bracing, rubbing, agitation, and restlessness. Often, changes in typical behaviors are the first indicators. Finding the cause of the pain is the first priority. Relaxation techniques, music, and touch may also be helpful in reducing pain intensity and pain perception. Prayer, particularly those that are familiar from an earlier time, can relax patients with cognitive impairments who are spiritually inclined. Because patients who are older are more likely to experience negative side effects from pain medications, they will need to be monitored more closely.

Evaluation of patient response to pain management interventions is accomplished by reassessing the signs and symptoms of pain with a 10-point scale or other standardized measurement. The psychiatric nurse examines pain relief among several dimensions to ensure that the patient

- Has not experienced injury,
- Accepts the diagnosis,
- Socializes appropriately,
- Understands the importance of medication adherence,
- Has improved with medication regimen,
- Has gained or nearly regained previous or optimal level of physical functioning,
- Exhibits improved cognition,
- Acknowledges problems and personal responsibility,
- Uses adaptive coping mechanisms when stressed,
- Eats well-balanced meals,
- Obtains adequate rest,
- Has gained education (along with family, if appropriate),
- Participates in treatment planning,
- Is willing to follow through on treatment plan, and
- Has improved relationships with family and significant others.

OVER-THE-COUNTER, COMPLEMENTARY, ALTERNATIVE, AND HERBAL AGENTS

As research evidence unfolds, many over-the-counter, complementary, alternative, and herbal agents are investigated as integrative therapies to supplement conventional medical treatments. The NCCIM is the research-based branch of the National Institutes of Health that provides information on a variety of complementary and alternative treatments. According to Results from the 2012 nationwide survey conducted by the National Center for Complementary and Integrative Health (NCCIH) revealed that more Americans of all ages are engaging in complementary health approaches, such as yoga, chiropractic or osteopathic manipulation, and meditation (NCCIH, 2015). Many over-the-counter and herbal supplements are poorly regulated or understood. Some believe that these supplements are safer because they do not require a prescription; however, that is not necessarily true. Some use the same liver CYP450 enzymes as prescription drugs and may, therefore, cause drug interactions by inducing or inhibiting those enzymes. It is important to educate patients to discuss their use with the interprofessional team, and for the team to discuss potential risks of using nonprescribed drugs.

St. John's wort is a plant-based supplement sometimes used to treat symptoms of depression, anxiety, and sleep difficulties. St. John's wort may cause increased sensitivity to sunlight. Other side effects can include anxiety, dry mouth, dizziness, gastrointestinal symptoms, fatigue, headache, or sexual dysfunction. It can interact with other antidepressants to cause potentially serious side effects. There is not enough research evidence to determine the efficacy of the supplement. The best approach is to advise patients to ask their physician or nurse practitioner before taking any nonprescribed drugs or supplements.

Biofeedback and the newer HeartMath systems (http://www.heartmath.org/) are instruments that monitor and feed back moment-to-moment changes in physiology. HeartMath is a computer-enhanced tool that generates graphs that a person can observe, and through behavioral and thought modification, can learn to self-regulate emotional state. Control may develop over time and experience that ultimately eliminates the need for biofeedback. Box 5–3 lists common complementary, alternative, and integrative mind-body practices that may be useful adjuncts to traditional psychopharmaceutical and psychotherapies.

> **BOX 5–3.**
> **COMPLEMENTARY, ALTERNATIVE, AND INTEGRATIVE THERAPIES: MIND-BODY PRACTICES**
>
> ▸ Biofeedback
> ▸ HeartMath systems
> ▸ Yoga
> ▸ Meditation
> ▸ Guided imagery
> ▸ Phototherapy
> ▸ Therapeutic touch
> ▸ Animal-assisted therapy
> ▸ Electroacupuncture
> ▸ Hypnotherapy (hypnosis)
> ▸ Sound/music therapy
> ▸ Prayer
> ▸ Acupuncture
> ▸ Aromatherapy
> ▸ Ambient therapy
> ▸ Herbal preparations
> ▸ Expressive/creative art and music therapy
> ▸ Reiki

SELECT SOMATIC THERAPIES: ECT, TMS, BRAIN STIMULATION, VNS, PHOTOTHERAPY

Electroconvulsive Therapy (ECT)

Electroconvulsive therapy (ECT) is a type of brain stimulation therapy that is reputed to be a fast and effective alternative treatment for persons with treatment-resistant major depression or who have other serious contraindications for using medication (e.g., pregnancy). ECT increases virtually every neurotransmitter system in the brain, and increases plasma prolactin levels, thyrotropin-releasing hormone, and brain-derived neurotrophic factor (BDNF; Rosedale, et al., 2013). The effects on the noradrenergic system resemble the changes that occur with antidepressant treatment. ECT involves the therapeutic induction of a bilateral generalized seizure. Although generally safe and effective, it is not a first-line treatment for psychiatric disorders because of the invasiveness of the procedure and the side effects. After the seizure induction, EEG shows about 60 to 90 seconds of postictal suppression, followed by the appearance of high-voltage delta and theta waves and a return to preseizure electroencephalogram (EEG) in about 30 minutes. After repeated treatments it may take 1 to 12 months for the EEG to return to pretreatment appearance. Notable side effects include reversible memory loss and confusion. Patients generally receive between 6 and 8 treatments, considered as one ECT course or series. ECT is provided to patient candidates in inpatient and outpatient treatment sessions. In the latter, ECT may be administered as a maintenance therapy.

Nursing care of a patient receiving ECT includes the following steps:

▸ Obtain informed consent. Explain and document consent related to beneficial and adverse effects, alternative treatments, natural course of the disorder, and the option of no treatment.

▸ Make sure that the patient remains NPO 6 hours before treatment.

▸ Remove dentures or anything in mouth.

▸ Establish IV line.

▸ Insert bite block just before treatment.

▸ Administer 100% oxygen at 5L per minute during procedure and until spontaneous respiration returns.

▸ Give an anticholinergic drug to minimize oral and respiratory secretions during the procedure.

▸ In addition to anesthesia inducement, the nurse may give a muscle relaxant, as prescribed, to minimize the risk of bone fractures or injuries.

▸ Observe seizure activity in the foot (fasciculation) that has been protected from the muscle relaxant (often a blood pressure cuff is inflated to keep the drug out of one limb).

▸ Monitor oxygen saturation with pulse oximeter.

▸ Observe vital signs.

▸ Observe mental status; patient may be confused and disoriented upon awakening.

▸ Continue observing at 15-minute intervals.

▸ After return of gag reflex, patient may resume eating meals.

▸ Common side effects include headache, confusion, nausea, short-term memory loss, and muscle aches.

▸ Reassure patient that most memory problems will resolve within several weeks.

Transcranial Magnetic Stimulation (TMS)

One of the newer treatments for stimulating the brain cells in persons with depression who have not responded to other therapies is transcranial magnetic stimulation (TMS) therapy. TMS uses magnetic fields to stimulate the nerve cells. A large electromagnetic coil is placed against the scalp and painless electric currents are produced. TMS is shown to increase cerebral blood flow in the prefrontal and paralimbic areas; increase dopamine, serotonin, glutamate, and GABA; and increases thyroid-stimulating hormone (Rosedale, et al., 2013). Common side effects from the treatment include headache, scalp discomfort, tingling of facial muscles, and lightheadedness. TMS is still considered an experimental treatment and the long-term risks are unknown.

Deep-Brain Stimulation (DBS)

Deep-brain stimulation is FDA-approved for treating the tremor associated with Parkinson's disease. Research is underway to determine whether it also might be effective for depression. Deep-brain stimulation requires surgery to implant electrodes deep into the brain. Wires from the electrodes are attached to a battery-operated stimulator implanted in the chest like a pacemaker. Risks include infection, bleeding, delirium, mood changes, lightheadedness, and insomnia. Recent studies point to the potential utility of DBS in treating severe cases of anorexia nervosa (Nestler, 2013). As with TMS, the long-term risks of this treatment are unknown.

Vagal Nerve Stimulation (VNS)

Vagal nerve stimulation was introduced in 2005 and is an additional option for treatment-resistant depression endorsed by the American Psychiatric Association. In this neuromodulation technique, a small wire lead device is implanted under the skin near the collarbone. The device emits regular mild pulses of electrical energy via the vagus nerve to the brain. Similar to phototherapy (see below), it is intended to normalize the body's internal clock, relieve depression, or both. Neither has shown reliable levels of efficacy.

Phototherapy

Phototherapy involves use of a portable lighting device known as a light box that may be prescribed primarily to treat seasonal affective disorder (SAD), a mood disorder that presents in the winter months. The bright light therapy, administered at home, may readjust the body's circadian (daily) rhythms or internal clock. Phototherapy may also trigger the production of serotonin and the hormone melatonin. Melatonin is the naturally manufactured hormone that eases insomnia.

REFERENCES

American Nurses Association, International Society of Psychiatric–Mental Health Nurses, and American Psychiatric Nurses Association. (2014). *Psychiatric–mental health nursing: Scope and standards of practice, 2nd ed.* Silver Spring, MD: Nursesbooks.org.

Bezchlibnyk-Butler, K. Z., & Virani, A. S. (Eds.). (2007). *Clinical handbook of psychotropic drugs for children and adolescents, 2nd ed.* Toronto: Hogrefe Group.

Boyd, M. A. (2007). *Psychiatric nursing: Contemporary practice.* Philadelphia: Lippincott Williams & Wilkins.

Carlat Psychiatry Report, (2013). What to remember about lithium. Psych Central Professional. Retrieved from http://pro.psychcentral.com/what-to-remember-about-lithium/001595.html.

Ciraulo, D. A., Shader, R. I., Greenblatt, D. J., & Creelman, W. (2006). *Drug interactions in psychiatry, 3rd ed.* Philadelphia: Lippincott Williams & Wilkins.

Crettol, J., de Leon, J., Hiemke, C., & Eap, C. B. (2014). Pharmacogenomics in psychiatry: From therapeutic drug monitoring to genomic medicine. *Nature, 95*(3), 254–257.

Deratnay, P., & Sidani, S. (2013). The effect of insomnia on functional status of community-dwelling older adults. *Journal of Gerontological Nursing, 39*(10); 22–30.

Flannery, R., & Everly, G. (2002). Crisis intervention: A review. *International Journal of Emergency Mental Health, 2*(2), 119–125.

Halter, M. J. (2014). *Varcolis' foundations of psychiatric mental health nursing: A clinical approach, 7th ed.* Philadelphia: Saunders.

HeartMath Institute. Retrieved from http://www.heartmath.org/.

Holloway, E. L., & Kusy, M. E. (2014). Toxic workers put organizations at risk. *Modern Healthcare, 44*(31); 25. Retrieved from http://www.modernhealthcare.com/article/20140802/MAGAZINE/308029979.

Institute of Medicine. Committee on Identifying and Preventing Medication Errors. (2007). *Preventing medication errors: Quality chasm series.* Washington, DC: National Academy Press.

Institute of Medicine. Committee on Quality of Health Care in America. (2000). *To err is human: Building a safer health system.* Washington, DC: National Academy Press.

The Joint Commission. (2005). *Official "Do Not Use" list.* Retrieved from http://www.jointcommission.org/assets/1/18/Do_Not_Use_List.pdf.

The Joint Commission. (2015). *National Patient Safety Goals.* Accessed February 23, 2015. Retrieved from http://www.jointcommission.org/assets/1/6/2015_BHC_NPSG_ER.pdf.

Lebovits, A. (2007). Cognitive-behavioral approaches to chronic pain. *Primary Psychiatry.* Retrieved from http://primarypsychiatry.com/cognitive-behavioral-approaches-to-chronic-pain/.

Matchar, D. B., Thakur, M. E., Grossman, I., McCrory, D. C., Orlando, L. A., Steffens, D. C., … & Gray, R. N. (2007). *Testing for cytochrome P450 polymorphisms in adults with non-psychotic depression treated with selective serotonin reuptake inhibitors (SSRI's).* Evidence Report/Technology Assessment No. 146. (Prepared by the Duke Evidence-based Practice Center under Contract No. 290-02-0025). AHRQ Publication No. 07–E002. Rockville, MD: Agency for Healthcare Research and Quality.

Mayo Clinic Staff. (2015). *Antidepressants: Safe during pregnancy?* Retrieved from http://www.mayoclinic. org/healthy-living/pregnancy-week-by-week/in-depth/antidepressants/art-20046420.

National Center for Complementary and Integrative Health. (2015). *Nationwide survey reveals widespread use of mind and body practices.* Retrieved from https://nccih.nih.gov/news/press/02102015mb.

National Institute of Mental Health. (2005). *Questions and answers about the NIMH clinical antipsychotic trials of intervention effectiveness study (CATIE) — phase 1 results.* Retrieved from http://www.nimh. nih.gov/funding/clinical-trials-for-researchers/practical/catie/phase1results.shtml.

Nestler, E. J. (2013). Brain surgery for anorexia nervosa? *Nature Medicine, 19*(6); 678–679.

Outcome Engenuity. (n.d.) *Getting to Know Just Culture.* Retrieved from https://www.justculture.org/ getting-to-know-just-culture/.

Peplau, H. (1988). *Interpersonal relations in nursing.* London: Macmillan.

Rosedale, M., Ecklesdafer, D., Kormos, T., Freedland, M., & Knapp, M. (October 9, 2013). *The significant promise of therapeutic neuromodulation: Implications for psychiatric mental health nurses.* Paper presented at the 27th Annual Conference of the American Psychiatric Nurses Association, San Antonio, TX.

Santaguida, P. S., Raina, P., Booker, L., Patterson, C., Baldassarre, F., Cowan, D., … Unsal, A. (2004). *Pharmacological treatment of dementia: Evidence report/technology assessment No. 97.* Prepared by McMaster University Evidence-based Practice Center under Contract No. 290-02-0020. AHRQ Publication No. 04–E018–2 Rockville, MD: Agency for Healthcare Research and Quality.

Smith, J. (2013). A randomized, double-blind, placebo-controlled, 6 month cross-over study to evaluate the efficacy of coconut oil (Fuel for thought) treatment for subjects with mild to moderate Alzheimer's disease. *Clinical Trials NCT01883648.*

Stahl, S. (2008). *Stahl's essential psychopharmacology: Neuroscientific basis and practical applications, 3rd ed.* New York: Cambridge University Press.

Stuart, G. (2009). *Principles and practice of psychiatric nursing, 9th ed.* St. Louis: Mosby.

Townsend, M. C. (2009). *Psychiatric mental health nursing: Concepts of care in evidenced-based practice, 6th ed.* Philadelphia: F. A. Davis.

Trigoboff, E., Wilson, B. A., Shannon, M. T., & Stang, C. L (2005). *Prentice Hall psychiatric drug guide.* Upper Saddle River, NJ: Pearson Education.

Wilson, B. A., Shannon, M. T., & Shields, K. (2012). *Pearson's nurse's drug guide 2012.* New York: Pearson Education.

Wise, D. (2014). Getting to know Just Culture. *Just Culture.* Retrieved from https://www.justculture.org/ getting-to-know-just-culture/.

Wong, D. & Baker, C. (1988). Pain in children: Comparison of assessment scales. *Pediatric nursing, 14*(1): 9–17.

CATEGORY III

NURSE-PATIENT (HEALTHCARE CONSUMER) RELATIONSHIP; PROFESSIONAL DEVELOPMENT AND LEADERSHIP

NURSING THEORISTS, THERAPEUTIC COMMUNICATION, DIVERSE POPULATIONS, AND DOCUMENTATION FORMATS

This chapter reviews professional nursing practices for the psychiatric–mental health nurse. Theoretical frameworks from nursing, psychology, sociology, and biology; cultural variations, similarities, and sensitivities; and nursing theories that guide the therapeutic interactions for derivation of optimal care strategies are addressed. The Professional Performance Standard 11 (ANA, 2014) states that the psychiatric–mental health nurse incorporates techniques related to verbal versus nonverbal communication; therapeutic versus nontherapeutic communication skills; appropriate use of self (derived from interpersonal theories); and active listening techniques. Relationship issues related to professional boundaries, patient (healthcare consumer)-centered care, attentiveness to cultural and spiritual variables, and communication in special circumstances are also presented in this chapter.

NURSING THEORIES AND THEORISTS

In addition to developmental, biological, psychological, and "use of self" theories, a variety of nursing theories assist in explaining the science of human behavior and help proscribe the nursing art of providing care to individuals. Nursing theories present a distinctive paradigm (world view) with related concepts that distinguish the nursing profession from other disciplines. Professional nurses should be familiar with major nursing theories and models (Fawcett, 2005). Application of nursing models provides a basis and direction for clinical nursing practice, education, and research (Fawcett, 2005). The four components of nursing's paradigm, which are addressed in all theories, include:

- **Person:** The recipient of nursing care; can refer to an individual, population, or community
- **Environment:** All the internal and external contextual factors that form the context of the person in the healthcare situation
- **Health:** A multidimensional concept referring to quality of life, health status, and well-being of individuals, families, and communities
- **Nurse:** The licensed professional providing the care

Florence Nightingale was the first nursing theorist, writing her first works on what constituted nursing in 1860 (Nightingale, 1980). She insisted that by providing a healthy environment with fresh air, cleanliness, and proper diet, nurses can influence a person's ability to get well again. Since Nightingale's time, a number of nurse theorists have proposed models, beginning in the 1950s, to guide nurses in applying nursing knowledge.

Nursing Theories

Nursing theories are classified according to their levels of abstraction, ranging from grand theories to mid-range theories to practice theories. Theories describe broad concepts relevant to nursing practice. Listed below are some of the better-known nursing theorists and the central focus of each theorist's model. It is important that, in preparation for the certification exam, the psychiatric–mental health nurse develop a working knowledge of the tenets of each of the nursing theorists. In addition to numerous texts on nursing theory (Sitzman & Eichelberger, 2011), there are websites dedicated to explaining nursing theories in more detail (http://www.nursing-theory.org/nursing-theorists/. Some of the more notable nursing scholarly theorists who contribute to psychiatric–mental health nursing practice include the following:

- Hildegard Peplau: Interpersonal Relations

- Imogene King: General Systems Framework—Goal Attainment

- Dorothea Orem: Self-Care Framework

- Ann Wolbert Burgess: Rape-Trauma Syndrome

- Gail Stuart: Stress Adaptation Model

- Dorothy Johnson: Behavioral Systems Model

- Madeleine Leininger: Culture Care Diversity and Universality

- Martha Rogers: Science of Unitary Human Beings

- Betty Neuman: Neuman Systems Model

- Margaret Newman: Theory of Expanding Consciousness

- Virginia Henderson: Basic Principles of Nursing Care

- Rosemarie Parse: Theory of Human Becoming

- Sister Callista Roy: Adaptation Model

- Myra Levine: Conservation Model

- Joyce Travelbee: Interpersonal Theory of Nursing

- Jean Watson: Theory of Human Science and Human Caring/Relationship-Based Care

- Josephine Paterson and Loretta Zderad: Humanistic Nursing Theory

- Kathryn Barnard: Child Interaction Model

- Nola Pender: Health Promotion Model

- Pamela Reed: Theory of Self-Transcendence

- Janet Younger: Mastery of Stress Theory

- Kristin Swanson: Theory of Caring and Healing

- Sharon Dingman: The Caring Model

Practice theories are the most concrete level of nursing theory, providing a specific outline for practice. Practice theories can focus on a single operationalized concept found in a specific population or nursing situation. Practice theories are helpful in a healthcare setting focused on developing evidence-based practice. One example is the From Novice to Expert Theory (Benner, 1984. As nursing continues to define itself as a profession, this assertion directs nurses to define nursing practice ourselves.

Hildegard Peplau: Interpersonal Relationship Theory

Hildegard Peplau, the mother of psychiatric nursing, defined the therapeutic (purposive and meaningful) relationship as a professional patient (healthcare consumer)–centered alliance in which a qualified nurse joins with a patient experiencing a mental healthcare need to meet health-related treatment goals. Peplau's theory of interpersonal relationships, first developed in 1952, is still considered the cornerstone of psychiatric nursing practice. Incidentally, 1952 was a transitional period for psychiatric practice; the first DSM was published and chlorpromazine (Thorazine) was introduced. Peplau's theoretical perspectives were derived from developmental, interpersonal, and learning theories, particularly the constructs presented by Harry Stack Sullivan. Heavily influenced by Sullivan's interpersonal framework, Peplau conceptualized the nurse's role in a therapeutic relationship as that of *participant-observer*.

In a therapeutic relationship, the nurse is an active participant and the primary tool psychiatric nurses use is "the self." As participants in the nurse-patient relationship, nurses share a partnership with their patients, and are focused on the patient's recovery. As observers, nurses consistently scrutinize the patient's behaviors, their own behaviors, and the nature of nurse-patient exchanges for interpersonal connections and disconnects. Nurses use active listening skills to deduce the meaning that communication content may have for the patient, engage in two-way communication to foster interpretation, and intervene appropriately.

Phases of the Therapeutic Relationship

Peplau identified four distinct sequential phases of the therapeutic relationship as part of her interpersonal theory: the orientation, identification, exploitation (working), and resolution (termination) phases. Ideally, the patient will demonstrate greater emotional stability and more effective coping skills as treatment outcomes resulting from effective therapeutic relationships. The phases are equally applicable in inpatient and outpatient settings. Each phase has specific therapeutic tasks or goals.

1. **Orientation phase** sets the stage for the relationship. Nursing tasks include:

   ▸ Establishing trust in the relationship

   ▸ Developing a therapeutic alliance

   ▸ Establishing therapeutic boundaries related to the structure of the relationship; confidentiality

   ▸ Mutually defining the therapeutic contract (time, place, duration of each meeting; length of relationship)

   ▸ Building rapport

- ▸ Assessing patient needs, strengths, and coping strategies

- ▸ Identifying nursing diagnoses based on assessment data

- ▸ Specifying treatment outcomes directly related to nursing diagnoses and initial treatment objectives

2. **Identification phase** occurs when expectations have been clarified, mutually agreeable goals have been set, and a realistic plan of action developed.

3. **Exploitation (Working) phase** is when most of the therapeutic work takes place; patient uses professional assistance for problem-solving alternatives and feels an integral part of the helping environment; may fluctuate on independence; can be more intense, focusing on:

- ▸ Teaching patients new skills

- ▸ Implementing a realistic plan of action related to identified therapeutic goals.

- ▸ Evaluating and modifying realistic goals, with related plans of action, to achieve identified treatment outcomes

4. **Resolution (Termination) phase** is the final stage of the process. No new work is begun in the termination phase. It occurs when mutually agreed-upon therapeutic goals are achieved, or the patient is discharged or transferred to another facility. Treatment outcomes relate to improving a patient's mental health and well-being (Peplau, 1997). Some patients demonstrate temporary regressive behaviors, hostility, or sadness that the relationship is ending. The work of this phase involves:

- ▸ Reviewing accomplishments and patient progress toward therapeutic goals

- ▸ Exploring the need for referrals post-discharge

- ▸ Establishing plans for long-term post-discharge functioning

- ▸ Moving towards closure of the relationship independent of the nurse

- ▸ Sometimes may be difficult for both as psychological dependence may persist

"Use of the Self:" Self-Awareness

Peplau noted that nurses must observe their own behavior, as well as the patient's, with "unflinching self-scrutiny and total honesty in assessment of their behavior in interactions with patients." Effective psychiatric nurses have a good sense of awareness about themselves—their strengths, weaknesses, actions, reactions, motivations, and personal beliefs. Self-awareness allows the nurse to act authentically and to remain centered, even in complicated situations. In addition to self-reflection, nurses can increase their professional self-awareness of issues affecting the nurse–patient relationship through regular peer supervision. It is also useful to seek consultation with expert nurses when confronted with transference or countertransference issues that threaten the integrity of the nurse-patient relationship.

FIGURE 6–1. JOHARI WINDOW

Box 1 Known to self and others	Box 2 Known only to others
Box 3 Known only to self	Box 4 Known neither to self nor to others

Note. Originally developed by Luft, J., & Ingham, H. (1955). The Johari window: A graphic model of interpersonal awareness. *Proceedings of the Western Training Laboratory in Group Development.* Los Angeles: UCLA.

Although no one has total access to his or her personality, it is possible, through communication with others, to know oneself and be known by others. The Johari Window (Figure 6–1) provides an interesting psychological tool for developing self-awareness. With this tool, one person (the participant learning self-awareness) is given a list of 55 adjectives and selects 5 or 6 that he or she feels describes his or her personality. A peer who knows this person does the same with the same list of adjectives. These adjectives are then mapped onto a grid. Adjectives selected by both are placed in Box 1 and represent traits that both are aware of about the participant; adjectives selected only by the participant are placed in Box 3; adjectives selected only by the peer are placed in Box 2; and adjectives selected by neither are placed in Box 4. The larger box 1 is, the greater the self-awareness. The best way to decrease the size of box 2 is to listen attentively to the feedback of others about their perceptions of you. Self-disclosure is a helpful way to decrease the size of box 3 (Stuart, 2009).

Self-disclosure: A deliberate, reflective interpersonal strategy in which the nurse may share personal information for the purpose enhancing the therapeutic relationship. When self-disclosure is brief, focused, and relevant to the goals of the relationship, it can be useful to the therapeutic relationship. It strengthens the bond between nurse and patient, and reassures patients that their problems are not unique. Self-disclosure should be used judiciously and sparingly, and only to meet an identifiable therapeutic patient need. Without a direct connection to meeting a patient's therapeutic need, self-disclosure by the nurse is ill-advised.

Giving gifts or accepting gifts from patients: Nurses should refrain from giving or accepting gifts unless it is an appropriate token gift that meets an identified therapeutic need and does not change the therapeutic dynamics of the relationship.

Touch and physical contact: Nurses should consider the possible meaning of touch and physical contact with mentally ill patients. Although limited touch may be helpful with dementia patients, children, or grieving patients, in general, it should be avoided because there is danger of misinterpretation.

Involvement in the patient's personal life: Nurses should not interfere in a patient's personal life. Meeting with patients outside of treatment sessions is not appropriate, and can sabotage the therapeutic work.

Dual relationships: Coexisting relationships can undermine the therapeutic judgment and objectivity needed for therapeutic care. Examples include providing professional nursing care to a relative or friend, engaging in business relationships with patients, and establishing outside relationships or friendships with patients.

"Use of the Self:" Professional Boundaries

Professional boundaries make the nurse–patient relationship safe. They clarify the nurse's role in the relationship and distinguish this relationship as a professional alliance that is separate and distinct from the patient's personal relationships. *Therapeutic boundaries* are the invisible interpersonal limits surrounding professional relationships that specify time, proximity, and distance between nurse and patient; informed consent; level of relationship; nontreatment meetings; clothing; language; gift-giving; touch; and professional self-disclosure. The most grievous boundary violation is that of a sexual nature, which is never permitted under any circumstance.

The nurse, not the patient, is responsible for establishing and maintaining the boundaries in the therapeutic nurse-patient relationship. *Boundary violations* occur any time a professional nurse enters into a social, financial, or personal relationship with a patient. *Boundary crossings* are lesser transgressions that can involve role, time, place, or financial boundaries. They generally fall in the realm of structuring the relationship, self-disclosure, gift-giving, touch, involvement in the patient's life outside of treatment, and involvement in dual relationships. Warning signs of boundary violations related to the structure of the relationship can include:

- ▸ Feeling that you understand the patient's problems better than other members of the healthcare team
- ▸ Giving certain patients extra time or attention
- ▸ Spending off-duty time with patients
- ▸ Giving patients personal contact information
- ▸ Failing to set limits with patients
- ▸ Giving patients money to buy snacks

THERAPEUTIC COMMUNICATION AND THE NURSE-PATIENT (HEALTHCARE CONSUMER) RELATIONSHIP

Standard 11 states that the psychiatric–mental health nurse communicates effectively in a variety of formats in all areas of practice (ANA, 2014; p. 75). Therapeutic (purposive and meaningful) communication is the primary strategy that psychiatric–mental health nurses use to implement all phases of the nurse-patient relationship. Therapeutic communication refers to goal-directed conversations with patients aimed at helping to sort through difficult issues and take thoughtful actions to improve their mental health and well-being. In the field of psychiatric and mental health nursing, communication moves to a deeper level as it becomes a primary therapeutic intervention in helping patients consider new, constructive perspectives that lead to a more productive and satisfying life. Communication occurs on many different levels, both conscious and unconscious. It is critical that nurses develop skills in therapeutic communication to lay the foundation for the patient to feel that he or she can trust the nurse to hear concerns that may be of a sensitive or personal nature. Trust in the relationship lays the foundation for open dialogue and rapport in the therapeutic relationship. Therapeutic communication includes the following factors:

- Culture, language, and ethnic values
- Perceptions of self and others
- Social class
- Developmental stage
- Intellectual processing abilities and skills
- Education
- Setting
- Relationship
- Choice of words and body language
- Timing
- Manner of presentation
- Level of anxiety

Functional Components of Communication

Communication is a two-way feedback loop. One does not merely give instruction or feedback; the circularity of communication means that the sender has to impart a message to the receiver. After this, there must be an opportunity for the receiver to process and express understanding for the sender to assess how the message was received. Feedback helps patients and the nurse become aware of how their behaviors and expressions are perceived by others and how others are interpreting their communications. People generally respond to the sum total of communication, taking into account the social context in which it is delivered and received. The context (time, place, and situational circumstances surrounding the communication) are important variables and the nurse uses concepts of milieu theory in deciding on the most appropriate the "stage" for exchange. The context includes the relationship dimension and how the participants are connected to each other, related to authority, attitudes, and roles. How communication is transmitted (pitch, tone, body language), and cultural and ethnic differences, age, gender, and social status can influence nonverbal communication and interpersonal distance requirements (e.g., hearing, touch, sight, direct discussion, emails, phone conversation; Arnold & Boggs, 2007).

Verbal Communication

Language is the crucial medium through which messages are conveyed orally (or visually in sign languages) and in writing. Conversing with others is a socially learned behavior, influenced by sociocultural values and perspectives. Variations in grammar and dialect can affect the meaning of a verbal message. Anxiety and loss of cognitive processing skills associated with several mental disorders can mean that messages are not fully understood. Psychiatric patients and patients from different cultures can understand concrete verbal messages in which the literal meaning of words is clear, direct, and easy to understand. Empathy, respect, therapeutic authenticity, and being concrete are important components of every therapeutic conversation. Words can both denote (provide literal meaning) and connote (imply or suggest a meaning that may or may not be the same as the literal meaning).

Nonverbal Communication

Universally, messages are conveyed through body language. *Metacommunication* is the term used for the nonverbal aspects of communication, such as gestures, facial expressions, and body movements. Nonverbal signals, transmitted through one or more of the human senses, can include body position, body movements, voice quality, and use of space, clothing, and personal mannerisms. Culture influences the meaning attributed to these signals, such that the same nonverbal symbol can convey entirely different messages in different cultures.

Congruent communication takes place when the words and nonverbal components of a personal message match. Incongruent communication occurs when they contradict each other. The nurse looking at her watch and telling the patient, "Tell me what is troubling you; I'm here for you," or asking the patient, "How are you feeling?" as he inserts the thermometer into the patient's mouth are examples of incongruent communication. An incongruent match between the words and nonverbal actions gives the patient a mixed message about the nurse's availability and intention.

The nonverbal elements express the relationship aspects of communication. They allow people to express their inner feelings without words, because they are not as easily controlled as the words we speak. Unfortunately, a nonverbal message is more open to misinterpretation than a verbal one. Concepts to be aware of when engaging in therapeutic communication include the following attending behaviors:

- **Paralinguistics:** Vocal cues, such as voice pitch, rhythm, pace of words, inflections, and intonations provide the listener with the emotions behind the words. *Example:* Saying "I will attend to it" or "May I help you?" with caring vocal cues is likely to be perceived differently than if the same statement is said with sarcasm or with an impatient intonation.

- **Body position:** Body position can be closed, with crossed legs, arms, or both, indicating that the person may feel threatened or is not open to conversation. An open body position, consisting of eye contact, sitting in a relaxed manner, and leaning forward, is indicative of acceptance and openness to conversation. Maintain an open, relaxed, attentive posture.

- **Kinesics:** Nonverbal communication involving muscle or body movement such as fleeting (not staring or glaring) eye contact, facial expression, head nodding, and smiling.

- **Proxemics:** The amount of physical space and distance needed for comfort in conversations between sender and receiver. Culture is an important variable in determining the amount of distance the patient needs to feel comfortable in a therapeutic interaction. Most therapeutic conversations take place within personal space. Sit facing and leaning slightly toward the patient; respect the interpersonal space of the patient—maintaining a distance of at least 18 inches; remove all unnecessary distractions.

- **Touch:** Physical contact can be very comforting to small children, frail older adults, and grieving patients. In such situations, light touch on the shoulder can be used to give encouragement or to show emotional support. However, the use of touch, with the exception of therapeutic touch, is largely contraindicated for use with mentally ill patients, because of the danger of misinterpretation, therefore is avoided unless the nurse has asked and been granted permission to touch sensitively.

▶ **Active listening:** Active listening responses are essential components of effective therapeutic communication, and the primary means of effectively responding to a patient's communication. Attending behaviors involve eye contact, posture, and verbal and nonverbal cues. Smiling, leaning forward, nodding, and using facial expression to demonstrate full attention are examples of facilitative, attending behaviors. These also include periodic use by the nurse of statements such as "Go on" or "I hear you, please continue." Sometimes referred to as *presence*, attending behaviors demonstrate the nurse's full involvement in "being with" the patient in a mutually interactive relationship.

Active Listening Response Strategies

Active listening is an interactive, reflective process in which the nurse actively focuses on what a patient is saying with an open attitude and uses a structured form of responses to fully understand the meaning of a communication.

Incorporating attending behaviors and active listening responses ensures mutual understanding of the communication. The nurse responds to the patient in such a way that the patient feels heard and understood. In addition to receiving the patient's message, the nurse examines his or her personal reaction to it, and asks for clarification or validation that the message received is the one the speaker intended. Nurses use nonverbal responses (eye contact, relaxed posture, gestures, leaning forward, facing the person) to display full attention.

In a therapeutic relationship, the patient should do more of the talking than the nurse. The nurse listens for themes, representing recurrent patterns or underlying central issues or problems requiring therapeutic intervention, especially during initial contacts, or during initial assessment collection so the nurse can formulate a baseline understanding of the patient and his or her chief complaint (major concern). Themes are usually expressed frequently during the course of the interaction and the psychiatric–mental health nurse is especially attuned to hearing where the patient is at that particular time.

Factors that enhance the effectiveness of a therapeutic relationship include consistency, pacing, encouraging active patient collaboration, and willingness to listen. Establishing and maintaining authentic, flexible professional boundaries in all phases of the therapeutic relationship helps protect the integrity of nurse-patient interaction. Finally, nurses play key roles in helping patients move in the direction of health and well-being. These roles include the following:

▶ **Stranger:** Meeting and accepting the patient as a unique person

▶ **Counselor:** Counseling patients related to current problems

▶ **Healthcare resource person:** Interpreting the treatment plan to the patient, and helping him or her access relevant treatment resources

- ▶ **Teacher:** Providing relevant information and helping the patient learn

- ▶ **Leader:** Mediating, acting as a safety agent

Regardless of which role the nurse assumes when providing care for patients, genuineness, respect, concreteness, and empathy should be basic features of every therapeutic conversation.

Therapeutic Communication Techniques

In addition to conveying interest and acceptance through attending behaviors identified above, the nurse incorporates listening responses to further enhance the depth and breadth of relevant information. These include the following therapeutic communication techniques:

- ▶ **Broad opening questions:** Questions that cannot be answered with a simple yes or no; open-ended questions should be neutral so the patient can set the direction of the conversation. *Example:* "Can you give me a picture of what a typical day would be like for you? Can you tell me what it (this experience) was like for you?"

- ▶ **Closed questions:** Require a one-word or specific answer; can be used to narrow the topic of discussion or get specific information, but should be used sparingly. *Examples:* "Are you sexually active?" or "Do you use tobacco or nicotine products?"

- ▶ **Minimum encouragers**: Offer encouragement with a general, minimum verbal lead, which encourages the patient to go into more detail. *Example:* Nodding or saying "Uh-huh," "I see," or "Go on." Refrain from suggesting or leading a patient on, to which they might easily respond affirmatively. *Example:* "Did you tell the sexual offender to stop?"

- ▶ **Restating:** Repeating the basic ideas or main thought in the communication by using the patient's own words. Usually only part of the statement is repeated. *Example:* Using opening phrases such as "If I understand you correctly..." or "So what you're saying is...," restate the core part of the patient's message. Restatement should be used sparingly.

- ▶ **Paraphrasing:** Recapping the core content components of a patient's message in your own words. The paraphrased message usually is shorter than the original message, and focuses on the *content* of the message. *Example:* Patient, "I am angry with my doctor; it just isn't right that I can't get my privileges." Nurse, "You believe your doctor shouldn't have done this."

▸ **Reflecting:** In a reflection response, the focus is on the feeling, rather than the content, of the communication. Expressing your perception of the patient's *feelings* in the communication is usually based on a combination of the patient's words, tone, and body language. Timing and respect for cultural differences are important when using reflection responses. *Example:* Patient, "I can't stand how dependent I am on my wife for her approval." Nurse, "It sounds like you feel frustrated by your level of dependence right now. Is that what you are feeling?"

▸ **Focusing:** Used to help patients examine relevant parts of their communication, usually related to treatment outcomes. A focused question asks the patient for more information about the central issues presented by the patient. It is different from a closed question in that it allows the patient a broader way of responding. *Example:* "I wonder if you could tell me more about how your illness is affecting your relationship with your wife and children."

▸ **Clarifying:** Listening response that signals the listener's need to understand the speaker's situation more fully; a way to check perceptions; indicates to the speaker that what he or she is saying is important. *Example:* Patient: "Jerry isn't honest with me. He promises me he will change, but it never lasts more than a few weeks." Nurse: "Marta, I'd like to understand better. Can you give me an example of what you mean by Jerry's being dishonest when he promises to do something, and then doesn't do it?" In addition to asking the patient to provide clarification, the nurse also uses consensual validation as a clarification strategy. *Example:* "It sounds as if Jerry's failure to follow through is very discouraging to you."

▸ **Empathizing:** Verbally acknowledges the patient's emotional state or frame of reference in ways that demonstrate to the speaker that the nurse fully understands and can related to the patient's situation. Empathy requires that the nurse put her- or himself in the patient's position with compassion and insight without losing her- or himself. Empathy can also be transmitted nonverbally through tone of voice, authenticity, and congruence among your words, body language, and the attending behaviors described above. *Example:* "I can see how difficult this conversation is for you."

▸ **Silence:** Appropriately timed, silence can be an effective listening response, particularly after expression of an important idea or feeling. The speaker can get significant thoughts together or correct a response as he or she reflects inwardly about it. Silence only should be used as a timely pause in relation to a significant communication. Lengthy silence can be awkward and uncomfortable.

▶ **Summarization:** This strategy is useful either at the end of the session or when the communication is moving to another topic. Effective summaries restate the most important points already covered. They also help the nurse and patient check and refine perceptions about what has been discussed and, in some cases, point out areas that need further exploration.

▶ **Sharing observations:** Nurses share their observations regarding the patient's behavior as a way to help the patient understand his or her emotions. For example: "Your hands are shaking." "You seem upset."

▶ **Verbalizing implied thoughts and feelings:** The nurse voices what the patient seems to have implied. *Example:* Patient: "It's a waste of time doing these exercises." Nurse: "You feel that they aren't benefiting you?"

▶ **Giving information:** As nurses, we educate and provide specific information. Studies have shown that a major cause of anxiety in hospitalized patients is lack of information or misconceptions about their conditions, treatments, or hospital routines. Education is a primary nursing function. Providing facts in an objective manner allows the patient to accept or reject them. It is up to individual patients how and to what extent they will use the information.

▶ **Giving feedback:** Feedback is an essential component of therapeutic communication. *Examples:* "It sounds as though you are saying that you have had enough;" "I hear you as saying…Is that correct?"

Effective feedback should be:

  ▸ Immediate, honest, reflective, constructive, and nonjudgmental

  ▸ Focused on the behavior, not the person or emotion

  ▸ Focused only on behaviors, which can be changed

  ▸ Given in a private setting

▶ **Questioning:** Open-ended questions are best ("How would you say you are doing at this time?"), unless the nurse needs to pinpoint a specific understanding ("Are you sexually active?").

▶ **Processing:** "Give me a minute to understand," or "Do you need a moment to understand?"

Barriers to Effective Communication

Anxiety

In addition to her seminal work detailing the nurse-patient relationship, Peplau developed a nursing model of anxiety in which she defined *anxiety* as a free-floating feeling of apprehension or dread related to a real or perceived threat to self-integrity. According to Peplau, anxiety can affect the development of the therapeutic relationship and be experienced on four different levels. Patient and nurse alike, each enters a new relationship with some level of anxiety as the unknown is faced. The psychiatric–mental health nurse recognizes this tendency and is accountable for his or her own level and transmission of anxiety. This is why the dynamic field of nursing is engaged in practices and continued education across multiple domains (health, social, cultural, crisis prevention, CPR, etc.) to improve, reflect, and promote self-confidence. Peplau's recognition of anxiety states on the interpersonal and therapeutic relationship can encompass one of these four levels:

1. **Mild:** Perceptual field widens; increased awareness, problem-solving, motivation

2. **Moderate:** Can attend to immediate tasks; difficulty with concentration; can be redirected

3. **Severe:** Significantly narrowed perceptual field; difficulty solving problems or completing tasks; difficulty learning

4. **Panic:** Closed perceptual field; inability to process environmental stimuli; irrational thinking and behavior; potential for self-harm.

Stress

Gail Stuart's (2009) Stress Adaptation Nursing Model examines stress from an integrated biopsychosocial perspective. Similar to anxiety, stress perceptions affect the patient's ability to corral adaptive coping resources. Specific components of her model include examining the following:

- **Predisposing factors:** Can be biological, psychological, or sociocultural risk factors such as genetic background, intelligence, age, self-concept, education, financial assets, belief systems, and past experiences.

- **Precipitating stressors:** Stimuli that require additional energy because they are challenging, threatening, or demanding to the person, such as stressful life events, life strains and hassles, or injury. The stimulus is not stressful in itself; it becomes stressful because of the interaction between the self and the stressful situation.

- **Appraisal of the stressor:** Includes a cognitive appraisal of the stressor's impact on a person's well-being. The person mentally and emotionally considers the stressor's meaning, intensity, social attribution, physiological impact, and feelings in evaluating the impact of the stressor.

▶ **Coping resources:** Includes an evaluation of the person's coping options or strategies related to what the person can do to resolve the stress (financial assets, social supports, knowledge, spiritual beliefs, and problem-solving skills).

▶ **Coping mechanisms:** Refers to efforts directed at stress management. Coping mechanisms can be problem-, cognitive-, or emotion-focused. They can be constructive, in which the person views the stressor as a challenge, or destructive, in which the person uses evasion or defense mechanisms to minimize anxiety without resolving the stressful conflict.

▶ **Continuum of coping responses:** Patient's coping responses are evaluated on a continuum of adaptation–maladaptation, with higher levels reflecting adaptive responses leading to personal growth and well-being and maladaptive responses requiring clinical or nursing diagnosis and treatment.

Stuart then identifies nursing goals, assessment focus, direction of nursing intervention, and expected outcomes of care for four different treatment stages. Identifying the treatment stage helps the nurse select the most appropriate nursing approaches and activities.

Nontherapeutic Communication

▶ **Giving false reassurance:** Statements such as "You're doing just fine" minimize the patient's concerns. Don't offer false reassurance. Share your observations instead and let the patient interpret their meaning.

▶ **Giving advice:** Direct advice imposes the nurse's own opinions and solutions on the patient and is inappropriate. Clarify and use other communication techniques to help patients come to their own solutions.

▶ **Making stereotypical comments:** Drawing a conclusion about a person based on general knowledge of ethnicity, gender, or social status detracts from considering each person's attributes. Regard each person as a unique human being. *Example:* "Those people like that…."

▶ **Changing the subject:** Arbitrarily changing the subject so the nurse directs the course of the conversation can make the patient feel unimportant and abandoned. Sometimes this occurs when the nurse is uncomfortable with the topic. Identify the source of your discomfort and work it through; then you will be able to use silence and really listen.

▶ **Moralizing or being judgmental:** Imposing of the nurse's values onto the patient implies that the nurse is entitled to make a value judgment regarding the patient's feelings or behavior. Keep an open mind and recognize that all behavior has meaning even if you don't understand it.

▸ **Minimizing or belittling the patient's feelings:** Statements such as "I know just how you feel" or "Everyone gets depressed sometimes" deny the importance of the patient's feelings and perceptions as unique. Each person reacts and responds differently. This approach shifts the focus from the patient to the nurse ("I know …") or others ("Everyone gets …"). Acknowledge the patient's feeling or information-sharing instead.

▸ **Disagreeing with the patient:** Although saying "You're wrong" or "That's not true" can be used appropriately as a reality check, it can indicate that what the patient said has not been accepted. Give correct information or offer reflective questions instead.

▸ **Tangential or irrelevant comment:** Trite sayings such as "You have a lot to be grateful for" or "Isn't it a beautiful day?" keep the conversation at a superficial level. Try starting with a broad opening statement instead.

▸ **Social responses:** "Oh well, that's just the way it goes."

Overuse of Freudian Defense Mechanisms

Defensive patient communication occurs when a person perceives or anticipates a threat as part of a conversation. As people become defensive, they are less able to accurately perceive the true motives or intent of a communication. Freud introduced the concept of ego defense mechanism as a form of defensive communication that patients use when they perceive threats to self-integrity.

Ego defense mechanisms are defined as unconscious methods that people use to protect themselves from consciousness of a threat to self. By distorting the meaning of the original threat, the defense mechanism makes it less anxiety-provoking to the person. The use of a defense mechanism distances the person from a full awareness of unpleasant thoughts, feelings, desires, or impulses. Common defense mechanisms include:

▸ **Denial:** Acting as though a painful circumstance, situation, feeling, or thought doesn't exist. *Example:* Denying that you are an alcoholic despite its negative impact on your marital relationship.

▸ **Rationalization:** Supplying a logical reason for a behavior to justify it. *Example:* Contending that the only reason you have two martinis for lunch every day is because you are a salesperson, and drinking at lunch is expected.

▸ **Displacement:** Directing unacceptable feelings, impulses, or thoughts onto a safer, less threatening target. *Example:* Being angry at your boss but not verbalizing or expressing it, coming home and getting angry at your wife for the way she handles the house.

- **Regression:** Reversion to an earlier stage of development. *Example:* Toddler who goes back to wanting a bottle or pacifier and soils his pants when his baby brother is born.

- **Repression:** An unconscious forgetting, usually of a traumatic event or feeling. *Example:* Forgetting being sexually abused as a child.

- **Reaction formation:** Taking on a position opposite to what one actually believes or perceives to be unacceptable. *Example:* A kidnap victim "falls in love" with the feared and hated person who has complete control over him or her.

- **Projection:** Attributing one's shameful or undesired impulses, thoughts, or feelings onto another. *Example:* An angry person who accuses her partner of being hostile.

- **Suppression:** The conscious dismissing from the mind of an unacceptable idea, desire, painful memory, and so on. Can be a positive defense mechanism, used to eliminate negative or thinking. *Example:* A person is thinking about the possibility of a promotion so much that it is compromising his work. He decides not to think about it and just go with the flow of his present job in the best way possible.

- **Undoing:** Trying to take back behavior, feelings, or thoughts that are unacceptable to a person by partially negating a previous communication or action. *Example:* When asked for a recommendation, a person makes derogatory remarks about a friend to her employer, but praises the good work her friend is doing for the company in the same interaction.

- **Sublimation:** This is actually one of the healthy defense mechanisms. It is defined as the channeling of unacceptable impulses into more acceptable outcomes. *Example:* A person with very aggressive tendencies becomes a butcher.

- **Dissociation:** Loss of track of time or sense of self.

- **Identification:** Looking up to someone so much that you don their style of dress, manner of speaking, and other visible attributes.

- **Introjection:** Taking on the beliefs and values of someone else.

- **Splitting:** Seeing everything as all good or all bad with nothing in between.

- **Compensation:** A counterbalancing technique. When told you cannot cook, you counter with "But I can dance."

- **Intellectualization:** Often used to distance oneself from entering into emotional responses or impulses. Instead of focusing on something that causes sadness, one focuses on minute details.

- **Acting out:** Engaging in extreme behaviors instead of language to express oneself.

Therapeutic Impasses and Problems

The key to handling a therapeutic impasse in the nurse-patient relationship is to acknowledge its existence, explore its role in stalling the relationship, and clarify relationship goals. If the nurse is experiencing counter-transference, seeking supervision from an expert nurse is advised.

The most common types of therapeutic impasses in nurse-patient relationships include resistance, transference, counter-transference, boundary violations, and cultural insensitivity.

Resistance refers to the patient's reluctance to reveal relevant information about his or her experience, feelings, or level of symptoms. It is an unconscious process that may reflect the patient's unwillingness to change, or fear of change. Resistance is most likely to occur in the working phase because this is the problem-solving phase associated with making therapeutic changes.

Transference (Freudian term) is the process where *a patient* inappropriately (and unconsciously) transfers attitudes and emotional reactions (positive or negative) originally linked with significant persons in the past onto current relationships. This stems from unresolved conflicts in past relationships.

> ▸ *Staff splitting* occurs when a patient displays a positive dependent transference toward one staff member, while demeaning the competence of other staff members.

Counter-transference (Freudian term) is *the nurse's (or other healthcare provider's)* unconscious displacement of feelings associated with past relationships onto the current relationship with a patient. Counter-transference feelings occur when the nurse feels very positive or negative feelings toward a patient that are not justified. This stems from unresolved conflicts in past relationships.

Boundary issues: There are major differences between personal and professional relationships. Boundaries are defined as the space between authority and vulnerability, formal and informal power differentials, rule definers and rule followers. Boundary concepts define healthy therapeutic relationships and lower risks to patients in the health exchange. Boundaries manage power differentials, protect the vulnerability of patients, protect staff from becoming over- or under-involved, and provides legal protection for both patient and nurse. Four main types of boundary issues are explored further:

> ▸ **Boundary challenges:** Your neighbor's mother is your patient, or you see your patient at church.

> ▸ **Boundary crossings** are contextual—rural and ethnic communities or going to court with your patient.

> ▸ **Boundary violations:** Maintaining contact after patient discharge, financial exploitation, nurse's needs met rather than patient's, sexualized touch, excessive self-disclosure.

> ▸ **Dual relationships:** Friend *and* physical therapist; nurse and business partner; volunteer and patient.

Cultural Insensitivity

Psychiatric–mental health nurses have a legal, ethical, and professional responsibility to respect, acknowledge, and incorporate knowledge of varying cultural attitudes, beliefs, values, and behaviors into their clinical practice. Culture is "the integrated pattern of human behavior that includes thoughts, communications, actions, customs, beliefs, values, and institutions of a racial, ethnic, religious, or social group" (Cross et al., 1989). Differences within cultures include age, gender, sexual orientation, religious and spiritual beliefs, social class, educational level, occupation, ability and disability. Ethnicity is defined as the shared feelings or identity among individual groups based on similar cultural patterns, values, beliefs, customs, and behaviors that create a common history. Race is a social construction (manmade) based on observations of physical markers, such as skin color, to identify group membership. Race is not a genetically defined category and racism is a real phenomenon that is linked to social inequalities and injustices.

Cultural and ethnic perspectives shape both the nurse's responses as well as those of the patient. Culture is a concept that helps explain a person's worldview, and provides significant resources and comfort to people in times of stress. Therefore, cultural sensitivity in care delivery supports health promotion and disease prevention. Yearwood (2006, p. 162) adds, "all healthcare providers would benefit from the knowledge exchange that occurs in environments that acknowledge and embrace diversity."

Culture is an important context from which to view a person or family. Cultural competence is defined as the "ability of individuals to establish effective interpersonal and working relationships that supersede cultural differences" (IOM, 2002, p. 554). The Surgeon General's report on *Mental Health: Culture, Race, Ethnicity* (2001) defines culture broadly as "a common heritage or set of beliefs, norms, and values." Cultural diversity finds expression in the patient's language, decision-making, food preferences, and ethnically influenced responses to stress, pain, sorrow, anger, bereavement, and the meaning of a mental illness.

The 2002 IOM report indicated that racial and ethnic minorities typically receive a lower quality of health care than nonminorities, even when the patient's insurance status and income are matched. Health disparities are defined as "the differences in care experienced by one population when compared to other populations." Kira and others (2014) suggest that cumulative effects of chronic identity traumatic discrimination, in the form of "chronic micro-aggressions (e.g., insults), intermittent macroaggressions (e.g., hate crimes), and proliferation, stress generation, and accumulative dynamics are inherent in discrimination" (p. 251) are often internalized and may facilitate the development of PTSD.

Federal initiatives to improve access to care and to help eliminate health disparities among different sectors of the population are found through the U.S. Department of Health and Human Services in the *Healthy People 2020* document (2015). This document identifies national priorities for the health care of the nation. Updated and revised every 10 years, the Healthy People document sets forth measureable objectives for the health of the nation. Several areas target mental health and cultural aspects of mental health. *Healthy People 2020* states that culturally competent health care is essential to eliminating health disparities. Common concepts related to culture include diversity, stereotyping, acculturation, and assimilation.

- **Diversity** refers to differences between cultures. Variation among members of the same culture is also the rule, rather than the exception. Factors such as urbanization, education, socioeconomic status, first-hand exposures, and religion all affect the variations found among persons within the same culture.

- **Discrimination** is defined as "differences in care that emerge from biases and prejudice, stereotyping, and uncertainty in communication and clinical decision-making" (IOM, 2002, p. 160).

- **Stereotyping** refers to oversimplified beliefs about a person or cultural group, often based on inaccurate data or overgeneralizations (e.g., all mentally ill persons are dangerous).

- **Ethnocentrism** refers to the belief that one's own culture is superior to all others. "Ethnocentric views and practices within the treatment team can result in misdiagnosis, conflict, and ultimately poor treatment choices" (Yearwood, 2006, p. 161).

- **Acculturation** refers to a socialization process in which a person from a different cultural group begins to learn and adopt the language and behavior patterns of the dominant culture as a result of firsthand contact. Questions to ask include: "Are you able to speak with me in English?"

- **Assimilation** refers to the adoption of the behavior patterns of the dominant culture to such an extent that the original ethnic identification disappears or is suppressed. It usually occurs over several generations. Questions to ask include: "How long have you lived in the United States?"

Attaining Cultural Competence

To become culturally competent, the nurse initially must be willing to do so, as opposed to "remaining distant from others due to anxiety about unpredictability, or fear of stirring up defensiveness (Yearwood, 2006). Leininger, the founder of the transcultural nursing movement in education and research posits that "cultural care preservation or maintenance refers to nursing care activities that help people of particular cultures to retain and use core cultural care values related to healthcare concerns or conditions; cultural care accommodation or negotiation refers to creative nursing actions that help people of a particular culture adapt to or negotiate with others in the healthcare community in an effort to attain the shared goal of an optimal health outcome for patients of a designated culture" (Sitzman & Eichelberger, 2011, p 95). Each person is first an individual, and second a member of a cultural or ethnic group.

In health care, culture is expressed at individual, interpersonal, and community levels related to perceptions of etiology, symptom expression, and treatment expectations. Psychiatric–mental health nurses need to be aware of cultural differences and the meanings of mental illness and treatment when assessing patient learning needs and readiness to plan culturally sensitive health teaching interventions. The nurse must be willing to learn about the customs, values, and beliefs of persons from diverse backgrounds and be willing to understand his or her own beliefs as they pertain to cultural nuances. A way for the nurse to begin this process is to participate in or attend the customs, practices, and rituals of colleagues. Attend a birth or death celebration; try a different food. Learn a different language. Invite diverse people to your gatherings. Metaphorically walk in someone else's shoes to strengthen empathic understanding.

Consider the level of patient involvement in formal healthcare systems and with traditional healers and healing rituals. Assess the meaning of mental health symptoms as they relate to cultural norms and are understood by various cultures. Elicit the patient's understanding and acceptance of biomedical models, including use of prescriptions, alternative forms of healing, effect of political and access factors on health practices, implications for taking medications (what this means to the patient and the patient's family). Gauge the patient's cultural heritage and belief systems. Doornbos and others (2014) point to the importance of attending to communication and patterns of interaction among diverse, impoverished, and underserved groups of women to solicit group and contextual understanding and meaning of shared personal stories. A mnemonic model that outlines elements that are important for engaging with patients from culturally diverse backgrounds is **LEARN**.

L = Listen with empathy.

E = Explain your perceptions of the patient's problem.

A = Acknowledge similarities and differences in perceptions.

R = Recommend treatment.

N = Negotiate treatment.

When constructing the most appropriate treatment formats for culturally diverse patients, psychiatric–mental health nurses take the following into consideration:

- The patient's language and ease of oral and written expression
- Differences in affective expression
- Meaning of nonverbal symbols, tone of voice, gestures, physical space
- Family structure, gender differences, family roles
- Rituals, particularly around births, deaths
- Religious practices and beliefs
- Level of self-disclosure permitted by culture
- Behavioral etiquette and taboo topics
- Social class distinctions
- Dietary taboos
- Meaning of space and distance
- Sexual orientation and preferences
- Comfort level with eye contact
- Time orientation (past, present, future)
- Comfort level with touch
- Observance of holidays

A cultural assessment would identify the following:

- Explanatory models of illness
- Traditional healing practices
- Lifestyle issues
- Types of family support and decision-making in health situations
- Spiritual healing practices and rituals
- Cultural norms about illness and modesty
- Truth-telling and level of disclosure about serious or terminal illness
- Ritual and religious ceremonies at time of death (Arnold & Boggs, 2007)
- How the person identifies him- or herself: "Can you tell me what race and ethnicity you belong to?"

- Immigration and degree of acculturation: How long has the person been in this country? Affinity of the person to the native culture or to the host culture.

- Experience with family deportation or threats of deportation

- Language use, abilities, and preferences: Does the person have a working or good command of the language?

- Cultural interpretations of functional levels: "How do you define health, or wellness?"

Cultural factors affect the expression and prevalence of mental disorders, as well as the interpretation of assessment data and treatment options. Several culturally specific formulations are listed within the *Diagnostic and Statistical Manual of Mental Disorders,* Fifth edition (DSM5; APA, 2013):

- **Acculturation problem:** The focus of clinical attention is a problem involving adjustment to a different culture.

- **Culture-bound syndromes:** Mental disorders particular to certain cultures.

  - *Examples:* Amok (Malaysia), Brain Fag (West Africa), Ataque de nervios (Latin America), and Evil Eye (Mediterranean cultures)

Communication With Special Population Groups

Effective communication requires that psychiatric nurses modify or adapt their communication styles to accommodate the specialized needs of patients they serve. This can include sensory alterations (visual, hearing impaired), speaking a different language, literacy level, developmental stage, or cognitive status (Potter & Perry, 2009). All communication strategies involve the psychiatric–mental health nurse decisively and deliberately reinforcing positive behaviors and communications.

Expressive language disorder, mixed receptive-expressive language disorder, phonological stuttering, and communication disorder not otherwise specified (NOS) are all classified as communication disorders. The most common expressive language disorder in younger children is *phonological disorder*, which is a failure to use developmentally expected speech sounds appropriate for the age and gender of the child. This involves failure to form speech sounds correctly—lisping is common. When there is a disturbance in fluency and language formulation, *cluttering*—an abnormally rapid rate and erratic rhythm of speech and disturbances in language structure—may occur. The developmental type of expressive language disorder is usually recognized by age 3. An essential feature in *stuttering* is a disturbance in the normal fluency and time patterning of speech that is appropriate for the child's age. It may be accompanied by motor movements and can be brought on by stress or anxiety. Male to female ratio is 3:1. Onset is usually between 2 and 7 years old. The acquired (functional) type of expressive language disorder because of strokes, brain lesions, head trauma, and so on, will have sudden onset and occur at any age. Communication modifications for different needs are described below.

Patients With Visual Impairments

▸ Make sure the patient has appropriate glasses or contacts.

▸ Use large print for visual instructions.

▸ Use a normal tone and pace for conversation.

▸ Orient the patient to the area, describing significant elements and boundaries.

▸ Identify yourself when entering the patient's space.

▸ Look directly at the patient when speaking.

Patients With Hearing Impairments

▸ Minimize background noise.

▸ Always face the patient when speaking.

▸ Speak slowly, in a normal tone; the tone can be slightly raised if the person is not completely deaf (do not shout).

▸ If the patient has a hearing aid, make sure the patient is wearing it, and that it is turned on.

▸ Rephrase, rather than repeat if the communication is not understood.

Patients With Cognitive Impairments

▸ Assess the patient's ability to communicate.

▸ Make adaptations with simpler, concrete words if needed.

▸ Speak slowly and clearly.

▸ Repeat or rephrase questions if the patient looks puzzled.

▸ Use simple questions and allow extra time for response.

▸ Look at and speak directly to the patient.

Patients Who Are Aggressive or Uncooperative

Aggressiveness in mental health settings has many possible causes, and can be exacerbated by comorbid substance abuse, impulsiveness, hallucinations (particularly command hallucinations), dementia, or antisocial personality traits. Patients with mental retardation can become violent when exposed to chaotic circumstances or overcrowding. Delirium and other forms of severe brain dysfunction caused by medical or psychiatric disorders can also stimulate aggressive episodes. Basically, any situation in which a patient feels loss of control can stimulate anger and potential aggression.

Most patients who are angry, manipulative, or uncooperative are extremely anxious and feel misunderstood. Addressing the deeper-rooted anxiety and validating the patient's feelings can help defuse a tense situation. Other facilitative strategies include expressing caring and empathy: "I can see that you are very upset. How can I help you?" or "I can see that you are angry; may I take your blood pressure and pulse because I am concerned about your heart; it must be beating so fast."

- Observe for prodromal signs of impending tension (eyes or mouth twitching, pacing, flinging arms, spitting, increased agitation).

- Check for nonverbal messages. Say "I notice that you are wringing your hands and you are pacing down the hallway. Can you tell me what you are feeling?"

- Be aware that the patient's words reflect his or her feelings about a stressful situation and are not directed toward you personally.

- Address the patient by name, and speak in a low, calm voice.

- Assess the environment and the patient for signs of escalating tension. Identify triggers. Remember that aggressive patients may be experiencing intense anxiety and may not be able to explain the cause of their agitation.

- Give the patient extra space; avoid crowding the patient; this may be misinterpreted as aggression or a desire to control.

- Use "I" statements, with concrete comments. *Example:* "I am concerned about your safety and the safety of others right now, because you are swearing and yelling loudly. I need for you to quiet down so we can figure this out."

- Own your own feelings.

- Criticize the behavior, not the person: "I want you to know that I care about your and others' health on this unit. However, your behavior of yelling and stomping around the unit is not acceptable."

- Do positive stroking: Find something genuinely positive to say, such as "I admire how you were able to calm down after your father came to visit. I am confident you can calm down today, as well."

- Point out what is in it for the patient: "I really can't help you, unless we can talk about it in a calmer way."

- Give a balancing message: "I know that what you are going through is very difficult for you. However, I know that you have the strength within you to cope in a manner that will help you in the long run."

- Summon extra help for a "show of support." Do not try to subdue an aggressive patient by yourself; use a planned team approach.

Communication in Conflict Situations

Conflicts are inevitable, and working through them can make a relationship stronger. Conflict resolution is a professional performance standard expected of the psychiatric–mental health nurse (see Chapter 7). Encourage collaboration, which stimulates cooperation.

- Both parties state their problem.
  - Use "I" statements.
  - Indicate a willingness to help resolve the problem.
  - Stick to the topic at hand.
- Hear the other person's point of view.
  - Acknowledge the other person' anger.
  - Don't interrupt unless patient is repeating him- or herself, then rephrase what was said.
- Acknowledge the patient's viewpoint.
  - Ask clarifying questions.
  - Use silence.
  - Rehearse.
- Look for areas of agreement.
  - Point out mutual interests.
  - Make an optimistic statement.
- Request behavior changes only.
- Help patients help themselves develop realistic solutions.
- Whenever possible, focus on solutions that satisfy the needs of both parties.

Patients for Whom English Is a Second Language

The Joint Commission mandates the use of a trained interpreter when necessary for patient-provider communication, with criteria published under Title VI of the Civil Rights Act. Nurses should learn simple words in the patient's language relevant to the treatment protocols. Often, however, this is not sufficient for patients with little or no fluency in English. There are federal mandates related to accommodation for language differences in providing culturally competent care. Every patient is entitled by law to have an interpreter, if needed to understand assessment or treatment protocols. Children and family members should not be used as interpreters. Compatibility between the ethnic backgrounds of the interpreter and patient is advised whenever possible, because persons from different regions in the same country may use different dialects. Guidelines for working with interpreters include:

▸ Get an interpreter. Provide the interpreter with a brief summary of the patient.

▸ Explain confidentiality and limits to confidentiality.

▸ Explain to the patient the role of the interpreter.

▸ Allow extra time for the translation and responses, particularly when word interpretation is not enough for understanding.

▸ Explain to the patient that you may need to ask additional questions for clarification.

▸ Provide opportunities to educate the interpreter about practices and technical terms.

▸ Ask for additional information about nonverbal cues, speech patterns, vocal tone, and other information needed to understand the patient or context of the communication.

▸ Avoid using family members as interpreters.

▸ Speak slowly and clearly.

▸ Use simple language and pause between sentences.

▸ Validate the patient's understanding by asking for frequent, brief summaries.

▸ Look at the patient when speaking, even when using an interpreter.

▸ Make allowances for differences in idioms, personal space, ritual, expression of emotions, parent-child interactions, customs, etc.

▸ Allow extra time for the interview.

Patients From a Different Culture

Communication is always to some degree culture-bound, and culture should be considered a critical component in professional therapeutic relationships. Because people respond to situations and experiences based on their worldviews and personal values, it is important for nurses to be aware of personal cultural orientations in therapeutic conversations with patients from different ethnic groups. Madeleine Leininger's Theory of Transcultural Nursing (Sunrise model) offers a good review of the areas of culturally sensitive beliefs, values, and practices that nurses need to incorporate as background information in therapeutic conversations with ethnically diverse patients. (Leininger, 2002).

At the same time, each patient is different. There is more variation in values within a culture than between cultures. Asking patients directly about cultural interpretations of mental illness and treatment is as important as having a basic cultural knowledge of ethnic values and behaviors. Incorporating ethnic values and paying attention to the cultural concerns of patients from different cultures are essential steps that increase understanding and make conversations go more smoothly. Other relevant communication strategies include:

▶ Keep questions simple, concrete, and specific.

▶ Choose unambiguous words with single, rather than connotative, meanings.

▶ Respect differences in the amount of interpersonal space and meaning of body language among different cultural groups.

▶ Ask only one question at a time.

▶ Use multiple methods to convey information (e.g., pictures, physical cues).

▶ Have the patient repeat back, in his or her own words, key ideas, and teaching content.

Patients With Different Spiritual and Religious Beliefs

Spirituality is defined as a person's values and beliefs about his or her place in the universe and the presence of a higher power in matters of life, health, and death. It is a state of wellness that may incorporate a sense of fulfillment and purpose in life. It may be expressed in terms such as peace, love, meditation, and joy. Spiritual orientation is often an important way for people to make sense of their illnesses and the things that are happening to them. Spirituality gives many patients a measured sense of control over their illnesses and has been associated with positive outcomes, such as a decrease in mental symptoms (Carson & Koenig, 2008).

Although religious content can be reflected as pathological symptomatology in persons with mental illness, nurses will need to be able to distinguish between pathologic religiosity and spiritual dependence on a higher power. Many persons with mental illness experience loneliness and isolation. Believing that a personal god is always with you can be comforting and strengthening. Basic concepts surrounding some of the major religious beliefs and practices are listed:

▶ **Christianity:** Offers healing prayers; receiving sacraments of Communion and the Anointing of the Sick for sick and dying persons.

▶ **Judaism:** Offers healing prayers; Kosher/Parve dietary practices; no shellfish, pork.

▶ **Hinduism:** One's beliefs determine one's thoughts and actions in life; Karma; vegetarian diet.

▶ **Jehovah's Witness:** Receiving blood or blood products is taboo.

▶ **Muslim:** Submission to God ideology; prayer beads provide comfort; halal dietary practices; no pork.

Spiritual worldviews, including atheism and agnosticism, develop over time. A person's spiritual orientation may or may not be tied to a defined religious framework. Nurses need to be aware of, objective, and nonjudgmental about a patient's religious and spiritual beliefs. Basic nursing actions that demonstrate spiritual support include encouraging hope, supporting religious or spiritual practices (prayer beads, rosaries, etc., at bedside).

The Joint Commission (TJC), formerly the Joint Commission on Accreditation of Healthcare Organizations, mandates that each person's psychiatric evaluation needs to include an assessment of spiritual needs, the role that spirituality plays in the patient's life, the patient's spiritual goals, and the types of supports the patient desires to help cope more effectively with his or her illness. The purpose of doing a spiritual assessment is to determine the most appropriate actions needed to address these issues. The spiritual needs assessment should include the patient's denomination, beliefs, and spiritual practices that are important to the patient, and information should be documented in the patient's plan of care. Assessment data with related actions must be documented in the patient's care plan. Even with mental illness, people seek to find a purposeful life. On its website, TJC includes sample questions to ask patients and their families about spiritual needs (TJC, 2008).

The language of faith is often learned before a mental illness develops. Some patients find spirituality painful because they view their illness as a punishment from God, or a betrayal of their adherence to religious beliefs. For these patients, helping them to correct or decrease the impact of painful feelings associated with negative spiritual images can be a useful intervention. Cognitive strategies can help these patients question the validity of their current thinking, and shift their negative spiritual images to more productive explanations of the role of a higher power in their lives.

WRITTEN COMMUNICATION AND DOCUMENTATION OF CARE

The Medical Record

Written documentation of the patient assessment, treatment, patient response, and progress is an important component of the communication process in psychiatric–mental health nursing. Documentation refers to the written legal recording of patient care. Unless care is documented in the patient's record, from a legal perspective, it is as though it was not done. The patient's medical record is often presented in court as evidence of assessment and treatment. In many instances, the written medical record is the sole informant about the care given to patients.

Written communication and documentation includes objective and subjective assessment data about the patient's condition or mental health issues, interprofessional plans and treatment, restrictive measures if used, treatment plan and outcome documentation, risk assessment documentation, mental status, occurrence reports, and treatment response.

Charted documentation is written in ink with no erasures. If there is a mistake in the documentation, the nurse should cross out the error with one line, insert the corrected information if needed, and initial the change. Charting should be completed after the care is given, not before. The three most common documentation methods include narrative documentation, SOAP notes, and focus charting. A fourth method, exception charting, is used in some agencies and institutions (Arnold & Boggs, 2007). Flowcharts and checklists are used by many agencies to document routine, ongoing assessments, and patient responses. Information recorded on flow sheets or checklists is not repeated in the progress notes.

Documentation Formats

Documentation Elements and Types

- ▶ Objective
- ▶ Subjective
- ▶ Interprofessional
- ▶ Restrictive measures
- ▶ Treatment plan and outcome documentation
- ▶ Risk assessment documentation
- ▶ Mental status
- ▶ Occurrence report

Narrative documentation reflects the format of the nursing process. It includes objective and subjective assessment data about the patient's condition or mental health issues, interprofessional plans and treatment, restrictive measures if used, treatment plan and outcome documentation, risk assessment documentation, mental status, occurrence reports, treatment response, and so on. The data is recorded in sequential order covering a specified time frame. Depending on the facility, flow sheets and checklists can be used to document routine care such as activities of daily living, personal care, vital signs, and so on, as well as standardized observations.

Problem-oriented charting (SOAP/SOAPIER) is a format in which the nurse lists patient problems in order of priority, followed by the plan, intervention, and evaluation, including any needed changes or revisions. The following headings are used in problem-oriented charting.

S = Subjective data: What patient says verbatim is placed in closed quotation marks.

O = Objective data: What the nurse can see or what data can be obtained (e.g., vital signs).

A = Assessment data: What the nurse finds that is important to the well-being or status.

P = Plan: What the nurse intends or anticipates needs to be done.

I = Intervention: What the nurse actually does.

E = Evaluation: Results of the intervention.

R = Revision: Modifications or changes necessary to promote well-being.

Focus charting requires the nurse to identify a particular focus based on a careful assessment of individualized patient behaviors or health concerns. The focus can be directly on a particular behavior or concern, such as aggressive or catatonic behavior, or it can reflect a change in a patient's condition or behavior, such as a delirium. It can also reflect a significant event in the patient's treatment, for example, an ECT treatment. With focus charting, the nurse documents:

- Subjective and objective data, supporting the stated focus.
- Actions: Completed nursing interventions related to the nurse's focused assessment.
- Response: Description of the patient's response, and the effect of interventions on patient outcomes.

Documentation by exception: Some clinical agencies use documentation by exception, a type of charting that assumes that assessment findings, nursing interventions, and clinical outcomes will follow the agency's established written standards of care. Charting by exception assumes that all relevant standards of care have been met with the expected treatment response, unless documented otherwise. The only other exclusion is for medication administration, which must be charted directly. *Example:* Check the "WNL" versus "not WNL" box. Formats:

- Flow sheets
- Clinical pathways

SBAR documentation: Standardized communication of expectations related to patient event.

Situation = statement of the problem

Background = brief, pertinent information related to situation

Assessment = what was found?

Recommendation = what recommendation is necessary?

Occurrence documentation: Document occurrences when care or patient response is outside of expected norms that may affect care quality or patient safety. Follow institutional policy and use appropriate forms. *Examples:*

- Sentinel events
- Quality variances
- Infectious disease
- Medication errors
- Patient harm

Use of Information Technology in Documentation

In an era when hospitals, agencies, and organizations are invested in protection of patients' personal health information (PHI) and moving towards the electronic medical record (EMR) or electronic health record (EHR) for record documentation and maintenance, nurses are seen as key stakeholders who possess the knowledge and clinical expertise to help systems with the translation of the current pen and paper format. Challenges lie in creating entities that can accurately describe clinical conditions, and simultaneously have the requisite "scrambling" and privacy elements to handle sensitive, personal, and potentially stigmatizing information. In this case, all the principles identified above for charting formats, access, storage, and retrieval of patient information are identical to those that govern paper-based documentation. Nurses must ensure the complete integrity of the electronic record. Of particular importance is the need to carefully protect personal identification numbers or passwords. Passwords should not be shared or revealed to others. They should not be easily decipherable. Nurses should always log off when leaving a terminal or otherwise not using the system, and protect patient information displayed on monitors while using the system. An additional concern is the potential for copying and pasting clinical summations derived from a different provider. This potential for cloning can be considered fraudulent documentation by compliance and legal experts (Repique, 2014). Workgroups are addressing these issues.

Use of Technology

The rise in Health Information Technology (HIT) services to facilitate care coordination, and integration of data systems, represent an initiative brought forward by "meaningful use" legislation. This legislation supports the mandate for electronic health records (EHR). *Telehealth* services that connect patient to provider by way of internet resources are additional methods for assessing and monitoring patients who live in distant or rural communities. The recent emergence of *textual healing* online therapy services connects patients with licensed therapists by way of smartphone technology (Fruhlinger, 2014). For a flat fee, online therapists provide texting services as a new way to connect with patients.

REFERENCES

American Psychiatric Association. (2013). *Diagnostic and statistical manual of mental disorders, 5th ed.* Arlington, VA: American Psychiatric Publishing.

American Nurses Association, International Society of Psychiatric–Mental Health Nurses, and American Psychiatric Nurses Association. (2014). *Psychiatric–mental health nursing: Scope and standards of practice, 2nd ed.* Silver Spring, MD: Nursesbooks.org.

Arnold, E., & Boggs. K. (2007). *Interpersonal relations in nursing, 5th ed.* Philadelphia: Elsevier.

Benner, P. (1984). *From novice to expert.* Baltimore: Wolters Kluwer Health.

Campinha-Bacote, J. (2011). Delivering patient-centered care in the midst of a cultural conflict: The role of cultural competence. *The Online Journal of Issues in Nursing, 16*(2), Manuscript 5. Retrieved from http://www.nursingworld.org/MainMenuCategories/ANAMarketplace/ANAPeriodicals/OJIN/TableofContents/Vol-16-2011/No2-May-2011/Delivering-Patient-Centered-Care-in-the-Midst-of-a-Cultural-Conflict.html.

Carson V & Koenig H. (Eds.). (2008). *Spiritual dimensions of nursing practice.* West Conshohocken, PA: Templeton Foundation Press.

Cross T. L., Bazron B. J., Dennis K. W., & Isaacs M. R. (1989). *Towards a culturally competent system of care: A monograph on effective services for minority children who are severely emotionally disturbed: Vol I.* Georgetown University Press.

Dillon, N. (2014). Risky business: *Walking the boundaries tightrope.* Paper presented at the 27th Annual American Psychiatric Nurses Association ATP Conference. Reston, VA.

Doornbos, M. M., Zandee, G. L., & DeGroot, J. (2014). Attending to communication and patterns of interaction: Culturally sensitive mental health care for groups of urban, ethnically diverse, impoverished, and underserved women. *Journal of the American Psychiatric Nurses Association, 20*(4), 239–249.

Fawcett, J. (2005). *Contemporary nursing knowledge: Analysis and evaluation of nursing models and theories, 2nd ed.* Philadelphia: F. A. Davis.

The Freeman Institute. (n.d.). *The Johari window.* Retrieved from www.joharigame.com.

Fruhlinger, J. (2014, October 18–19). Textual healing. *Wall Street Journal*; p. D11.

Gutheil, T., & Gabbarad, G. (1993). The concept of boundaries in clinical practice: Theoretical and risk management dimensions. *American Journal of Psychiatry, 150,* 188–196.

Institute of Medicine. (Smedley, B. D., Stith, A.Y., & Nelson, A.R., Eds). (2002). *Unequal treatment: Confronting racial and ethnic disparities in health care.* Washington, DC: The National Academies Press.

Jackson, J. S., Knight, K. M., & Rafferty, J. A. (2009). Race and unhealthy behaviors: Chronic stress, the HPA axis, and physical and mental health disparities over the life course. *American Journal of Public Health; 99*(12), 1–7.

The Joint Commission. (2008). *Spiritual assessment.* Retrieved from http://www.jointcommission.org/mobile/standards_information/jcfaqdetails.aspx?StandardsFAQId=290&StandardsFAQChapterId=29.

Kira, I. A., Lewandowski, L., Ashby, J. S., Templin, T., Ramaswamy, V., & Mohanesh, J. (2014). The traumatogenic dynamics of internalized stigma of mental illness among Arab American, Muslim, and refugee clients. *Journal of the American Psychiatric Nurses Association; 20*(4); 250–266.

Leininger, M. (2002). Culture care theory: A major contribution to advance transcultural nursing knowledge and practices. *J Transcult Nurs, 13*(3); 188–192.

Lipson, J. G., & Dibble, S. L. (Eds.) (2005). *Culture and clinical care, 2nd ed.* San Francisco: UCSF Nursing Press.

Luft, J., & Ingham, H. (1955). The Johari window: A graphic model of interpersonal awareness. *Proceedings of the Western Training Laboratory in Group Development.* Los Angeles: UCLA.

Marrs, J., & Lowery, L. (2006). Nursing theory and practice: Connecting the dots. *Nursing Science Quarterly, 19*(1), 44–50.

Newman, C. (2005). Too close for comfort: Defining boundary issues in the professional-client relationship. *Rehabilitation & Community Care Medicine, Spring;* 7–9.

Nightingale, F. (1980). *Notes on nursing: What it is, and what it is not.* New York: Appleton & Co. Retrieved from http://digital.library.upenn.edu/women/nightingale/nursing/nursing.html.

Office of the U.S. Surgeon General: Center for Mental Health Services: National Institute of Mental Health. (2001, Aug.). Mental health: *Culture, race, and ethnicity: A supplement to mental health: A report of the Surgeon General.* Rockville, MD: Substance Abuse and Mental Health Services Administration.

Peplau, H. E. (1997). Peplau's theory of interpersonal relations. *Nursing Science Quarterly, 10*(4), 162–167.

Peterneij-Taylor, C. A., & Yonge, O. (2003). Exploring boundaries in the nurse-client relationship: Professional roles and responsibilities. *Perspectives in Psychiatric Care, 39*(2), 55–66.

Potter, P. & Perry, A. (2009). *Fundamentals of nursing, 7th ed.* St. Louis, MO: Mosby Elsevier.

Repique, R. J. R. (2014). Cloning in electronic mental health record: Understanding the perils and suggested safeguards. *Journal of the American Psychiatric Nurses Association, 20*(4), 268–270.

Sitzman, K. & Eichelberger, L. W. (2011). *Understanding the works of nurse theorists: A creative beginning, 2nd ed.,* (pp. 101–108). Boston: Jones & Bartlett.

Stuart, G. W. (2009). *Principles and practices of psychiatric nursing, 9th ed.* Philadelphia: Mosby.

U.S. Department of Health and Human Services (2015). *Healthy people 2020.* Retrieved from http://www.healthypeople.gov/sites/default/files/DefaultPressRelease_1.pdf.

Yearwood, E. L. (August, 2006). The "problem" of cultural diversity. *Journal of Child and Adolescent Psychiatric Nursing;* 19(3), 161–162.

CHAPTER 7

ELEMENTS OF PROFESSIONALISM IN NURSING PRACTICE

The registered nurse who practices psychiatric–mental health nursing at the basic level has demonstrated the skills outlined in *Psychiatric–Mental Health Nursing: Scope and Standards of Practice, 2nd ed.* (ANA, 2014) as addressed in earlier chapters. The *Scope and Standards of Practice* represents a consensus document among three professional groups: American Nurses Association (ANA), International Society for Psychiatric Nursing (ISPN), and American Psychiatric Nurses Association (APNA). The publication delineates the scope and standards of clinical practice across clinical healthcare settings, incorporating a nursing process format at both basic and advanced practice levels to identify a competent, safe level of care for patients with psychiatric and mental health issues. It provides six standards of professional nursing practice and nine standards of professional performance. For quick reference, the *Scope and Standards of Psychiatric–Mental Health Nursing Practice* are listed below.

Professional Practice Standards

Standard I. Assessment
The Psychiatric–Mental Health Registered Nurse collects and synthesizes comprehensive health data that are pertinent to the patient's health and/or situation.

Standard 2. Diagnosis
The Psychiatric–Mental Health Registered Nurse analyzes the assessment data to determine diagnoses, problems, and areas of focus for care and treatment, including level of risk.

Standard 3. Outcomes Identification

The Psychiatric–Mental Health Registered Nurse identifies expected outcomes and the patient's goals for a plan individualized to the patient or to the situation.

Standard 4. Planning

The Psychiatric–Mental Health Registered Nurse develops a plan that prescribes strategies and alternatives to assist the patient in attainment of expected outcomes.

Standard 5. Implementation

The Psychiatric–Mental Health Registered Nurse implements the identified plan.

> ▸ **Standard 5A. Coordination of Care**
>
> The Psychiatric–Mental Health Registered Nurse coordinates care delivery.

> ▸ **Standard 5B. Health Teaching and Health Promotion**
>
> The Psychiatric–Mental Health Registered Nurse uses strategies to promote health and a safe environment.

> ▸ **Standard 5C. Consultation**
>
> The Psychiatric–Mental Health Advanced Practice* Registered Nurse provides consultation to influence the identified plan, enhance the abilities of other clinicians to provide services for patients, and effect change.
>
> *No additional information is discussed in this chapter because this standard applies only to Advanced Practice nurses.*

> ▸ **Standard 5D. Prescriptive Authority and Treatment**
>
> The Psychiatric–Mental Health Advanced Practice* Registered Nurse uses prescriptive authority, procedures, referrals, treatments, and therapies in accordance with state and federal laws and regulations.
>
> *No additional information is discussed in this chapter because this standard applies only to Advanced Practice nurses.*

> ▸ **Standard 5E. Pharmacological, Biological, and Integrative Therapies**
>
> The Psychiatric–Mental Health Registered Nurse incorporates knowledge of pharmacological, biological, and complementary interventions with applied clinical skills to restore the patient's health and prevent disability.

> ▸ **Standard 5F. Milieu Therapy**
>
> The Psychiatric–Mental Health Registered Nurse provides, structures, and maintains a safe, therapeutic, recovery-oriented environment in collaboration with patients, families, and other healthcare clinicians.

▶ **Standard 5G. Therapeutic Relationship and Counseling**

The Psychiatric–Mental Health Registered Nurse uses the therapeutic relationship and counseling interventions to assist patients in their individual recovery journeys by regaining and improving their previous coping abilities, fostering mental health, and preventing mental disorder and disability.

▶ **Standard 5H. Psychotherapy**

The Psychiatric–Mental Health Advanced Practice* Registered Nurse conducts individual, couples, group, and family psychotherapy using evidence-based psychotherapeutic frameworks and nurse-client therapeutic relationships.

No additional information is discussed in this chapter because this standard applies only to Advanced Practice nurses.

Standard 6. Evaluation

The Psychiatric–Mental Health Registered Nurse evaluates progress toward attainment of expected outcomes.

In addition, this chapter examines the 10 *Standards of Professional Performance* outlines of nursing action steps that demonstrate professional behavior enhancement. The standards describe a competence level of professional role behaviors in professional psychiatric–mental health nursing practice. Application of professional standards promotes high-quality nursing care, which helps to advance the purposes of the profession and the healthcare of the nation. Professional standards also have significance as a resource for personal development, peer review, and work performance appraisal processes and are an important means of evaluating and improving care through the implementation of quality improvement programs. The 10 *Standards of Professional Performance* are identified are described below.

Professional Performance Standards

Standard 7. Ethics

The Psychiatric–Mental Health Registered Nurse integrates ethical provision in all areas of practice.

Standard 8. Education

The Psychiatric–Mental Health Registered Nurse attains knowledge and competence that reflect current nursing practice.

Standard 9. Evidence-Based Practice and Research

The Psychiatric–Mental Health Registered Nurse integrates evidence and research findings into practice.

Standard 10. Quality of Practice

The Psychiatric–Mental Health Registered Nurse systematically enhances the quality and effectiveness of nursing practice.

Standard 11. Communication

The Psychiatric–Mental Health Registered Nurse communicates effectively in a variety of formats in all areas of practice.

Standard 12. Leadership

The Psychiatric–Mental Health Registered Nurse provides leadership in the professional practice setting and the profession.

Standard 13. Collaboration

The Psychiatric–Mental Health Registered Nurse collaborates with the patient, family, interprofessional health team, and others in the conduct of nursing practice.

Standard 14. Professional Practice Evaluation

The Psychiatric–Mental Health Registered Nurse evaluates his or her own practice in relation to the professional practice standards and guidelines, relevant statutes, rules, and regulations.

Standard 15. Resource Utilization

The Psychiatric–Mental Health Registered Nurse considers factors related to safety, effectiveness, cost, and impact on practice in the planning and delivery of nursing services.

Standard 16. Environmental Health

The Psychiatric–Mental Health Registered Nurse practices in an environmentally safe and healthy manner.

FACTORS AFFECTING SCOPE OF PRACTICE

Nurses can be held liable for failing to perform nursing care in accordance with state laws and within the scope and standards of professional nursing practice (e.g., failure to obtain informed consent, report a change in the patient's condition, take appropriate action to provide for a patient's safety). Several factors affect the actual scope of practice for psychiatric–mental health nurses, including licensure and allowable practices within particular clinical settings. The American Nurses Association's *Nursing's Social Policy Statement* (2003) and Institute of Medicine's (2001; 2011) recommendations for patient-centered care, transformative care at the bedside, and accountabilities for nurses to practice to their full scope broaden the nurse's understanding of published professional standards of psychiatric nursing practice and professional performance.

TABLE 7-1.
SELECTED STATEMENTS FROM NURSING'S SOCIAL POLICY STATEMENT

Values and Assumptions
Humans manifest an essential unity of mind, body, and spirit.
Human experience is contextually and culturally defined.
Health and illness are human experiences.
The presence of illness does not preclude health, nor does optimal health preclude illness.
Essential Features of Professional Nursing
Attention to the full range of human experiences and responses to health and illness without restriction to a problem-focused orientation.
Integration of objective data with knowledge gained from an understanding of the healthcare consumer's or group's subjective experience.
Application of scientific knowledge to the processes of diagnosis and treatment.
Provision of a caring relationship that facilitates health and healing.

© 2003 American Nurses Association. Reprinted with permission.

American Nurses Association's Social Policy Statement

Nursing's Social Policy Statement (ANA, 2010) is a document that nurses can use as a framework for understanding the profession's relationships to society and its obligation to those who receive nursing care. Nursing is dynamic, not static, and reflects the changing nature of societal needs. Table 7–1 presents the ANA *Social Policy Statement* for the nursing profession.

State Licensure

The overarching scope of practice for psychiatric–mental health nurses is established by the profession and is published through the professional association for nurses, the ANA. Specific guidelines and licensure requirements are state-regulated through each state's Board of Nursing. "Boards of Nursing are state governmental agencies that are responsible for the regulation of nursing practice in each respective state. Boards of Nursing are authorized to enforce the Nurse Practice Act, develop administrative rules and regulations and (carry out) other responsibilities per the Nurse Practice Act" (National Council of State Boards of Nursing, 2008). Each state has its own requirements, rules, and regulations for nursing practice. Nurses need to consult the latest versions, because these documents are regularly revised and updated. Scope of practice regulations differ for basic and advanced practice nurses in most states. Nurses are responsible for practicing in accordance with state laws. Just as a driver's license is attainable when standardized practices are recognized, applied, and adhered to, a nursing license is granted when compliance is demonstrated to provisions of safe and accountable quality care. Either could be revoked by failing to maintain safe, quality practices.

Multistate (Compact) Licensure

Registered nurses legally residing in a nurse licensure compact state are eligible for multistate professional licenses. A mutual recognition model of nurse licensure, multistate licensing is the result of legislative action to allow professional nurses to practice across state lines without having to secure a separate license in each state. This model allows a nurse to have one license (in his or her state of residency) and to practice in other compact states (both physically and electronically) without having to secure an additional RN license. The nurse is subject to each state's practice laws and discipline. Under mutual recognition, a nurse may practice across state lines unless otherwise restricted. The state of residence, not the state of practice, determines the licensure-granting state. Over the past few years, more than half the nation's states have enacted the RN and LPN/LVN nurse licensure compact.

Nursing staff at all levels and in all settings are being called upon to practice to the fullest extent of their license (Institute of Medicine [IOM], 2011). This invitation is extended to the most honest and ethical healthcare providers—nurses (Gallup Poll, 2013)—owing to our broad insight into, and far-reaching effect on, not only patients and families, but the entire system as well. Psychiatric–mental health nurses are in positions to identify system strengths and constraints given our unique perspective that can only be provided by 24/7 caregivers. It is time, in this currently fragmented healthcare system, to step forward, assure accountability, and voice collective insights. Standing tall and responsibly on professional performance standards provides the nursing profession with latitude and leverage to assume our part in improving the health opportunities for all patients. Examples of how Professional Performance Standards 7 through 15 may be addressed are detailed below.

PSYCHIATRIC–MENTAL HEALTH PROFESSIONAL PERFORMANCE STANDARD 7. ETHICS

Ethics and legal protections that apply to care for the psychiatric patient often intersect. Nurses are primary partners for serving on ethics committees established by various healthcare organizations and systems. Again, the nurse's unique perspective adds a dimension to the equation as it relates to basic rights of persons to be educated, and to be cared for. The ANA Code of Ethics provides a framework for ethical decision-making. The American Nurses Association's *Code of Ethics for Nurses With Interpretive Statements* (2001) consists of nine provisions or proclamations describing the principled behaviors and professional attributes expected of professional nurses (see Table 7–2). These ethical provisions require that nurses uphold each patient's right to self-determination and extend entitlement to be treated with respect regardless of age, race, ethnicity, beliefs, type of illness, sexual orientation, or social status. This means that nurses should promote a healthcare environment that takes into account and respects the human values, cultural customs, and spiritual beliefs of their patients. Nurses also should maintain ethical standards of personal conduct compatible with the expectations of the profession and public confidence in the integrity of professional nurses. The values and obligations expressed in the ANA's Code of Ethics apply to all nurses in all roles and settings. Having a written professional code of ethics is particularly important at a time when the nation is undergoing fundamental changes in delivery of care that create important ethical dilemmas. Ethical standards are founded on the following assumptions:

▸ Ethical concepts cannot be considered apart from the social contextual environment in which they occur.

▸ Factors of family, religious, and cultural standards and beliefs are important determinants of ethical standards.

▸ Expected socialized behaviors of the profession serve to influence the nurse's understanding of ethical behavior.

TABLE 7-2.
NINE PROVISIONS OF ANA'S CODE OF ETHICS WITH INTERPRETIVE STATEMENTS

1	**Respect for the Individual** The nurse, in all professional relationships, practices with compassion and respect for the inherent dignity, worth, and uniqueness of every individual, unrestricted by considerations of social or economic status, personal attributes, or the nature of health problems.
2	**Commitment to the Patient** The nurse's primary commitment is to the patient, whether an individual, family, group, or community.
3	**Advocacy for the Patient** The nurse promotes, advocates for, and strives to protect the health, safety, and rights of the patient.
4	**Responsibility and Accountability for Practice** The nurse is responsible and accountable for individual nursing practice and determines the appropriate delegation of tasks consistent with the nurse's obligation to provide optimum patient care.
5	**Duties to Self and Others** The nurse owes the same duties to self as to others, including the responsibility to preserve integrity and safety, to maintain competence, and to continue personal and professional growth.
6	**Contributions to Healthcare Environments** The nurse participates in establishing, maintaining, and improving healthcare environments and conditions of employment conducive to the provision of quality healthcare and consistent with the values of the profession through individual and collective action.
7	**Advancement of the Nursing Profession** The nurse participates in the advancement of the profession through contributions to practice, education, administration, and knowledge development.
8	**Collaboration to Meet Health Needs** The nurse collaborates with other health professionals and the public in promoting community, national, and international efforts to meet health needs.
9	**Promotion of the Nursing Profession** The profession of nursing, as represented by associations and their members, is responsible for articulating nursing values, for maintaining the integrity of the profession and its practice, and for shaping social policy.

Theoretical Approaches to Ethics

Ethics is a formalized area of study that examines a person's values, beliefs, choices, and actions. Two prominent approaches provide guidelines for use in ethical decision-making:

1. **Utilitarianism (Teleology or Situational Ethics)**

   ▸ This approach focuses on the consequences of actions; the end justifies the means.

   ▸ Risk- or cost-benefit analysis is the basis for making ethical decisions.

   ▸ Ethical decisions reflect actions that would result in the greatest good for the largest number of people.

2. **Deontology**

   ▸ Actions can be evaluated ethically in and of themselves as being intrinsically right or wrong.

   ▸ Ethical decisions should be based on duty and obligation to others, absolute moral rules and principles that are fixed and do not change.

Key Components of Ethical Decision-Making

Ethical decision-making is based on professional values articulated in the *ANA Code of Ethics With Interpretative Statements* (2001). Key components of ethical decision-making are based on the following:

▸ **Justice:** Fairness to everyone, sound reason, rightfulness of decisions and actions

▸ **Beneficence:** The duty to do good, not harm, to others

▸ **Nonmaleficence:** The duty to do no harm to others, and to protect from harm those who cannot do so for themselves (e.g., children, mentally incompetent persons, survivors of abuse)

▸ **Fidelity:** The duty to be true and loyal to others

▸ **Autonomy:** The duty to protect the rights of a person to self-determination (i.e., to make decisions and take actions without external control)

▸ **Veracity:** The duty to tell the truth, and not to lie or deceive another

Basic ethical responsibilities of the psychiatric nurse are to

▸ Honor patient's confidentiality,

▸ Practice within area of expertise and competence,

▸ Maintain accurate patient records,

▸ Clarify nursing responsibilities to patients and families,

- Serve as a patient advocate,

- Maintain a therapeutic (purposeful) nurse-patient relationship,

- Demonstrate a commitment to self-care, and

- Participate on committees that determine ethical outcomes for patients, organizations, self.

An *ethical dilemma* is a situation in which a choice must be made between two or more potentially justifiable ethical choices. Examples seen in recent years include issues such as those listed below:

- Who has the rights to cells and body tissue excised during surgery? (Skloot, 2010)

- Eugenics

- Personal genetic mapping

- Treatment for uninsured

- Who gets the available heart or liver?

- Oral contraception for intellectually disabled

- Involuntary commitment

- Insanity defense

- What are the rights of same-sex couples to adoption, insemination? Should gender rules for children of same-sex parents be imposed?

- Allocation of resources in a hospital

- Right to refuse treatment

- Cultural conflicts between provider and patient regarding treatment

- Advocacy for patient rights to gender reassignment

PSYCHIATRIC–MENTAL HEALTH PROFESSIONAL PERFORMANCE STANDARD 8. EDUCATION

The psychiatric–mental health nurse is accountable for the ongoing acquisition of continued education to support improvements in care delivery and care delivery systems. As a member of a profession, the nurse leader examines trends in health care, attends professional meetings, and participates by sharing knowledge and information. Aiken, et al. (2014), a nurse leader and researcher, finds that when increased numbers of nursing staff are educated at the baccalaureate degree and higher, inpatient mortality is lower. Aiken's study examined this hypothesis, looking at staffing and education in nine European countries.

The Future of Nursing: Leading Change, Advancing Health (IOM, 2011) is an important and timely collaborative publication of the IOM and the Robert Wood Johnson Foundation (RWJF) that comprised experts from healthcare policy arenas, medicine, nursing, and academia. This report lays out some directive guidance for the nursing profession and professionals to steer the course forward in a rapidly changing healthcare environment. Four key messages for a fundamental transformation of the nursing profession are summarized below (pp. 28–34):

1. Nurses should practice to the full extent of their education and training.

2. Nurses should achieve higher levels of education and training through an improved education system that promotes seamless academic progression.

3. Nurses should be full partners, with physicians and other health professionals, in redesigning health care in the United States.

4. Effective workforce planning and policy-making require better data collection and an improved information infrastructure.

Eight specific recommendations are concluded by the committee (pp. 278–284):

1. Remove the scope-of-practice barriers.

2. Expand opportunities for nurses to lead and diffuse collaborative improvement efforts.

3. Implement nurse residency programs.

4. Increase the proportion of nurses with a baccalaureate degree to 80 percent by 2020.

5. Double the number of nurses with a doctorate by 2020.

6. Ensure that nurses engage in lifelong learning.

7. Prepare and enable nurses to lead change to advance health.

8. Build an infrastructure for the collection and analysis of inter-professional healthcare workforce data.

PSYCHIATRIC–MENTAL HEALTH PROFESSIONAL PERFORMANCE STANDARD 9. EVIDENCE-BASED PRACTICE AND RESEARCH

The professional performance standards specifically direct a role in research for registered nurses in nursing practice across all settings. Research is defined as the systematic gathering of information to gain, expand, or validate knowledge about health and responses to health problems. It follows, then, that *Research Utilization* is the use of research findings in practice. Like steps of the nursing process, the term *Outcome Evaluation* is the final activity of evidence-based practice that examines whether the application of evidence-based care resulted in an improvement or met expected treatment goals. Nurse leaders participate in the process of translating relevant and current clinical research into patient care. Participating in panels and presenting posters, symposia, or clinical outcome data aids the process of translation.

Essentially, the registered nurse conducts research studies from a unique perspective. The SQUIRE (Standards for Quality Improvement Reporting Excellence; n.d.) guidelines provide an outline of the important elements necessary to follow in planning and conducting a research project from inception to end. The registered nurse integrates research findings into practice by using the best available evidence, including research findings, to guide practice decisions. No longer can a response such as, "We've always done this way" be an appropriate answer to nursing practice at any step in the nursing process. Today, the registered nurse actively participates in research activities at various levels appropriate to the nurse's level of education and position. This includes activities such as the following:

▸ Identifying clinical problems that can be translated into a nursing research question

▸ Participating in data collection activities

▸ Participating on formal committees, such as the Institutional Review Board (IRB) at your organization or academic department

▸ Sharing research findings with peers and others through formal presentations at unit, agency, organization, or professional conferences

▸ Conducting research studies as Principal Investigators (PIs)

▸ Analyzing and interpreting (clinically) research findings to practice (called translating "bench to bedside" activities)

▸ Using research findings in the development of policies, procedures, and standards of practice across various settings

▸ Incorporating research as a basis for learning

Evidence-Based Practice

Evidence-based nursing practice has evolved as the gold standard for health treatment. Stuart (2009) defines evidence-based practice as "the conscientious, explicit, and judicious use of the best evidence gained from systematic research for the purpose of making informed decisions about the care of individual patients" (p. 58). Evidence-based practice consists of finding and using (Standard 14: Resource Utilization) the best available evidence to guide our practice. That does not mean that the nurse has to conduct research studies to find the evidence, but it does mean that nurses are charged with keeping up to date and using the best available evidence to guide practice and evaluate patient care outcomes. Incorporation of this evidence, combined with the nurse's clinical expertise, consensus recommendations of psychiatric experts, and knowledge of the patient, provides the strongest basis for achieving effective, efficient treatment outcomes.

The five steps of evidence-based-practice are:

Step 1.
Ask an Answerable Clinical Question

Both research and research use requires the identification of a relevant clinical question. The "PICO" (Oxman et al., 1993) mnemonic can be used to guide the process of developing a question that can be answered by reviewing the literature:

- ▸ Patient population

- ▸ Intervention or area of interest

- ▸ Comparison interventions

- ▸ Outcome measures

Step 2.
Collect the Most Relevant and Best Evidence

It is not enough to simply read one glowing article about a particular intervention and take it as evidence. Reviewing the literature for the most relevant and best evidence is a systematic process that involves searching for the following:

- ▸ Systematic reviews of the literature or as many single studies as possible

- ▸ Best practice guidelines

- ▸ Clinical pathways

The best evidence hierarchy can be used to evaluate the strength or validity of the identified literature and is ranked from best (highest level) to lowest level.

Systematic review or meta-analysis represents an evaluation and synthesis of all available literature on a particular topic, and is therefore considered to be the highest level of evidence. Systematic review articles can be found by searching online databases. The Cochrane Library, of the Cochrane Collaboration (www.cochrane.org), provides a database of current systematic review articles on all the major mental disorders. The Cochrane Collaboration is dedicated to the dissemination of up-to-date information to inform evidence-based practice in the broader healthcare arena. Additional sources for nurses include the Joanna Briggs Institute (http://joannabriggs.org) and the Agency for Healthcare Research and Quality (AHRQ; www.guidelines.gov).

Randomized controlled trials (RCTs), especially if they have been replicated, are considered to be strong evidence because of the way the studies are designed. RCTs control variables (such as age, race, gender, comorbidities) in determining participant eligibility. Participants are randomly assigned to the group receiving the intervention of interest (e.g., the drug) or to the group receiving either the usual treatment or placebo. Controlling variables and randomly assigning the participants, rather than letting them pick their own groups, minimizes the possibility that the two groups are somehow different before the intervention and makes findings of posttreatment differences much more interpretable. RCTs can answer research questions about cause and effect. A double-blind RCT, the strongest research design, is designed so both the study participants and the study designers (principal investigator and clinical research assistants) are unaware of (i.e., kept blinded to) which participants receive the particular treatment (e.g., medication) being studied. RCTs and results are referred to as the "gold standard" for high confidence in their conclusions because of the double-blinding and randomization of study participants.

Quasi-experimental studies compare two naturally occurring groups of interest. For example, a researcher could implement a new treatment (e.g., communal dining) on one unit of a treatment center, but not another, and then compare patient satisfaction between the two units. The problem with quasi-experimental designs is that the differences between groups could be the result of some unknown variable (e.g., staff turnover).

Case control studies are retrospective observational studies used to determine factors that may contribute to a medical condition by comparing patients who have the condition with persons who do not. Case control studies have helped us understand certain risk factors (e.g., smoking) associated with the development of illnesses (e.g., lung cancer); however, they are subject to confounding because the researcher has little knowledge of other factors that may have influenced the outcome.

Cohort studies are prospective observational studies that are used to examine variables that might be relevant to the development of a condition. For example, a researcher might choose to study children of depressed mothers to determine whether they develop any behavioral or emotional problems over time. The problem with this type of design is again, the lack of control and the possible effects of some unknown variable. Studies examining relationships between variables cannot answer cause and effect questions.

Single descriptive (cross-sectional) or qualitative studies add to our knowledge about a condition, but must be replicated to provide reliable evidence. For example, if the prevalence of schizophrenia is found to be 1% in many different countries, and in urban and rural sites, this would provide strong evidence for a prevalence of 1%, but it would not provide any further information concerning the contributions of nature versus nurture or other factors potentially leading to schizophrenia. Qualitative studies are important in helping to understand the lived experience of illness. They are frequently based upon the analysis of interview data and the identification of themes.

Expert opinions are also important and need to be considered in relation to available evidence.

Step 3.
Critically Appraise the Evidence

Individual research study reports are usually organized in the same order. The title is brief and refers to the population of interest and major variable(s). The abstract is a brief summary with approximately one sentence describing each section of the paper. The literature review provides the background for the study, the conceptual framework, and the hypotheses to be tested. The methods section describes the participants, instruments, and the procedure. The intervention or manipulated variables are labeled "independent" and the outcome variables are called "dependent." The results section reports the findings. The discussion section presents the researchers' interpretations of the findings. The references section includes all cited studies.

Important statistical concepts should be understood when psychiatric–mental health nurses are critically appraising the literature. These include terms that relate to statistical measurement levels, sample size, control of variables, generalizability, reliability, validity, probability, research design and methodology, findings, implications for practice, and conclusion. Several concepts will be briefly reviewed in an attempt to establish a working knowledge level; nursing research textbooks should be consulted for a deeper understanding of these concepts. Consider the elements of a study described below.

Sample size: The larger the sample, the more generalizable the results or findings. A general rule is that a sample size of 30 or more is necessary for generalizable results, but the number of participants needed to interpret findings is actually based upon the number of variables in the study and the type of statistical analysis.

Generalizability: Can the results of the study be applied to other groups or populations who were not actually participants in this study? Generally, it's hard to make a case that concludes that all nurses feel one way or another, if you only asked nurses from one hospital.

Control of variables: The more control over the independent variable, the more confidence one can have in interpreting the findings. Descriptive studies do not exercise any control. RCTs exercise the most control, with one group receiving the intervention or new treatment and another receiving a placebo or standard treatment and serving as a comparison control group.

TABLE 7–3.
LEVELS OF MEASUREMENT

LEVEL	DEFINITION	EXAMPLES	RESEARCH MEASURES
Nominal	Categorical, named variables Red, white, blue Race, religion	Group 1, Group 2, Group 3	Count Frequencies
Ordinal	Rank order	Rankings 1st, 2nd, 3rd Grades A, B, C Likert and psychometric scales	Count Frequencies
Interval	Divided by equal differences between values, but no true starting point	Days, education, temperature (a temperature of zero is not an absence of temperature)	Can be added, subtracted, multiplied and divided
Ratio	Ratios between measurements, meaningful with a set zero point (1:1 for example).	Age, weight, number of children	Can be added, subtracted, multiplied and divided; ratios are meaningful

Major types of studies include: *descriptive, quantitative, qualitative,* and *inferential.* The level of measurement adopted in a research study determines or constrains the types of descriptive and inferential statistics that may be applied to the variable (Table 7–3).

Descriptive statistics are used to describe the basic features of the data in a study. The majority of nursing studies are descriptive. When reporting descriptive findings, the researcher reports numerical values that summarize, organize, and describe the observations. Descriptive studies tend to be hypothesis-generating. Certain measures (below) show how the focus of interest in the study falls out along the normal bell-shaped curve (Figure 7.1 below). Terminology important in understanding descriptive study designs includes:

▸ **Frequency:** How often a particular finding occurs. Frequencies are useful for describing nominal or ordinal data.

▸ **Mean:** A measure of central tendency derived by summing all scores and dividing by the number of participants. Means can be found for interval and ratio data.

▸ **Standard deviation:** A measure of the distance of a measure from the group mean. Based upon the formula for calculating the standard deviation, approximately 68% of the scores will fall within one standard deviation from the mean, approximately 95% will fall within two standard deviations, and approximately 99% will fall within three standard deviations—the normal population distribution (see Figure 7.1). Interval and ratio level data are normally distributed.

▸ **Variance:** A measure of variation derived by squaring each standard deviation in a set of scores and then taking the mean of the squares. The larger the variance, the greater the dispersion of scores.

FIGURE 7-1.
THE NORMAL DISTRIBUTION

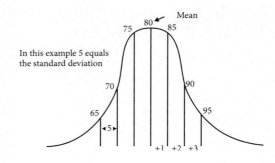

In this example 5 equals the standard deviation

Quantitative studies use quantities, metrics, and numbers to describe a phenomenon. Results are described according to the strength of the numbers and inferences are obtained that suggests a result.

Qualitative studies use observations, interviews, or both as the data collection foci. The methods of phenomenological, grounded, or lived experiences are some of the methods for collection. The researcher will transcribe actual study participant responses and *code* these responses into themes, which are then grouped and interpreted.

Inferential statistics are used to reach conclusions that extend beyond the immediate data alone. They are used to infer something about a population based upon sample data. For example, a researcher might want to make a judgment of the probability that a new medication will be efficacious for treating persons with bipolar depression. The use of an experimentally controlled research design, interval or ratio level variables, and the calculation of inferential statistics would allow the test of a null hypothesis of no difference between the two populations of interest. Studies using inferential statistics allow us to test hypotheses and make conclusions about a population from a sample. A result is considered to be statistically significant if the probability result reveals that it (the phenomenon of interest) is unlikely to have occurred by chance. Statistical significance, however, does not necessarily mean that a result is clinically relevant. Terminology important in understanding inferential study designs includes:

▸ **Probability:** A statement of the likelihood that an event will occur. A probability of 0 means that the event is certain not to occur; a probability of 1 means that the event will occur with certainty.

▸ **Probability value (P-value):** Inferential statistics tests the hypothesis that there will be no difference between groups (e.g., the experimental and control group). A *P-value* for a hypothesis test is the probability of obtaining, by chance alone, a value of the test statistic as extreme or more extreme than the one actually computed when the null hypothesis is true. The convention for judging the *statistical significance* of a *P-value* is the significance level that we set. In most studies, a P-value less than 0.05 ($p \leq 0.05$) is considered statistically significant.

▶ **Analysis of variance:** A set of statistical procedures designed to compare two or more groups of observations. It determines whether the differences between groups are because of experimental influence or chance alone. A simple t-test can be used to test differences between two groups.

▶ **Validity:** Are the conclusions valid? In other words, are the conclusions right or true? Types of validity include:

> ▶ **Internal validity:** Is there a relationship between the intervention and the outcome? Did the treatment cause the outcome?

> ▶ **External validity:** Can we *generalize* the findings? Was the sample large enough, representative enough, etc.?

▶ **Reliability:** Are the conclusions reliable? In other words, were the measures consistent?

> ▶ **Test/retest:** Assuming there is no change in the underlying condition (e.g., trait or personality), does the measurement tool obtain the same result on repeated measures? That is, when it is administered again?

Potential Bias in Research: Who Were the Study Participants?

▶ Were women, children, minorities, and older adults included? If not, why not? The researcher, typically called the Principle Investigator, has to address this question. In the past, most healthcare research was conducted using healthy white men as participants. Today's standards of research require that diverse groups be included as study participants; otherwise, the investigators have to present good justification for why not. Determine whether best evidence for excluded subgroups is available.

▶ Were there conflicts of interest on the part of the investigators? Drug companies fund many randomized control trials (RCTs). Was there inappropriate involvement of research sponsors in the design and management of the RCT? Drug company sponsors stand to profit from favorable outcomes.

▶ Was there a publication bias in the dissemination of results? Were financial incentives given? Are the bar or line graphs depicting the results based upon using equivalent dosages of comparison drugs, with equivalent age groups, etc.?

Findings, Results, and Conclusions: Findings are statements derived from statistical analysis of the data. The conclusions drawn from research depend upon the design of the study and the questions asked or hypotheses tested. The results, findings, and conclusions of a study do not prove anything; they merely offer a *suggestion* (for example: "the research findings suggest that olanzapine offers improved outcomes, as compared to chlorpromazine") as to what the researcher has determined according to their interpretation. The critical reader may not draw the same conclusions as the researcher. This is one of the beauties of systematic research and publication of results and conclusions. They point a direction for subsequent researchers to pick up where someone left off because of missing an important or relevant piece, or because the particular focus was not examined in relevant or generalizable populations.

Step 4.
Synthesize and Integrate With Professional Experience, Patient Preferences, and Values in Making a Practice Decision or Change

Research findings cannot be helpful unless they are translated into practice ("bench to bedside"). The length of time between the completion of research studies and the translation of their findings into clinical practice is often many years. Nurses have a great deal of practice-based knowledge that they can draw upon from experience. This experience and knowledge should be considered in combination with utilization of research-based results or findings to determine the best plan of care for individual patients.

We can further evaluate the *strength* of the evidence by the study design, using the best evidence hierarchy. We evaluate the *quality* of the evidence from individual studies based upon sample size, experimental control, and the conclusions of the findings. If we are evaluating the evidence of a systematic review, we would also want to note whether the reviewed studies found consistent results.

Step 5. Evaluate the Practice Decision or Change

The last step of evidence-based care is to evaluate the response to the practice decision or change in care (outcomes evaluation). Change can only be measured if baseline levels are known. For example, to evaluate the efficacy of a preventive exercise plan on depression, it would be essential to take baseline as well as periodic depression surveys. To measure response to care, outcomes indicators must be specified. Types of outcome indicators include:

- **Clinical outcomes:** Health status, relapse, recurrence, readmission, number of episodes, symptomatology, coping responses, high-risk behaviors, incidence reports

- **Functional outcomes:** Functional status (e.g., DSM5 Global Assessment of Functioning), social interaction, activities of daily living, occupational abilities, quality of life, family relationships, housing arrangements

- **Satisfaction outcomes:** Satisfaction with treatment, treatment outcomes, treatment team or organization. *Example:* Press Ganey Healthcare Consumer Satisfaction Scores.

- **Financial outcomes:** Cost-effective, revenue-generating, reduced length of stay, efficient use of resources, good returns on investments (ROIs)

Ethical Considerations in Research

Ethics involves doing what is right, because it is right. The psychiatric–mental health nurse is bound to a code of ethics. Investigators or others who are involved in conducting research studies must take and pass a required test on the protection of human participants based on the *Belmont Report* (National Commission for the Protection of Human Subjects of Biomedical and Behavioral Research, 1979). This requires researchers to meet the criteria of

- ▶ **Beneficence** (do no harm),
- ▶ **Respect** for human dignity (right for self-determination), and
- ▶ **Justice** (fair treatment and nondiscriminatory selection).

The U.S. Office for Human Research Protections (OHRP), through the Code of Federal Regulations (45 CFR 46), requires that research involving human participants assures certain information be addressed before enrolled in a study, including:

- ▶ Description of the nature and purpose and procedures
- ▶ Description of any reasonably foreseeable risks or discomforts; potential consequences, side effects, complications
- ▶ Description of any benefits
- ▶ Duration of the study
- ▶ Disclosure of appropriate alternative procedures or courses of treatment
- ▶ Statement describing the extent, if any, to which confidentiality of records and identity will be maintained
- ▶ Description of any treatments or compensations for injury
- ▶ Statement of how and with whom the participant may make contact with questions
- ▶ Statement that participation is voluntary and additionally, that refusal to participate, or decision to discontinue participation, will involve no penalty or loss of benefits to which the participant is otherwise entitled.
- ▶ How the data will be collected, used, and reported

Institutional Review Boards (IRBs)

Nurses are frequently asked to voluntarily serve on formal review boards. Again, the nurse's expertise and clinical understanding of patient actual and potential problems along the healthcare continuum makes for an unparalleled perspective in assuring good patient and research participant outcomes. IRBs exist within most healthcare and academic institutions to review all study plans and protocols to ensure that:

- ▸ Risks to participants are minimized.

- ▸ Participant selection is equitable and without coercion.

- ▸ Informed consent is obtained and documented.

- ▸ Data and safety monitoring plan is implemented when indicated.

Informed Consent

Informed consent is a communication issue as well as a legal and ethical one. Every patient and research participant must have the capacity to understand the nature of the proposed treatment, receive adequate information to make an informed decision, and be presented with options to make an informed choice. This is especially of concern for patients with serious mental disorders because they often have more difficulty understanding a proposed treatment or have diminished capacity to fully comprehend its meaning. For this reason, psychiatric–mental health nurses must be extremely attentive to the psychological and cognitive barriers these patients present to ensure accurate comprehension. Additional patient characteristics or situations that preclude adequate understanding or comprehension of the information required to complete an informed consent process include cognitive deficits, primary language differences, literacy level, fatigue, and level of psychological stress. In most states, patients must give informed consent for clinical treatments, such as acceptance of psychotropic medications. The only exception is for emergency treatment in which the risk to health or life requires that treatment be given immediately, and then only on a one-time basis.

Voluntarily hospitalized patients must sign consent for treatment at the time of admission. Involuntary patients cannot give informed consent. In this case, the guardian for the involuntary patient, court-appointed administrative treatment protocol, or an advance directive for mental health can override the patient's objection. Informed consent for psychiatric treatment requires that each person adequately understand the essential information needed to give informed consent. Informed consent also represents an ongoing communication process between nurses and patients receiving the medication or treatment, including the opportunity to ask questions and to have relevant provider contact information for further questions or dialogue. Information the patient needs to provide informed consent includes:

- The diagnosis and target symptoms for which the medication or treatment is being prescribed

- Trade and generic names of all medication

- The benefits or intended effects of the treatment or medication(s)

- The risks and side effects of each medication or treatment

- Significant drug-drug and food-drug interactions

- Information on appropriate dosing and administration of medications

- The possible results of not taking the recommended medication as prescribed

- The possibility of needing to make changes in medication dosages based on the patient's condition

- Alternatives to the proposed medication or treatment

- A statement of the person's right to withdraw voluntary consent for medications or treatment at any time (unless the medication or treatment is mandated as part of court-ordered treatment or there is a significant change in the person's condition requiring one-time emergency treatment)

- If medication treatment is provided as a result of an emergency situation without obtaining the consent of the person, the nurse needs to document the emergency situation and the rationale for the one-time emergency use of a medication or treatment, and the time the medication was administered, in writing. Thereafter, informed consent must be obtained voluntarily from the patient for further administration of the medication or treatment.

Patients must give informed consent to receive ECT and to participate in research studies. The law requires true informed consent by any person before becoming a participant in a research project. Potential participants must sign and understand a written informed consent to participate in any research protocols. They can never unknowingly participate in research. Children under the age of 18 can give assent, but only a legally responsible adult can give official consent. Documentation of the information given to the patient and the patient's consent should be included in the medical record.

PSYCHIATRIC-MENTAL HEALTH PROFESSIONAL PERFORMANCE STANDARD 10. QUALITY OF PRACTICE

The nurse leader participates in the process of continuous quality improvement (QI). High-quality health care is care that is safe, effective, patient-centered, timely, and equitable (IOM, 2001). Risk managers, who may be nurses, work to decrease the probability of adverse outcomes related to patient care. They identify patient and organizational risk factors and coordinate corrective actions and strategies to prevent negative outcomes. Continuous QI strategies minimize patient and organizational risk. QI frameworks are called by different names, but the goal is always to assure that quality of patient care is maintained in an organization through an ongoing, continuous, effort:

- Quality assurance (QA)

- Performance improvement (PI)

- Total quality management (TQM)

- Continuous improvement (CI)

- Continuous quality improvement (CQI)

The QI process is a problem-solving process that starts with the assembly of a QI infrastructure. This would include determining the leadership, membership, and meeting structure. To facilitate collaboration in QI, staff involvement on the QI team is very important. The QI team identifies annual quality goals, outcome monitoring and evaluation processes, and participates in the development of performance appraisals. (See Table 7–4 for facilitation and barriers to successful QI.)

TABLE 7–4.
FACILITATORS OF AND BARRIERS TO SUCCESSFUL QUALITY INITIATIVES (QI)

QI FACILITATORS	QI BARRIERS
▸ Perceived relevance	▸ Lack of system support
▸ Sufficient expertise	▸ Lack of financial resources
▸ Motivational (transformational) leadership:	▸ Lack of time
▸ Conveys the importance of QI	▸ Conflicting organizational goals
▸ Organizes educational activities to promote quality	▸ Insufficient expertise
▸ Commits resources to support QI program	▸ Information overload
▸ Acts as clinical champion, keeping the team on track	▸ Lack of understanding regarding purpose
▸ Recognizes staff for their QI efforts	▸ Lack of feedback to staff
▸ Institutionalizes QI	
▸ Demonstrates program successes	
▸ Shares outcomes with staff	

- Plan priorities and goals.
    - Define the mission statement and goals.
    - What are the patients' expectations?
    - What criteria define quality?
    - What are the expected outcomes of this service?
    - How will outcomes be monitored?
- Identify processes or services that need improvement and design solutions.
    - Describe current processes, identify data that are needed.
    - Localize problems: sentinel events, incident reports, and chart audits.
    - Conduct a root cause analysis to specify the organizational underlying causes, not just the immediately obvious errors or incidents.
    - Generate solutions to root causes and develop a pilot study.
- Measure performance.
    - Test the pilot and collect outcome data.
    - Outcome measures may include medication errors, functional outcomes, patient satisfaction, intervention times, or costs per capita.
- Analyze data.
    - Evaluate the pilot data; compare with baseline data.
    - Determine whether the change was effective.
- Improve practice.
    - Standardize the new process or repeat the problem-solving process.
    - Disseminate the results to the organizational leaders and staff.

Organizational quality improvement frameworks are based upon having defined missions and values, professional standards for providers, and guidelines for the provision of care. Major organizations assist healthcare organizations in maintaining safety and quality of care through healthcare accreditation. The Joint Commission (TJC; formerly the Joint Commission on the Accreditation of Health Care Organizations), accredits hospitals, healthcare agencies, and behavioral healthcare organizations. The Commission on Accreditation of Rehabilitation Facilities (CARF) provides accreditation standards for rehabilitation, substance abuse, home and community services, retirement living, and other health and human services. The National Committee for Quality Assurance (NCQA) is the leader in accrediting managed care organizations. The psychiatric–mental health nurse should review the mission, vision, and value statements of outlined by his or her employer. These tenets lay out the basic direction of service orientation and focus adopted by the organization or agency. The employed professional, by virtue of his or her employment, tacitly adopts this direction as well.

- ▶ **Mission, Vision, and Value Statements**

    - ▶ Brief statement of the purpose and values of an organization

    - ▶ Defines the types of patients are served by the organization

    - ▶ Defines the responsibilities of the organization toward the patients

- ▶ **Professional Standards**

    - ▶ Authoritative statements that include position descriptions, performance skills, and institutional policies

    - ▶ An organization's interpretation of professional's competency

    - ▶ Measurement through professional outcomes

- ▶ **Care Guidelines**

    - ▶ Systematically developed (evidence-based) statements to assist in determining appropriate care

    - ▶ Institutional protocols and procedures, care plans, and pathways

    - ▶ Measured though patient outcomes

Quality Improvement (QI) Processes

Nursing is faced with many current challenges: the nursing shortage, an aging population, continued health disparities, and increasing social problems. The IOM's 2001 landmark report, *Crossing the Quality Chasm: A New Health System for the 21st Century*, recommended that all healthcare organizations promote healthcare that is safe, effective, patient-centered, timely, efficient, and equitable. Specific recommendations for ensuring quality patient-centered care is care that

- ▶ Respects and is responsive to individual patient preferences, needs, and values;

- ▶ Is available in many forms other than face-to-face contact, such as the Internet and telephone;

- ▶ Makes the patient the source of control in his or her own care, and incorporates shared decision-making;

- ▶ Provides patients with free access to their personal medical information;

- ▶ Provides full clinical knowledge that is evidence-based and reflective of the best available scientific knowledge;

- ▶ Ensures patient safety from injury caused by the healthcare system;

- ▶ Maintains efficiency in terms of resources, energy, ideas, and patient time;

▸ Equitably provides care for all patients regardless of ethnicity, geographic location, or socioeconomic status; and

▸ Reduces medication-related errors.

The roles of the leaders of quality improvement processes include the following:

▸ Conveying the importance and relevance to colleagues about the need for QI

▸ Organizing educational activities to promote quality

▸ Motivating and recognizing colleagues for their QI efforts

▸ Institutionalizing QI

▸ Committing monies, time, and sufficient expertise

▸ Providing feedback in the form of data (metrics) to demonstrate program successes and further improve performance

▸ Committing resources to support QI programming

▸ Acting as a clinical champion, keeping the team motivated and on track

In recognition of evidence on the key role of nurses, the IOM (2004) conducted a study to identify aspects of the work environment for nurses that are likely to have an impact on patient safety, and developed the following goals for transforming the work environment:

▸ Transformational leadership

▸ Evidence-based management

▸ Maximizing workforce capability

▸ Redesigning work and workspace to prevent and mitigate errors

▸ Creating and sustaining a culture of safety

PSYCHIATRIC–MENTAL HEALTH PROFESSIONAL PERFORMANCE STANDARD 11. COMMUNICATION

Chapter 6 reviewed therapeutic and nontherapeutic communication strategies. As an educator, the nurse leader uses appropriate communication, teaching principles, and strategies to teach patients, precept students, and mentor other healthcare professionals under his or her supervision. Becoming an educator or mentor depends upon having expert knowledge and skills. Brenner (1984) introduced the framework of "novice to expert" to describe the process by which novice nurses can develop into experts over time as clinical practice experiences provide opportunities to apply knowledge and develop more proficient skills.

Standard 11 states that the professional mental health nurse communicates effectively in a variety of formats and works to continuously assess and improve upon his or her personal level of communication skills. Communication forums include patient and family, interdisciplinary, and peer conveyances of accurate and timely information; contributing in professional meetings; questioning rationale of treatment decisions when appropriate; disclosing hazards, concerns, and errors to appropriate levels; and documenting referrals, updates, revisions, and changes to the care plan.

Mentoring is an important leadership role that requires, in addition to clinical expertise and knowledge, interpersonal communication skills that inspire and facilitate personal growth. The nurse leader commits as a lifelong learner and actively pursues new knowledge and skills as her or his role and needs of the healthcare system evolve. A helpful resource for psychiatric–mental health nurses is Medscape's psychiatric and mental health nursing section (http://www.medscape.com/resource/Psychiatric–nursing). The Institute for Healthcare Improvement (IHI) is another influential force in health and healthcare improvement offering webinars and on-site presentations on various topics (www.ihi.org).

Attendance at national conferences (such as those of the American Psychiatric Nurses Association, International Society of Psychiatric Nurses, International Nurses Society on Addictions) and memberships in nursing organizations (such as the American Nurses Association, state-level nursing associations), and participation in workshops, targeted courses, web-based resources, and webinars and reading professional journals all enhance the individual nurse. For example, the psychiatric–mental health nurse would do well to read the article (http://jap.sagepub.com/content/19/4/205) published in the *Journal of the American Psychiatric Nurses Association* about the APNA's position paper on suicide prevention. Additional ways to enhance one's own education and elevate the entire nursing field is by engaging in any of these professional performances:

- Maintain and demonstrate competency
- Role-modeling
- Orient new staff or student nurses
- Conduct peer reviews and appraisals
- Gain specialty certification
- Engage in public speaking about mental health and illness in churches and community centers
- Prepare abstracts and present at local, state, national, and international conferences

The nurse, as leader, plans, coordinates, integrates, and evaluates patient care that is delivered by nursing ancillary staff. This includes delegating nursing tasks, supervising personnel carrying out the tasks, and evaluating the outcomes of care. *Delegation* of nursing tasks to appropriately supervised nursing assistive personnel (the delegator to delegatee) is one way of addressing shortages in nursing and maximizing workforce capacity. Legal limits for delegation are specified by State Nurse Practice Acts and state laws; job descriptions and institutional policies may place further limits or include detailed guidelines for delegation. In 2005, the National Council of State Boards of Nursing (NCSBN) and the American Nurses Association issued a joint statement on delegation that was developed to support practicing nurses in using delegation safely and effectively.

- ▶ **Delegation:** The process for a nurse to direct another person to perform nursing tasks and activities.

- ▶ **Supervision:** The provision of guidance and oversight of a delegated nursing task.

The joint statement on delegation principles specifies that only nursing *tasks*, not nursing *practice*, can be delegated. The nurse takes the responsibility and accountability for delegating nursing tasks to team members. Only those tasks within the ancillary staff's scope of practice can be transferred, and only to those team members with appropriate skill and sufficient knowledge and judgment to complete them. Table 7.5 outlines the elements and rights of delegation.

TABLE 7–5.
THE ELEMENTS AND RIGHTS OF DELEGATION

The 4 Elements of Delegation
1. Assess and plan: Act based on patient needs and available resources.
2. Communicate directions: Include any unique patient requirements and characteristics as well as clear expectations regarding what to do, what to report, and when to ask for assistance.
3. Surveillance and supervision: Provide oversight at the level of supervision needed, and clarification as needed.
4. Evaluation and feedback: Assess effectiveness and adjust the plan of care as needed.
The 5 Rights of Delegation
1. The right task
2. Under the right circumstances
3. To the right person
4. With the right direction and communication
5. Under the right supervision and evaluation

Adapted from *Joint Statement on Delegation* by the American Nurses Association and the National Council of State Boards of Nursing, 2005, retrieved from https://www.ncsbn.org/Delegation_joint_statement_NCSBN-ANA.pdf

PSYCHIATRIC–MENTAL HEALTH PROFESSIONAL PERFORMANCE STANDARD 12. LEADERSHIP (AT EVERY LEVEL)

Leadership and Management Competencies

Nursing leadership is essential to promoting safe health care. Leadership is the explicit use of one's abilities to direct and influence others to perform to the best of their abilities. The nurse leader is both transactional and transformational, simultaneously stabilizing and effecting change in the work culture when appropriate. Nurses at all levels function in leadership roles. Leadership roles are available to all nurses who have the knowledge, competence, affiliation, and desire to take such a role. Most nurses are leaders in one aspect or more of their work. The management role is focused on handling the day-to-day operations of a work group to achieve a desired outcome. Both roles require a set of broad and specific competencies that evolves over time.

Nurse leaders, as stipulated by the ANA Code of Ethics (2008), advocate for and strive to protect the health, safety, and rights of the patient. Nurse leaders advocate for patients by assuring a safe healthcare environment. The rights of the patient, formerly specified by the *Healthcare Consumer Bill of Rights,* are now detailed in a new brochure published by the American Hospital Association (2008) called *A Healthcare Consumer Care Partnership*. Nurse leaders advocate for patients by ensuring that patients, families, and communities are well-informed and included in healthcare planning. Advocacy can also take the form of working with organizations, such as the National Alliance for the Mentally Ill, on issues relevant to persons and families with mental disorders. By staying informed of national and local healthcare issues and policies, working on task forces, or voicing concerns to policymakers, the nurse leader advocates for populations of persons with mental disorders.

Nurse leaders use information technology systems to gain access to current research and provide evidence-based care. The Institute of Medicine's (2006) report on *Improving the Quality of Health Care for Mental and Substance-Use Conditions* called for improved technology related to healthcare benefits for improved access to care. Automation of patient-specific clinical information leads to better-organized and retrievable records. In addition, nurse leaders use technology to coordinate care between providers and systems.

The nurse leader as team manager is able to properly delegate and manage nursing team resources (human and fiscal) and serve as a leader of and partner in the interdisciplinary healthcare team. Managerial roles include:

- **Staffing:** Choosing the management structure; coordinating people, time, task assignments
- **Recruiting:** Hiring, training, scheduling, ongoing staff development

▸ **Planning:** Defining goals, objectives, policies, procedures; resource allocation

▸ **Conducting:** Evaluating performance, analyzing financial activities, monitoring quality of care

▸ **Supervising:** Directing, guiding, and influencing a staff member's performance

Nurse leaders display collaboration abilities, effective communication, clinical competence, and organizational and time management skills. Good leader attributes include being consistent, responsible, calm, articulate, fair, objective, a good problem-solver, and organized. It requires a level of open-mindedness, flexibility, and tact. The nurse leader is a role model who displays decisiveness, clinical competence, and a sense of humor. These attributes convey and model the expectation among staff for collegial trust, respect, warmth, and rapport. The best leadership style depends upon the setting, expertise of the staff, and needs of the organization. Box 7–1 describes different styles of leadership.

BOX 7-1.
LEADERSHIP STYLES

Autocratic
▸ Leader retains all authority, makes all decisions, and establishes one-way communication with the work group.
▸ Can be effective in crisis situations

Democratic
▸ Leader focuses on teamwork and workgroup participation in decision-making.
▸ Leader collaborates with others in making decisions.
▸ Can be effective with mature staff

Laissez-faire
▸ Leader gives up control with free-run or permissive style.
▸ Can only be effective with highly motivated staff

Situational
▸ *Situation* is the major determinant of leader's behaviors.
▸ Flexible and adapts to needs of person or work group
▸ *Directing* is most important with new staff.
▸ *Coaching* involves interpersonal processes with those who are more experienced but still need some guidance.
▸ *Supporting* assists in problem-solving.
▸ *Delegating* transfers responsibility while retaining accountability, promotes staff development.

Transformational
▸ Leader inspires and motivates others to follow.
▸ Leader has vision, passion, enthusiasm and energy.
▸ Leader creates and communicates shared vision and values.
▸ Leader champions solutions to patient and organizational challenges.
▸ Leader provides intellectual stimulation.

Leadership Power

Leaders have power that allow them to accomplish goals. Marquis & Huston (1992) describe the following types of nursing leadership power:

- **Reward:** Obtained by the ability to grant favors or reward others with whatever they value

- **Coercive:** Based on a person's real or perceived fear of punishment by another person

- **Legitimate:** Derived from a person's organizational title or position rather than from a personal quality

- **Expert:** Gained through knowledge, expertise, or experience

- **Referent:** Given by others because the leader is perceived as powerful

- **Informational:** Result of one person having, or being perceived to have, special information that another desires

Leader Conflict Resolution Skills

Leaders need conflict resolution skills to foster healthy communication among staff. A conflict, in and of itself, need not be viewed as a negative experience. A conflict might arise when staff members present interpersonal conflicts to the leader, or present different ideas about solving a problem. In both cases, a nurse leader might look upon this challenge as an opportunity to closely examine some ambivalent aspect of an interpersonal or decision issue. People may have strong differences of opinion on some issues.

Before attempting any conflict resolution strategies, the leader needs to know his or her own role and response to conflict, and manage any uncomfortable feelings. Ideally, the leader prepares for the meeting and selects an optimal time for all parties. It is important for the leader to separate the problem from the persons involved, stay focused on the issues, and work on one problem at a time. The next step is to identify available options and attempt to mediate a solution. The goal is to agree on an outcome based upon fair, objective criteria. Evaluating the outcomes by checking back in with the parties is important. Keep in mind cultural differences and individual conflict resolution styles (Box 7–2). The ultimate goal in conflict resolution is to engender a supportive work environment where all staff and colleagues learn that they have valuable input in positive outcomes and shared governance within the employment milieu.

Conflict resolution principles involve a series of process steps:

- Identify conflict issue.

- Know your own response to conflict.

BOX 7-2.
CONFLICT RESOLUTION STYLES

▸ **Avoidance:** Pick your battles.

▸ **Accommodation:** Focus is on the present situation.

▸ **Coerciveness:** Focus is on convincing others of your position to the exclusion of "hearing" other's perspectives. Selective listening is evident.

▸ **Competition:** Focus is on being heard and being seen as right. Selective listening behaviors evident.

▸ **Compromise:** Resolution is the priority, not winning the battle, or being seen as right.

▸ **Collaboration:** Being willing to forgive; trying out the alternative approach.

▸ Separate the problem from the persons involved.

▸ Stay focused on the issue and the underlying motivations of stakeholders.

▸ Identify available options.

▸ Mediate (settle differences).

▸ Search for an outcome based on the fair, objective criteria.

PSYCHIATRIC-MENTAL HEALTH PROFESSIONAL PERFORMANCE STANDARD 13. COLLABORATION

In today's managed care environment, it is imperative for nurses to work collaboratively with patients and families with a shared responsibility for assessing and treating healthcare problems and for promoting their own health and well-being. Today, consumers of healthcare expect a patient-centered approach. Issues of importance to the development of shared responsibility between healthcare providers and patients include the following:

▸ Incorporating patient family values, beliefs, and knowledge backgrounds into planning and delivery of care (Healthcare Consumer and Family Centered Care Models)

▸ Communicating and sharing comprehensive information with patients

▸ Involving patients and families in patient-centered discussions of unified care planning activities and anticipated outcomes

▸ Encouraging patients and families to participate in all aspects of their care and clinical decision-making

▸ Collaborating in policy and program development to facilitate quality care

Gardner (2005) defines collaboration as "a process and an outcome in which shared interest or conflict that cannot be addressed by any single individual is addressed by key stakeholders (p. 1)." A collaborative outcome involves the development of integrative solutions that go beyond an individual vision to a productive resolution that could not be accomplished by any single person or organization. Interdisciplinary collaborative practices bring together multiple providers to achieve objectives aimed at meeting the mental health needs of patients and their families.

The nurse collaborates with the interdisciplinary healthcare team to insure a seamless transition of care from admission through treatment and back to the community by promoting prompt referrals and timely communication. This may be fostered by including representatives of other disciplines in practice meetings (e.g., conferences, rounds, in-service programs, staff meetings) and by meeting or communicating with alliance groups and referral sources. Consultation-liaison teams composed of multidisciplinary partners, including nurses, can be effective in caring for patients in larger systems who might be housed on more medical or critical care units before a formal admission to psychiatric inpatient settings.

Building collaborative relationships among and between the nurse, psychiatrist, clinical specialist or nurse practitioner, social worker, occupational therapist, recreational therapist, case manager, psychologist, physical therapist, nutritionist, occupational therapist, substance abuse counselor, law enforcement and security providers, peer counselors, and spiritual advisors who are directly involved with a patient's care (and have a need to know) in face-to-face meetings enhances and extends care provision. All can contribute to identifying and monitoring safe, quality care for patients with mental illness. Collaborative discussions can include developing and sharing comprehensive treatment plans, making treatment decisions, resolving patient issues, setting treatment goals, and coordinating care within a cooperative, integrated framework. External collaborations can help hospitals and clinical agencies share information and resources with the community, and important supporters of mental health such as religious leaders and traditional healers. Remember that collaboration is not required for all decisions. Collaboration is not a panacea, nor is it needed in all situations. Gardner lists 10 ideas the nurse can use to become an effective collaborator with other interdisciplinary healthcare providers:

1. Know thyself. Many realities exist simultaneously. Each person's reality is based on self-developed perceptions. Requisite to trusting self and others is knowing your own mental model (biases, values, and goals).

2. Learn to value and manage diversity. Differences are essential assets for effective collaborative processes and outcomes.

3. Develop constructive conflict resolution skills. In the collaborative paradigm, conflict is viewed as natural and as an opportunity to deepen understanding and agreement.

4. Use your power to create win-win situations. Sharing power and recognizing one's own power base is part of effective collaboration.

5. Master interpersonal and process skills. Clinical competence, cooperation, and flexibility are the attributes most frequently identified as important to effective collaborative practice.

6. Recognize that collaboration is a journey. The skill and knowledge needed for effective collaboration take time and practice. Conflict resolution, clinical excellence, appreciative inquiry, and knowledge of group process are all skills that can be improved throughout one's lifetime.

7. Leverage all multidisciplinary forums. Being present both physically and mentally in team forums can provide an opportunity to assess how and when to offer collaborative communications for partnership-building.

8. Appreciate that collaboration can occur spontaneously. Collaboration is a mutually established condition that can happen spontaneously if the right factors are in place.

9. Balance autonomy and unity in collaborative relationships. Learn from your collaborative successes and failures. Becoming part of an exclusive team can be as bad as working in isolation. Be willing to seek feedback and admit mistakes. Be reflective and willing to seek feedback, and admit mistakes for dynamic balance.

10. Remember that collaboration is not required for all decisions. Collaboration is not a panacea, nor is it needed in all situations.

PSYCHIATRIC–MENTAL HEALTH PROFESSIONAL PERFORMANCE STANDARD 14. PROFESSIONAL PRACTICE EVALUATION

Accreditation and Regulatory Organizations

The psychiatric–mental health nurse observes political, social, and environmental trends that affect the dynamic healthcare marketplace. Ever since findings from the 1999 publication of the IOM's *To Err is Human* which revealed that upwards of 100,000 Americans die each year as a result of medical errors (subsequent publications raised that estimate to 200,000+), the U.S. public and accreditation and regulatory organizations emphasize that healthcare providers examine practices, behaviors, and processes for the purpose of institution of quality improvements and error reduction. The advent of transformational leadership, use of evidence-based interventions, refocus on maximizing workforce capacity, a redesign of the work environment to detect and prevent errors, and creation of a culture of safety have taken center stage at the forefront. This, along with the IOM's *The Future of Nursing:*

Leading Change, Advancing Health (2011), recommends that Nurse-Residency: Transitions to Practice solutions be put in place, similar to Physician-Residency Models, so new nurses have increased opportunity for preceptorship and mentoring from seasoned nurses before assuming independent nursing activities. This collaboration additionally outlays support for the elevation of nursing where 80% have BSNs and DNPs by the year 2020.

Knowledge of various bodies that evaluate professional practice environments is important. Accreditation is a voluntary process through which national government and nongovernment accrediting bodies grant recognition to designated schools and universities of nursing education, and to healthcare institutions that meet defined quality and safety standards in the care of patients and organizational management. Accreditation provides solid, consistent structural guidelines for professional development in various entities. Accreditation provides a standard mark that indicates conformance with a core set of standards, beliefs, values, and behaviors. It assures accountability for quality initiatives, and in the case of the nursing profession, attests that graduates have been introduced to core curricula across national criteria.

Accreditation processes in healthcare settings are designed to encourage continuous improvement in patient care processes and outcomes, improve upon the management and delivery of services, and provide recognition for excellence in providing safe, effective, quality, and cost-effective healthcare services. Reimbursement by governmental agencies such as Medicare, third-party payers, and vendors requires accreditation approval.

Key Regulatory Organizations for Nursing Education

The National League for Nursing Accrediting Committee (NLNAC) accredits various levels of post-secondary and higher nursing degrees, including practical, diploma, associate, baccalaureate, and master's programs. This accreditation assures a common core of standards and criteria of education. The Commission on Collegiate Nursing Education (CCNE), offered by the American Association of Colleges of Nursing, ensures the quality and integrity of baccalaureate, graduate, and residency programs in nursing. Both the NLNAC and the CCNE "should require that all nursing students demonstrate a comprehensive set of clinical performance competencies that encompass the knowledge and skills needed to provide care across settings and the lifespan" (IOM, 2011, pp. 13–14), and endorsement of a nursing program by either entity is accepted in every U.S. state.

Key Regulatory Organizations for Healthcare Settings

Key organization accreditation bodies include the Joint Commission, Health Insurance Portability and Accountability Act (HIPAA), Centers for Medicare and Medicaid Services (CMS), and the Commission on Accreditation of Rehabilitation Facilities (CARF). TJC is the oldest and largest national healthcare accrediting body in the United States. The mission of TJC is to continuously improve the safety and quality of care provided to the public by providing healthcare accreditation and related services that support performance improvement in patient care organizations. TJC's standards and performance measurements, which are reasonable expectations and able to be surveyed, provide a standardized objective evaluation process for healthcare organizations. TJC standards are updated at least annually and include sentinel event and root cause analyses.

National Committee for Quality Assurance (NCQA) is a private, nonprofit agency that is the leader in health maintenance organization (HMO) accreditation. This agency provides information to employers, federal and state agencies, and consumers to assist them in selecting among competing health plans. This organization focuses on accreditation and performance measures related to access and service.

Health Plan Employer Data and Information Set (HEDIS) is the interactive tool implemented by NCQA and used by more than 90% of America's health plans to measure performance on important dimensions of care and service. NCQA's Health Plan Report Card is a written compilation of clinical quality, member satisfaction, and comprehensive evaluation of key systems and processes.

TJC, with the National Association of Psychiatric Health Systems (NAPHS), National Association of State Mental Health Program Directors (NASMHPD), and NASMHPD Research Institute, Inc. (NRI), developed a national database of core standardized screening and evaluation measures for hospital-based patient psychiatric services (HBIPS). This initiative will be useful for quality improvement, benchmarking, accountability, decision-making, accreditation, and research. Additionally, national websites (www.hospitalscompare.gov) are arming the public with important sources for examining health outcomes among different hospitals and providers.

PSYCHIATRIC–MENTAL HEALTH PROFESSIONAL PERFORMANCE STANDARD 15. RESOURCE UTILIZATION

Resource utilization is a practice standard and an essential component of evidence-based practice. Keeping up with every change in psychiatric and mental health nursing is impossible; however, attending professional conferences and workshops, reading selected journals, and maintaining specialty certification are a few ways of remaining competent in our highly complex healthcare environment.

On the national level, the psychiatric–mental health nurse uses resources from Substance Abuse and Mental Health Services Research (SAMHSA), Brain and Behavior Research Foundation, Mental Health America (MHA), National Alliance for the Mentally Ill (NAMI), Suicide Prevention Lifeline (800-273-TALK/800-273-8255), ANA's Ethnic and Minority Fellowship Program, and the branches of the National Institutes of Health (such as National Institutes of Mental Health (NIMH), National Institute on Drug Abuse (NIDA), National Institutes on Aging (NIA), National Institute of Nursing Research (NINR), National Institute on Alcohol, Abuse and Alcoholism (NIAAA), National Center for Complementary and Integrative Health (NCCIH), National Institute of Neurological Disorders and Stroke (NINDS), National Institute on Minority Health and Health Disparities (NIMHD), National Institute of Child Health and Human Development (NICHD) (http://nih.gov/icd/). Opportunities generated from the U.S. Department of Housing and Urban Development (HUD) and the U. S. Department of Agriculture (USDA) additionally set some standards for the quality of basic care that needs to be available for all of us.

Best practice models for specific care points and specific healthcare problems are available in the literature and frequently revised when new information is disseminated in the field. Evidence-based models of care are best practices. Best practice models require the synthesis and translation of relevant research findings into guidelines for practice.

Practice guidelines provide detailed specification of the methods and procedures for treating an identified healthcare problem. These represent the synthesis of systematic literature reviews and knowledge into a set of guidelines that can be used for prevention, case-finding, diagnosis, and treatment. Many different agencies publish best-practice guidelines for treating persons with psychiatric disorders, including the National Guideline Clearinghouse (www.guideline.gov), American Psychiatric Association, and Agency for Healthcare Policy and Research.

Clinical pathways are practice guidelines that identify key clinical processes and corresponding timelines. They are generally developed by healthcare professionals within patient settings and serve as a shortened version of the multidisciplinary care plan. Clinical pathways include the following specifications (Stuart, 2009):

- Identification of target population based on diagnoses (DSM5 or nursing), conditions, treatments, interventions, or behaviors.

- Expected outcome described in a measurable, realistic, and patient-centered way.

- Specified treatment strategies and interventions.

- Documentation of patient care activities, variances, and goal achievement. This might be in the form of checklists.

Clinical algorithms represent a sequential flowchart of possible treatment options, use of medications, and progress assessment. The chart is presented as a set of guidelines, which "make explicit the art of diagnostic reasoning" (Stuart, 2009, p. 62). Each algorithm uses a decision tree format featuring decision points requiring a *yes* or *no* response, or range of lab values. This offers the advantage of providing clinicians with evidence-based standards for sound clinical practice in a timely manner. Clinical algorithms provide a standardized way to compare a patient's actual progress with expected progress guidelines. Computerized clinical algorithms are increasingly being used in mental health settings to improve clinical decision-making.

PSYCHIATRIC–MENTAL HEALTH PROFESSIONAL PERFORMANCE STANDARD 16. ENVIRONMENTAL HEALTH

Safety Across the Life Span

One way the psychiatric–mental health nurse can address environmental health involves a focus on deterrence of potential problems, before there is any real evidence of a problem (primary prevention). By facilitating primary prevention activities in healthcare or community-based settings, the nurse conveys relevant education based upon knowledge of risk factors that are pertinent to that patient or group. Some examples of safety-related targeted prevention-based information for disparate age groups are listed below:

Parents With Infants

- Choking
- Sudden Infant Death Syndrome (SIDS)
- Falling
- Drowning
- Car accidents

Parents of Young Children and the Children

- Drowning
- Pedestrian accidents
- Sharp object injuries
- Poisoning
- Falls
- Getting stuck in play objects (car trunk, refrigerator)

Parents of School-Age Children and The Children

- Equipment accidents
- Bicycle injuries
- Sports injuries
- Electrical injuries
- Firearms

Parents of Adolescents and the Adolescent

- Motor vehicle accidents

- Safe, protected sex

- Binge-drinking

- Sexually transmitted infections

- Drug and substance curiosity and experimentation

Older Adults

- Falls

- Accidents

- Fatigue-related problems

Environments that may be directly affected by psychiatric–mental health nurses include short-term and long-term inpatient consumer facilities, community-based outpatient locations, social service agencies including shelters and soup kitchens, healthcare clinics, church-sponsored activities, halfway and residential or group housing, correctional institutions, and Therapeutic Community Models. The goal is to achieve a state of balance or stability in the environment that promotes optimal health and healing. A caring-healing framework, recognized by Jean Watson and others, incorporates attending to the whole person, and is within the purview and scope of practice of the field of professional nursing. An experience of health can take form in many dimensions (Swanson & Wojnar, 2004). Health may be defined as any of the following:

- Absence of illness

- Capacity to adapt

- Functional, emphasizing role fulfillment

- Eudaimonistic (*eu* = good attention, happy; *demon* = spirit)

Several additional strategies are considered in environmental health practice promotion (ANA, 2014; pp. 84–85) and includes the identification of

- Sounds, odors, noises, and lights that threaten health,

- Caustic and toxic chemical solutions in use,

- Appropriate personal protective equipment,

- Sustainable environmental policies and conditions,

- Ergonomic tools, and

- Tobacco-free environments (healthcare settings, schools, restaurants, etc.).

Tobacco-Free Environments

Care delivery in tobacco-free environments is an important support for patients who are regular nicotine users. The American Psychiatric Nurses Association (APNA) and other organizations, such as the American Lung Association, provides training to nurses and other clinicians on tobacco cessation strategies and nicotine replacement therapies. Tobacco-Free Nurses (http://www.tobaccofreenurses.org) is a body of nurses who work to build capacity among peers to assist them with cessation strategies for patients and nurses themselves. The organization exists, also, to facilitate nursing's involvement in tobacco control policies, research, and promotion in nursing academic curriculum.

Clinical practice guidelines initially published in 2000 by the U.S. Public Health Service (2014) recommend that all healthcare providers conduct the 5 action "A's" (Table 7.6) for tobacco assessment at every clinical encounter. Tobacco dependence is a chronic condition that often requires repeated intervention. The 5 A's recommend that nurses (and other providers) **A**sk about tobacco use (smoking, chewing, dipping), **A**ssess frequency and type of use, **A**dvise

TABLE 7-6.
THE FIVE A'S FOR ADDRESSING NICOTINE (TOBACCO USE)

5 A'S	ACTIONS	STRATEGIES AND TIPS
1. Ask about use and ETS exposure.	Identify and document tobacco use with every patient at every visit.	As part of the routine assessment
2. Advise to quit.	Use clear, strong, personalized messages.	"We will help you quit; your health is important; you will save money and prevent future illnesses."
3. Assess willingness to quit.	Willing to quit now?	Provide motivational video, information on aids to quitting.
4. Assist with quit attempt.	Use counseling, pharmacotherapy, refer for cessation treatment.	Strategies: ▸ Set a quit date contract within 2 weeks. ▸ Tell family and friends—arrange new social network. ▸ Anticipate challenges and withdrawal symptoms. ▸ Prepare the home, workplace setting, and car. ▸ If smoking 10 or more cigarettes a day, recommend OTC or prescription aid.
5. Arrange a follow-up.	Office visit or telephone 1 week after quit date.	▸ Arrange second follow-up within 1 month. ▸ Expect a relapse; use it as a learning experience. ▸ Problem-solve. ▸ Inquire about pharmacotherapy side effects, if appropriate.

U.S. Public Health Service. (2014). *USPHS Clinical Practice Guidelines: Tobacco Use and Dependence: Overview of Best Practices.* Retrieved from http://www.rchsd.org/documents/2014/02/clinical-practice-guideline-treating-tobacco-use-dependence-overview-of-best-practice.pdf.

person that quitting is possible and quit-lines are available, **A**ssist person with identifying their readiness to change and learning styles and needs, and **A**rrange follow-up for continued support and nicotine replacement therapies. Nurses have great advocacy opportunities to lead their organizations in planning and implementing strategies to retain patients in care environments that are tobacco-free.

PATIENT LEGAL PROTECTIONS

Civil (Involuntary) Commitment (5150; pink slip, etc.): Laws spell out legal processes leading to involuntary commitment. They are also used to determine the legal declaration of mental illness and provide guidelines for when people can be placed in in-patient settings without their consent. Civil commitment procedures allow states to involuntarily commit a patient to a mental health facility or hospital when the patient is unable to take care of him- or herself because of mental illness. *Involuntary admission* does not originate with the patient, but is initiated by the hospital or court. Depending on individual state laws, patients may lose some or none of their civil rights during the time of involuntary confinement. A petition for involuntary admission can be placed by a police officer, a psychiatrist, or other designees appointed by the state, or the patient's family. Specific state mandates vary, but usually one or two physicians are required to medically certify that the patient is in need of involuntary confinement based on their examination of the patient's mental status. In some states, a psychiatric–mental health nurse clinician has this authority.

An initial confinement in a medical facility can be ordered for up to 72 hours. If the person is still considered a danger to self or others or is gravely disabled after the 72-hour period, he or she can usually be legally placed on an additional 14-day certification, but a court hearing must be held to uphold the confinement of persons beyond this time. People are entitled to have their commitment reviewed every 6 months. Specifics of civil commitment laws vary from state to state, although the criteria commonly involve:

- Having a serious mental illness that creates a lack of insight about the need for hospitalization
- Being an immediate danger to self or others because of a mental illness
- Being unable to care for him- or herself because of a mental illness

Civil law: A breach of civil law by nurses most frequently involves a violation of a patient's legal rights or a wrongful act that causes a patient injury. A *tort* is defined as a wrongful act committed against a person or his or her property that involves a violation of a patient's legal rights, or of a standard of care that causes patient injury. Intentional torts include assault and battery.

Common law: Common laws involve negligence and malpractice. They evolve from previous legal decisions, which form a precedent over time.

Competence and incompetence: Psychiatric–mental health nurses must understand the concept of competency because patients must be competent to give informed consent to their treatment plan. Competency is not necessarily a fixed idea; incompetence can be episodic with some mental disorders. As in the case of bipolar disorder, or major depressive episodes, competence can be re-established during remissions. A person under the influence of psychoactive drugs or severely stressed may not be competent at one point, yet fully competent at another. Competency also is an issue in a court of law, where it is used to determine whether a person with mental illness is able to aid his or her defense attorney and to understand the charges in a court of law and therefore able to proceed to trial.

If a competency evaluation determines that a person is incompetent, an appropriate mental health provider has diagnosed a person to be physically or mentally unable to make a well-reasoned, deliberate, and knowledgeable healthcare decision. In this situation, a guardian or conservator is legally appointed to make healthcare decisions for the patient until such time as he or she is judged to be competent. Guardianship or conservatorship refers to a prescribed legal process in which a person or agency is appointed by the court to act on behalf of the disabled person. The guardian or conservator can make decisions on behalf of the patient, as well as provide informed consent for the identified patient when the patient is unable to do so. This person also has the authority over the patient's finances. Competence has implications in determining issues such as healthcare power of attorney (HCPOA), advance directives, etc. Competence involves the patient's ability to

▸ Understand the information provided,

▸ Reason the implications logically through to making a decision,

▸ Appreciate the consequences of making one choice over another, and

▸ Clearly express a reasonable choice.

Custody Issues: When parents divorce or die, the court establishes legal arrangements to provide for the care of minor children. The parent or caregiver who is awarded custody has the decision-making responsibility regarding healthcare, education, and religious upbringing. There are different types of custody.

▸ **Joint custody:** Both parents hold physical and legal custody equally. Joint physical custody means that the child will physically live at both parents' homes with an equal amount of scheduled time spent at each parent's residence. Legal custody means that both parents are involved in making decisions and fulfilling financial obligations.

▸ **Sole legal custody:** One parent has the right and responsibility to make decisions relating to the health, education, and welfare of the child. The other parent generally is awarded defined visitation rights.

▸ **Joint legal custody:** Both parents have the right and responsibility to make decisions relating to the health, education, and welfare of the child.

▸ **Sole physical custody:** The child resides with and under the supervision of one parent, subject to the court's power to order visitation by the other parent.

▸ **Joint physical custody:** Both parents have significant periods of physical custody to assure a child of frequent and continuing contact with both parents.

Duty to Warn (Tarasoff's Law): Healthcare professionals have responsibility for assessing threats of violence, identifying persons being threatened, and implementing some affirmative, preventive actions. For the psychiatric–mental health nurse, this may involve deliberate and decisive reporting of elicited threats up the chain of command.

Insanity Defense: Two types of insanity defenses are used when persons with mental illnesses commit a criminal act: (1) not guilty by reason of insanity, or (2) guilty but mentally ill. Successful defenses can result in confinement in a state hospital for treatment rather than in a prison. The burden of proof is on the defense to determine if a person is competent to stand trial or engage in legal processes. Two legal standards are most frequently used to determine criminal responsibility:

▸ **M'Naghten Rule:** The person lacks the mental capacity to understand that his or her actions were legally wrong, or is mentally unable to understand the physical nature or quality of his or her act.

▸ **Irresistible Impulse Test:** The person was impulsively driven to commit the criminal action and could not control his or her actions because of lack of mental capacity, even if he or she knew the actions to be wrong.

Malpractice: Malpractice is a type of negligence for which the nurse can be sued in court. To meet the criteria for malpractice in a court of law:

▸ The duty was obligated to the patient because of the professional relationship.

▸ There was a breach of duty in which the actions of the nurse violated this duty, failed to adhere to appropriate standards of care, or both.

▸ The breach of duty was the immediate cause of the resulting injury.

▸ Substantive damages or injury resulted directly from the breach of duty.

Negligence: Negligence is the commission or omission of an act that falls below the accepted standard of care. In a court of law, negligence is judged based on what a reasonable and prudent nurse would ordinarily do, or would not have done, in a similar situation. Basic issues of nurse negligence would be failing to report

▸ Child and elder abuse (sexual, physical, emotional, exploitative) and neglect;

▸ Contagious diseases; or

▸ Gunshot wounds and stabbings.

Patient Rights Covered by General Statute: Patients have both specific and general rights. The specific rights can vary from state to state. Rights of institutionalized patients are established by state statutes and vary greatly. Any time any of these rights are denied, there must be a sound reason and it must be documented. Denial of rights can never be punitive. In general, patients have the right to adequate, appropriate treatment, which includes the following at the basic level:

- A humane psychological and physical environment
- Qualified personnel to provide individualized care and individualized treatment plans
- The right to be released if not dangerous
- The right to aftercare
- Confidentiality
- Issues related to being involuntary detained
- Send and receive mail
- Consult with personal physician, attorney, or clergy
- Visitation, unless there are documented reasons for denial
- Use allowable (safe) personal possessions
- Privacy and private storage space
- Self-determination
- Refuse treatment or medication. All patients have the right to refuse medication, except for limited use during emergency situations or when they are court-ordered to take the medication.
- Refuse psychosurgery or electroconvulsive therapy (ECT)
- Receive help from patient advocates
- Least restrictive treatment environment—a balance between maintaining highest level of patient freedom and providing appropriate behavioral emergency treatment

Privileged Communication: Privileged communication does not fall under HIPAA supervision. It refers exclusively to court proceedings, and is designed to protect the provider from having to reveal in court a patient's communication without the patient's written permission. This means that the nurse cannot be called to testify as a witness in a court procedure without the patient's written permission to release information about him- or herself.

Protected Health Information (PHI) and Health Insurance Portability and Accountability Act (HIPAA): HIPAA is a federal law that went into effect in April 2003 and places restrictions on the use of a patient's "protected health information" by covered entities such as individual healthcare providers, hospitals, nursing homes, clinics, mental health centers, and researchers. HIPAA defines protected health information (PHI) as any identifiable health information, including the name and contact information of a patient, that is or can reasonably be linked to that patient. Release of such information is prohibited unless it is explicitly allowed by the privacy rule or the patient gives written consent. HIPAA

▸ Defines who may see or use health information, and what they can do with it;

▸ Limits uses and disclosures of health information to the minimum amount of information needed for care; and

▸ Establishes broad patient rights related to seeing and asking for corrections of their own health information.

PHI includes all identifiable patient information related to past, present, or future physical or mental health needs, treatment provision, or payment for providing mental health care of patients. For example, PHI would include who provided the care, what type of care was provided, where the care was given, when the care was provided, and the rationale for providing the care. This information can only be transmitted when the patient, or someone legally acting on the patient's behalf, provides written permission to do so. Potential sources of HPI appear in the form of written or oral communication (e.g., charts, letters, notes, reports, phone calls, meetings, informal conversations), computerized or electronic communication (e.g., email, computer records, faxes, voicemail, laptop and tablet computers, personal devices, smartphones, Google glasses).

Privacy maintenance of PHI in patient records requires that nurses use and do not share computer passwords, keep records behind locked doors in locked file cabinets, and limit access to workspace where health information is stored or used and printers or fax machines where health information is printed to only those professionals who need the information for a specific function or health-related care task. Allowable disclosures according to HIPAA:

▸ Judicial and administrative proceedings in response to a written order of the court or an administrative tribunal, or in response to subpoena, discovery request, or "other lawful process." The requester or healthcare provider must give notice to the patient or get a protective order from the court first.

▸ To avert serious threat to the health or safety of a person or the public, disclosures must be only to the person reasonably able to prevent or lessen the threat, or only when it is necessary for law enforcement personnel to identify or apprehend a person.

Rights of Minors: Only parents or legal guardians have the legal right to make treatment decisions for minors, unless they are emancipated. Minors are defined as all persons under the age of 18 years. The authority of a parent can come to an end for minors upon the appointment by a court of a guardian for the minor, or through a legal process in which the adolescent requests a court to declare him or her emancipated. The Emancipation of Minors Act allows for a legal process in which a mature minor, demonstrating the ability and capacity to manage his or her own affairs and living independently of parents or guardian, may obtain the legal status and power to enter into valid legal contracts. There is some variation among states as to exact protocols, but, in general, criteria for emancipation include one or more of the following: marriage of the minor, enlistment of the minor as a member on active duty in the U.S. military, living independently and able to maintain financial independence.

▸ **Confidentiality:** Parents or legal guardians have the legal right to review their minor child's record unless there is legal documentation that the court has terminated parental rights. At the beginning of treatment this should be discussed with the minor and the parents, defining what information will be shared and what will be kept private. The minor also can authorize release of medical records.

▸ **Privilege:** Confidentiality relates to legal matters; parents usually hold the privilege to disclose or not to disclose information in a court of law.

▸ **Exceptions to parents:** The provider or therapist can refuse to allow parents to inspect the records when the minor is the victim of a crime or when there is a court-appointed guardian or custodian holding privilege.

▸ **No parental consent:** When the minor is 12 or older, presents good reason not to involve parents, and is mature enough to participate intelligently in outpatient treatment, parental consent need not be obtained. Clinical issues that can be treated without parental consent include help for substance abuse and prevention or treatment of pregnancy; when the child has been the alleged victim of incest or child abuse (including rape); and when the minor might be a serious threat, mentally or physically, to self without treatment.

▸ **Fees for treatment of a minor:** Parents are not held responsible for payment for treatment of their minor child when the parent has not been contacted and has not given consent for treatment.

▸ **Assent:** A minor can generally *assent*, not *consent*, to treatment or participation in a research study. A minor's assent must be followed by obtaining required consent from the parent or legal guardian before treatment or participation begins.

▸ **Therapist responsibility:** Involve parents in treatment of a minor unless the therapist believes it is not in the best interest of the minor. The therapist must note in the record if or when the parents were notified or, if not notified, why it was considered inappropriate to notify.

Voluntary admission to a hospital or treatment center begins with the written application of the patient **(informed consent),** or patient's guardian in the case of a minor. The patient or guardian can initiate discharge and the patient retains all civil rights. Voluntary patients who elect to leave the hospital against medical advice must sign a form indicating that this is their intent.

REFERENCES

Agency for Healthcare Quality and Research. (2008). *Healthcare consumer safety and quality handbook: An evidence-based handbook for nurses.* Publication #08–0043. Retrieved from http://www.ahrq.gov/qual/nursehdbk.

Aiken L. H., Sloane D. M., Bruyneel L., Van den Heede, K., Griffiths, P., Busse, R., … Sermeus, W., RN4CAST consortium. (2014). Nurse staffing and education and hospital mortality in nine European counties: A retrospective observational study. *Lancet, 383*(9931): 1824–30.

American Hospital Association. (2008). *A healthcare consumer care partnership. Understanding expectations, rights and responsibilities.* Retrieved from http://www.aha.org/aha/issues/Communicating-With-Healthcare consumers/pt-care-partnership.html.

American Nurses Association. (2001). *Code of ethics for nurses with interpretive statements.* Silver Spring, MD: Nursesbooks.org.

American Nurses Association. (2010). *Nursing's social policy statement.* Silver Spring, MD: Nursesbooks.org.

American Nurses Association, International Society of Psychiatric–Mental Health Nurses, and American Psychiatric Nurses Association. (2014). *Psychiatric–mental health nursing: Scope and standards of practice, 2nd ed.* Silver Spring, MD: Nursesbooks.org.

Barloon, L. (2000). Legal aspects of psychiatric nursing. *Nursing clinics of North America, 38*(1), 9–19.

Boyd, M. A. (2007). *Psychiatric nursing: Contemporary practice, 4th ed.* Philadelphia: Lippincott Williams & Wilkins.

Brenner, P. (1984). *From novice to expert: Excellence and power in clinical nursing practice.* Menlo Park, CA: Addison-Wesley.

Commission on Accreditation of Rehabilitation Facilities. (2015). *CARF accreditation focuses on quality, results.* Retrieved from http://www.carf.org/home/.

Gardner, D. (2005). Ten lessons in collaboration. *Online Journal of Issues in Nursing, 10*(1). Retrieved from www.nursingworld.org/MainMenuCategories/ANAMarketplace/ANAPeriodicals/OJIN/TableofContents/Volume102005/No1Jan05/tpc26_116008.aspx.

Gallup Poll. (2013, December 5–8). Honesty and ethics rating of clergy slides to new low. Retrieved from http://www.gallup.com/poll/166298/honesty-ethics-rating-clergy-slides-new-low.aspx.

Halter, M. J. (2014). *Varcolis' foundations of psychiatric mental health nursing: A clinical approach, 7th ed.* Philadelphia: Saunders.

Hutchinson, K. M., & Froelicher, E. A. (2003). Populations at risk for tobacco-related diseases. *Seminar in Oncology Nursing, 19*(4), 276–283.

Institute of Medicine. (2001). Committee on Quality of Health Care in America. (2000). *To err is human: Building a safer health system.* Washington, DC: National Academy Press.

Institute of Medicine. (2011). *The future of nursing: Leading change, advancing health.* Washington, DC: The National Academies Press.

Institute of Medicine: Smedley, B. D., Stith, A. Y., & Nelson, A. R. (Eds.). (2002). *Unequal treatment: Confronting racial and ethnic disparities in health care.* Washington, DC: The National Academies Press.

Institute of Medicine's Committee on Crossing the Quality Chasm: Adaptation to Mental Health and Addictive Disorders. (2006). *Improving the quality of health care for mental and substance-use conditions: Quality chasm series.* Washington, DC: The National Academies Press.

Institute of Medicine's Committee on Quality of Health Care in America. (2001). *Crossing the quality chasm: A new health system for the 21st century.* Washington, DC: The National Academies Press.

Institute of Medicine's Committee on the Work Environment for Nurses and Healthcare Consumer Safety. (2004). *Keeping healthcare consumers safe: Transforming the work environment for nurses and healthcare consumer safety.* Washington, DC: The National Academies Press.

Marquis, B., & Huston, C. (1992). *Leadership roles and management functions in nursing and healthcare.* Philadelphia: J.B. Lippincott

Melnyk, B., & Fineout-Overholt, E. (2004). *Evidence-based practice in nursing and healthcare: A guide to best practice.* Baltimore: Lippincott Williams & Wilkins.

National Commission for the Protection of Human Subjects of Biomedical and Behavioral Research. (1979). *The Belmont report.* Retrieved from http://www.hhs.gov/ohrp/humansubjects/guidance/belmont.htm.

National Council of State Boards of Nursing. (2005). *Joint statement on delegation: American Nurses Association and the National Council of State Boards of Nursing.* Retrieved from https://www.ncsbn.org/Delegation_joint_statement_NCSBN-ANA.pdf.

National Council of State Boards of Nursing. (2008). *Boards of nursing.* Retrieved from https://www.ncsbn.org/boards.htm.

Newhouse, R., Dearholt, S., Poe, S., Pugh, L., & White, K. (2007). *Johns Hopkins nursing evidence-based practice model and guidelines.* Indianapolis: Sigma Theta Tau International.

Oxman, A., Sackett, D., & Guyatt, G.; Evidence-Based Medicine Work Group. (1993). Users' guides to evidence-based medicine. *Journal of the American Medical Association, 270,* 2093–2095.

Polit, D. F., & Beck, C. T. (2011). *Nursing research: Generating and assessing evidence for nursing practice, 9th ed.* Philadelphia: Lippincott Williams & Wilkins.

Potter, P., & Perry A. (2009). *Fundamentals of nursing, 7th ed.* St. Louis: Mosby Elsevier.

Puntil, C., York, J., Limandri, B., Greene, P., Arauz, E., & Hobbs, D. (2013). Competency-based training for nurse-generalists: Inhealthcare consumer intervention and prevention of suicide. *Journal of the American Psychiatric Nurses Association, 19*(4), 205–210.

Quinn, F., & Hughes, S. (2000). *The principles and practice of nurse education.* Kingston upon Thames, UK: Nelson Thornes.

Sarna, L., Bialous, S. A., Hutchinson, K. M., Williams, B. S., Froelicher, E. S., & Wewers, M. E. (2003). Views of African American nurses about tobacco cessation and prevention. *Journal of the National Black Nurses Association, 14*(2), 1–8.

Skloot, R. (2010). *The immortal life of Henrietta Lacks.* New York: Crown Publishers.

SQUIRE guidelines summary. (n.d.) Retrieved from http://www.squire-statement.org/guidelines.

Stein, K. F. (2014). Why use publication guidelines in JAPNA? *Journal of the American Psychiatric Nurses Association, 20*(5), 305–306.

Stuart, G. (2009). *Principles and practice of psychiatric nursing, 9th ed.* St. Louis: Mosby Elsevier.

Swanson, K. M., & Wojnar, D. M. (2004). Optimal healing environments in nursing. *The Journal of Alternative and Complementary Medicine, 10*(supplement 1), S-43–S-48.

Townsend, M. C. (2009). *Psychiatric mental health nursing: Concepts of care in evidence-based practice, 6th ed.* Philadelphia: F. A. Davis.

U.S. Department of Health and Human Services: Office for Human Research Protections. Human subjects research (45 CFR 46). Retrieved from http://www.hhs.gov/ohrp/humansubjects/guidance/45cfr46.html.

U.S. Public Health Service. (2014). *USPHS clinical practice guidelines: Tobacco use and dependence: Overview of best practices.* Retrieved from http://www.rchsd.org/documents/2014/02/clinical-practice-guideline-treating-tobacco-use-dependence-overview-of-best-practice.pdf.

Wysoker, A. (2003). HIPAA and psychiatric nurses. *Journal of the American Psychiatric Nurses Association, 9*(5), 173–175.

CATEGORY IV

PATIENT EDUCATION AND POPULATION HEALTH

CHAPTER 8

PATIENT EDUCATION, POPULATION, AND ENVIRONMENTAL HEALTH

This chapter focuses on various teaching and learning strategies, counseling approaches, and other individual psychoeducational techniques that support patient- and family-centered mental health promotion across the life span. Standard 5A of the ANA's (2014) *Scope and Standards of Psychiatric–Mental Health Nursing Practice* pertains to care delivery and coordination models, and 5B addresses the health teaching and health promotion responsibilities of the psychiatric–mental health nurse. Issues pertinent across the life span related to individual, family, group, community, and national health models are outlined in this chapter. The chapter concludes with various roles of the professional registered nurse in advocating for process and policy change to eliminate stigma, discrimination, and criminalization experiences among persons with mental illness.

PSYCHIATRIC–MENTAL HEALTH PRACTICE STANDARD 5A: COORDINATION OF CARE

All therapeutic (purposeful) treatment approaches try to help patients use their own mental processes, adaptabilities, strengths, and personal internal and external supports to bring about desired changes. In some states, nurses with advanced preparation can perform psychotherapy, but all psychiatric and mental health nurses should be familiar with relevant treatment models used in psychiatric settings across the life span care continuum. Care delivery models incorporate needs of the individual and family throughout the lifecycle from "womb to tomb."

Case management is a collaborative process to assess, plan, implement, coordinate, monitor, and evaluate patient options and services. Case management includes developing a plan of care to meet identified needs, ensuring access to care, and implementing a method of monitoring care. It is a unique form of treatment management that nurse case managers coordinate between and within systems, connecting services, and acting as important safety nets in the event of service gaps. Designed toward improved patient outcomes, the enlisted strategies support closer communication and connection to available high-quality, cost-effective resources. The case manager may advocate for use of medications on formulary and works with community agencies to ensure high-quality coordination of follow-up care. Case managers help in determining the best location for care and avoiding duplication of services and use of unnecessary resources.

The Joint Commission (TJC) sets standards for admission and discharge that require attention. Prior to admission, the nurse identifies and uses information about patient needs that may come from collateral sources or communication from other care settings and organizations. During the admission process, service provisions are consistent with the hospital, organization, or agency's mission, and facilitation from one setting to another is arranged. Medication reconciliation must occur across settings; and formal consultations, contractual arrangements, or referrals are used to support the transfer of patient care from one level to another. While the patient is hospitalized, service flow continues for the patient, care is individualized and coordinated among providers, and appropriate age, developmental level, and family-centered care is collaborated and delivered across the healthcare continuum. Before discharge, TJC requires that the need for discharge planning is determined; the patient and family have received education in preparation for the discharge and an understanding of early signs and symptoms of relapse, as well as strategies to address safety issues (safety plan, suicide hotlines, provider contact information) is articulated and signed. At discharge, the patient's individual needs are reviewed and reassessed, and referral or aftercare arrangements are made and communicated orally and in writing to the patient and signed.

Discharge Planning

Discharge planning is a patient-centered, cost-effective interdisciplinary process that helps the patient receive additional necessary mental and community-based health care, and follow-up care and case management once discharged from the hospital. Effective discharge planning requires ongoing collaboration among the patient, patient's family, and the interdisciplinary team to assure informed decision-making. Discharge planning and teaching should begin with the patient's admission and be continually documented and updated based on changes in patient status. The discharge plan should relate to the initial assessment of the patient's potential needs identified on admission to the setting. For maximum effectiveness, discharge plans should be written and orally conveyed to the patient and patient's family. Written instructions should be clear, simple, and easy to understand. Each discharge plan contains common elements, as well as others tailored to the individualized needs of the patient. For example, discharge plans should include a summary that details the following:

▸ Patient's physical, mental, cognitive, economic, and emotional strengths and abilities

▸ Patient's functional status

▸ Patient's support system and its availability

▸ An identified safety plan

▸ Emergency contact numbers

▸ Resolution of any medication reconciliation issues

▸ Whether the patient needs post-hospital services and, if yes, whether these services are available, and who will provide them

▸ Available community resources and public benefits, including financial assistance

▸ Early signs of relapse and risky behaviors that can lead to relapse

▸ Medical and psychological strategies for handling early warning signs, including whom to contact if reemergence of symptoms is suspected

▸ Details of medication adherence, including medication name, dosage, treatment effects, and potential side effects; whom to call and for what reasons

▸ An individualized recovery plan including biopsychosocial treatments, informal and formal community-based support systems

▸ Referrals for case management and other essential social and financial supports

▸ Provider contact phone numbers with emergency contact numbers should be given to patient and family caregivers

Service providers, case managers, and other agencies involved in the ongoing care of the patient should be contacted. Discharge summaries and follow-up actions should be clearly spelled out in writing to all involved professionals (with the patient's knowledge and written permission). Some communication, general or specific, about patient needs may have to be shared with primary providers, again, with the patient's knowledge and written permission. Because psychiatric and substance abuse disorders tend to be persistent and recurrent, many persons with serious and persistent mental illnesses (SPMI) or chronic substance abuse problems require a continuous, integrated, and comprehensive approach of assessment and treatment to function effectively and to maintain self-sufficiency in the community.

Patient Strengths and Assets (Protective Factors) and Liabilities (Risk) Factors

Health education and prevention efforts target social, environmental, and personal variables that may affect the development or expression of mental disorders. Often described as risk and protective factors, personal variables contribute to a person's resilience (protective) in the face of challenges to mental health, or increase a person's susceptibility (risk) to developing a mental disorder. An important goal of health promotion and disease prevention activities is to decrease risk factors and increase protective factors implicated in the development of mental disorders and behavioral problems. The Joint Commission advises (Schyve, 2014) that screening for violence risk, psychological trauma history, substance use, and patient strengths be demonstrated. Knowledge of patient strengths is essential for developing and delivering comprehensive patient-centered care.

Protective factors may include the following:

- Social and community supports
- Strength-based personal competencies
- Knowledge and education
- Culture and spirituality
- Access to care
- Supportive relationships
- Healthy lifestyle
- Safe living environment
- Access to nutritious foods

Risk factors for mental disorders and behavioral problems represent a complex interplay of biopsychosocial and spiritual variables. Identifiable risk factors include the following:

- Gender, ethnicity, and age
- Residence in food deserts
- Lack of access to, or inadequate, health care
- Poverty and homelessness
- Substandard housing
- Significant losses
- Family or personal history of mental illness or substance abuse
- History of trauma or exposure to violence

- Limited social and financial resources

- Family or marital discord

- Neglect and abuse during childhood

- Weak social ties to the community or cultural group

- Lack of supportive relationships

- Developmental, intellectual, neurodevelopmental, and learning disorders

- Genetic vulnerability

- Poor sleep hygiene

PSYCHIATRIC-MENTAL HEALTH PRACTICE STANDARD 5B: HEALTH TEACHING AND HEALTH PROMOTION

Levels of Prevention

Illness (disease or disorder) prevention activities target three levels of prevention: primary, secondary, or tertiary strategies. At each level, education is an essential methodology for achieving health-related goals.

Primary prevention actions are taken before a mental disorder develops to minimize risk factors and health-related threats to vulnerable populations. From an epidemiological perspective, primary prevention strategies emphasize reducing the *incidence* of mental disorders. Health teaching focuses on helping patients develop skills and knowledge related to controllable risk factors and promoting a healthy lifestyle. In assessing patient learning needs for primary prevention actions, the nurse considers three areas for primary prevention foci. *Examples:* parenting classes for expectant families, stress management skill training.

- **Universal prevention** strategies target the general public or an entire population group.

- **Selective prevention** strategies target only those individuals or subgroups of a population whose risk factors for developing a mental disorder are significantly higher than that of the general population.

- **Indicated or targeted prevention** strategies specifically target persons at highest risk for development of mental disorders.

Secondary prevention actions and interventions promote early diagnosis of symptoms and timely treatment near the beginning of a disorder or disease. From an epidemiological perspective, secondary prevention strategies are designed to reduce the number of current cases of mental disorder (prevalence). *Examples:* blood pressure screening; screening for cognitive impairment among older adults, screening for depression or substance use.

Tertiary prevention refers to rehabilitation efforts and strategies designed to minimize the handicapping effects of a mental disorder and problem behaviors. Tertiary preventive teaching includes helping patients to cope more effectively with the necessary adjustments that a serious mental disorder may impose. Other tertiary prevention strategies are designed to address challenging behaviors that can be dangerous or disruptive enough to impair education or job achievement and quality of life. Supports for rehabilitative efforts in tertiary prevention often are provided through case management. Patient and family engagement with Assertive Community Treatment Teams (ACCT) teams is an example of a tertiary prevention intervention.

Considerations in Patient Education, Teaching, and the Learning Process

Patient education refers to any type of planned educational activity developed for the purpose of empowering an individual and family to participate in improving health status, health promotion behaviors, health self-management, or general well-being. Patient education is a collaborative, interactive process between nurse and patient in which:

- Instruction and skill demonstration is presented formally or informally, depending on the individualized learning needs of the patient and family.

- Skill development is based on cognitive understanding according to ability, readiness, and motivation to learn.

- Instruction and skill development is age- and developmentally appropriate and culturally sensitive.

- The desired outcome is to produce an observable change in the learner's health knowledge, attitude, and behavior related to an identifiable mental healthcare need.

The Learning Process

Learning is defined as an active and continuous process of acquiring knowledge and skills, manifested by growth and changes in behavior. Health teaching should incorporate recognition and acknowledgment of spiritual values, especially those that are part of the person's cultural heritage. The goal of any health learning engagement is to change behaviors by acquiring appropriate knowledge, skills, and attitudes. The nurse demonstrates the therapeutic (purposive) nature of interactions with patients and families. Teaching interventions that help provide meaning and hope are more likely to be accepted by patients and their families.

Children and adults learn differently. Pedagogy refers to the art and science of teaching children. Andragogy is defined as the art and science of teaching adults. Understanding the specific learning needs of the learner and the level of the patient's knowledge are necessary components of effective psycho-education or health teaching efforts. Adult learning principles and developmentally appropriate educational strategies to use with children and adolescents are important variables that influence teaching and learning.

Teaching Children: Pedagogy

Recognizing the child's cognitive, developmental, and psychosocial stages of development and incorporating this knowledge into a teaching plan are important dimensions of effective health teaching for children. The most effective teaching approaches include describing each behavioral skill, followed by activities that teach and allow the child sufficient time to practice those skills (serial or sequential learning). Role-playing and discussion about choices that allow children to think through options are important components of this form of health teaching for school-aged children, as well as adolescents.

In contrast to adult learners, children are much more dependent on the educator for direction. The health educator serves as a role model for the child. Children have much less life experience that can be tapped as a resource for the current learning. They learn more effectively when the presentation is lively and interactive and when the nurse has taken the time to establish a relationship with the child. Games, simple activities, and stories can be used to teach children important concepts about ways to enhance their health and well-being.

Teaching content and presentations should be culturally appropriate and geared to the developmental age of the child (e.g., therapeutic play with puppets or dolls for preschoolers). Pictures and telling stories are useful strategies in helping children tell you what they need and how they feel, and engaging them in a learning environment. Diagrams and models can be used to teach school-aged children. Children learn best in short sessions, because their focused attention spans may be shorter than an adult. They are eager to learn things, but content must be presented in a concrete, interesting manner and in shorter segments. Children also need consistent, positive feedback and reinforcements to learn appropriate behavior.

Psychiatric–mental health nurses working with children having a clinical or behavioral mental disorder need to be familiar with the Individuals with Disabilities Education Act (IDEA) (U.S. Department of Education, 2004) and Section 504 of the Rehabilitation Act of 1973 (USDHHS, n.d.). These federal laws require that schools provide equal opportunities to succeed in the classroom. Nurses can advise parents of these laws, because their child, if he or she qualifies, will be eligible for planned special accommodations and individualized behavioral support necessary to promote succeed in the classroom. Test scores, school performance, and parental involvement largely determine eligibility. Each child who qualifies is entitled to have an individualized education plan (IEP), which mandates and describes the specific teaching accommodations required by the child.

Teaching Adults: Andragogy

Malcolm Knowles (2005) is recognized as a pioneer in describing the characteristics of the adult learner using principles of andragogy, writing "Adults need to know why they need to learn something before undertaking to learn it" (Knowles, Holton, & Swanson, 2005, p. 64). With adults, learning is intended to build on life experience, skills, attitudes, and competencies already achieved. According to Knowles, adult learners

- Value self-directed learning;
- Are motivated to learn new things that will help them function more effectively;
- Want to be active participants in all aspects of the learning process;
- Want guidance, but not an authoritarian teaching style;
- Want their previous life experiences to be respected as a resource and integrated into their learning process;
- Want variety in learning experiences;
- Want to be immediately able to apply learning to real-life contexts;
- Respond best to pragmatic, problem-centered learning; and
- Want to learn at their own speed and in their own style.

Facilitating the learning process for adults requires that

- Information is relevant;
- Information progresses from simple to complex, from the known to the unknown;
- The facilitator is open to prompt and frequent feedback;
- The facilitator allows the learner to test ideas, analyze mistakes, take risks, and be creative;
- Feedback is optimized to provide personal knowledge of the learner's progress toward the goal;
- Information is satisfying;
- Information is comparable to similarities and differences between past experiences and present situations that can be recognized and incorporated;
- Information is immediately applicable;
- Information can be integrated patient's own areas of interest within the learning content;
- Information is attainable for assimilation at one's own rate; and
- The teacher acts as a guide, but learners are encouraged to find answers to questions on their own.

Teaching Older Adults: Special Considerations

Older adults may need modifications in the learning environment for maximum learning effectiveness. The speed of learning tends to decrease with age, but the depth of learning may increase. Although it may take people longer to learn as they get older, older adults can grasp what is learned at a deeper and more relevant level. Physical factors should be considered as well to maximize learning; for example, using larger print, making sure the patient has the appropriate hearing aids or corrective lenses if needed. Additional strategies that can be helpful with older adults:

- Keep explanations brief, but accurate.
- Use analogies to illustrate abstract information.
- Speak slowly and distinctly.
- Minimize distractions.
- Use concrete examples in the environment.
- Build on past life experiences.
- Make information relevant and meaningful.
- Present one concept at a time.
- Allow time for processing.
- Repeat and reinforce information.

Ability to Learn

Effective teaching plans recognize that one size does not fit all. In addition to assessing patient readiness to learn, psychiatric nurses need to consider the patient's ability to learn.

- **Developmental level:** Personality and cognitive development variables affect learning readiness and ability, but are not always completely correlated with chronological age. Patients at different cognitive and psychosocial developmental levels require different learning strategies to maximize learning.

- **Cognitive ability** is the extent to which a person can gain knowledge, understand, and process information. Cognitive factors that can affect the learning process include thought-processing deficits associated with schizophrenia, cognitive disorders, and distortions relative to being under the influence of psychoactive drugs or alcohol. Other factors include cognitive ability gauged by IQ levels and level of health literacy. Learning disabilities, intellectual disability, low reading skill levels, and low health literacy are factors that need special considerations. Without individualized disability-related accommodations, patients may struggle to attain or practice new or complex health-promoting information.

Health Literacy

Health literacy is the degree to which persons are able to attain and understand health information to the extent that they can make appropriate personal health decisions. (Ratzan & Parker, 2000). In 2004, the Institute of Medicine issued a landmark *Report on Health Literacy*, taking the position that health literacy occurs through a combination of education, health services, and cultural factors. Although people may be functionally literate, they may not be health-literate. Health literacy is obtained by people who are specially educated in the various health sciences or have health-related exposure or knowledge from courses taken in primary or secondary schooling, or by way of direct involvement because a close family member or significant other has been diagnosed or hospitalized with an illness. It is important that the nurse acknowledges his or her own critical understandings of health information owing to acquisition of formal education, practice, and continued education. As a professional registered nurse, you have a deep appreciation for physiological, biochemical, and psychosocial connections to state of health and well-being. Other factors affecting health literacy include the following:

- Language barriers of either patient or family
- Health topics that are taboo or interfere with strongly held beliefs
- Vocabulary: most instructional materials should be geared to a 6th grade reading level
- Differences between the clinical and human experience of illness
- Health beliefs and health behaviors that may have culturally relevance and tradition
- Ability to learn
- Motivation to learn
- Developmental level
- Stage of change level

Potential indicators of low health literacy include the following:

- Difficulty in engaging fully with the healthcare provider
- Difficulty understanding medical problems
- Lack of follow-through with medications, tests, or appointments
- Inability to describe how to take medication, or when to get help
- Reluctance in asking clinically relevant questions, or asking only general basic questions

Patient education topics that promote health literacy can focus on the following:

- ▸ Promoting health literacy

- ▸ Skills in coping with the disorder itself

- ▸ Increasing medication and treatment compliance

- ▸ Mental and physical exercises that promote cognitive and physical optimization

- ▸ Problem-solving and decision-making about coping with the situational and relationship consequences of having a mental disorder

- ▸ Increasing confidence in successfully managing day-to-day life experiences through coaching and role-playing

- ▸ How to access help in the community

Readiness to Learn

Prochaska and Velicer's (1997) model to determine learning readiness is useful. Readiness to learn refers to the learner's willingness to invest time and energy in the learning process because he or she perceives it as being important. Individual differences in patient readiness to learn can influence the effectiveness of health teaching efforts. Factors that can influence a person's readiness to engage in a learning process include:

- ▸ **Life experiences:** People enter a learning situation with different cultural, educational, and environmental resources to draw from in learning health-related material. Positive experiences can enhance learning readiness; negative experiences can negatively reduce learning readiness.

- ▸ **Psychological processes:** Transference, counter-transference, or resistance in the therapeutic relationship can stifle nurse-patient interactions.

- ▸ **Complexity of the learning task:** Self-efficacy (see Albert Bandura's theory below) and confidence in being able to learn new material enhances learning readiness. When the learning tasks are within the patient's abilities or can be broken down into concrete terms or smaller, achievable steps, a significant barrier to learning is removed.

- ▸ **Language** is an important factor affecting learning readiness if the educator and learner are not equally fluent in the same language. By law, patients who are not able to comprehend health teaching because of language differences are entitled to have an interpreter. Patient education and socioeconomic variables can influence the use and comprehension of language. The nurses' skill in framing content with that understanding is key to patient learning success.

- ▸ **Culture:** Learning topics and presentation that are consistent with cultural beliefs and values boost learning readiness, whereas those in opposition decrease readiness. Using culturally relevant examples and anecdotes can facilitate acceptance. Patients can be encouraged to share examples from their cultures with the nurse. This type of interaction helps to personalize learning and validates the cultural values of the learner.

- ▸ **Values, beliefs:** Attitude toward education, self-direction, and beliefs about the capacity to affect health issues through education influences readiness to learn. The cues to action outlined by Pender (et al., 2006) can be useful in creating teachable moments.

- ▸ **Level of anxiety:** High anxiety can compromise the patient's ability to focus attention and comprehend material; mild anxiety can enhance learning. A key to the success of health teaching is reducing a patient's anxiety so learning can take place.

- ▸ **Maslow's Hierarchy of Needs:** Consideration of meeting lower-level needs, such as relief from fatigue, hunger, and fear, and safety while communicating a sense of acceptance and belonging promotes opportunities for successful exchanges.

- ▸ **Social support** provides motivation and encouragement during the learning process. When family social support is missing, the nurse can and should provide social and educational encouragement during the learning process.

- ▸ **Patient health status:** To learn effectively, people must have the physical strength, endurance, and ability to focus attention. Timing teaching to those periods when the patient has more energy and capacity to focus attention is critical to success.

- ▸ **Environment** should also be made conducive to learning; that is, a quiet, well-lit, ventilated space that is free from distractions.

Transtheoretical Model of Behavior Change: Stages of Change Theory

Prochaska and Velicer's model of change (1997) is particularly useful in helping to identify when people are apt to learn new behaviors that involve a change in lifestyle from that which currently helps to maintain problem behaviors. It provides a framework for assessing a person's *readiness* to change or learn, and then matching the specific treatment to the patient's state of readiness. This strategy allows the person more control over the pace of the learning and in exerting choice in which behaviors they wish to tackle, and in what order. The theory describes five stages of change and learning suggestions:

1. **Precontemplation:** Patient does not see there is a problem, and is not considering change. *Example:* "I never thought about quitting smoking." Nursing approach: Raise doubt, give information to raise awareness of health risk. The strategy here is to try to engage the patient to give it a thought.

2. **Contemplation:** Patient sees there is a problem, is thinking about but not committed to changing behavior. *Example:* "I have thought about quitting smoking...maybe someday soon." Nursing approach: Promote discussion of pros and cons of change, give detailed information about possible actions and solutions.

3. **Preparation:** Patient sees there is a problem and is willing to make a change within the next 30 says. *Example:* "I will put a quit-date on my calendar." Nursing approach: Help patient choose a realistic course of action.

4. **Action:** Patient takes concrete actions to make needed changes. *Example:* "I will toss my ashtrays and lighters, and plan to take a walk outside after meals." Nursing approach: Support active steps to change behavior, give feedback, review progress.

5. **Maintenance:** Patient perseveres with consolidated actions to sustain positive behavior change. Nursing approach: Continue support to sustain progress, accept relapses as temporary, use steps in preparation stage to resume progress. This is probably the hardest stage; relapses are common. Inform patient of this reality and provide encouragement to "get back in the saddle."

Motivational Interviewing

Motivational Interviewing techniques developed by Miller & Rollnick (1991) are an outgrowth of the stages of change theory. This counseling style uses communication designed to strengthen one's personal motivation to change. It directly poses back to the patient his or her ambivalence about change, offered in an atmosphere of acceptance and compassion (Motivational Interviewing Network of Trainers, 2013). Motivational interviewing techniques help the patient to "discover the advantages and disadvantages of their behaviors for themselves" (Rusch & Corrigan, 2002; p. 28).

Social Learning Theory

Albert Bandura's (1977) theory of social learning proposes that *self-efficacy*, defined as the person's perception of his or her ability to perform an action successfully and the belief (confidence) that such action will have a desirable effect or outcome, is an important correlate of learning behavior and success outcomes. If a person does not feel capable or believes that he or she is not able to learn the appropriate skills, the person is unlikely to try. The importance of this theory for patient education and related skill development is to break down desired learning tasks into manageable segments that can lead to learner success. When this occurs, the person begins to develop an internal sense of competence (self-efficacy), which stimulates the desire to learn more and to attempt more complex learning tasks. The importance of this theory for nurses pursuing specialty certification is, likewise, to break down learning tasks into manageable segments that can lead to board certification (*prepare well, anticipate success!*). Bandura described three types of motivators that help people consider learning new behaviors necessary for their health and well-being.

▸ **Physical motivators,** such as memory of previous discomfort or current symptoms

▸ **Social incentives,** such as praise and encouragement

▸ **Cognitive motivators,** such as perceived self-efficacy and self-determination

Health Promotion Model

Nola Pender's health promotion nursing model (Pender et al., 2006) asserts that perceptual health beliefs differ from person to person and affect patient compliance with treatment and with making effective lifestyle changes. In general, the stronger the health belief about the severity of a disorder or the eventual consequences of not taking a particular action, the more likely the person is to engage in health education programs. Pender describes enhancing the level of well-being and self-actualization of individuals and groups as relevant to health promotion activities. Pender describes *modifying factors* that can serve as "cues to actions" in encouraging people to engage in health-promoting activities. Cues to action can include interpersonal reminders from friends or family, mass media, previous experience with the healthcare system, and preventive health education. Pender's model posits that people are willing to engage in health teaching based on their perceptions and beliefs about

▸ Their susceptibility to disease,

▸ A disease's severity or consequences, and

▸ The potential effectiveness of preventive actions in minimizing health risks.

Lifestyle modifications can be fostered through passive or active strategies. An example of a passive strategy would be the establishment of no smoking policies in hospitals. An active strategy might be offering a community health fair or event. Health promotion and wellness standards involve activities supporting self-care behaviors (e.g., psychoeducation groups, encouraging positive self-talk, eating foods that supply good nutrients, getting adequate sleep and exercise). Examples of health promotion and health maintenance opportunities include providing parenting classes for adolescent mothers, reminiscence groups for older adults living in long-term-care facilities, rewarding self for achievements, following age-appropriate recommended health screenings.

LEARNING ENGAGEMENT PROCESSES: NURSE AND PATIENT MUTUAL TEACH AND LEARN

Domains of Learning

There are three primary domains of learning: cognitive, affective, and psychomotor. Each of the domains should be incorporated in creating and delivering comprehensive learning formats.

The *cognitive domain* is concerned with content knowledge and the recall or recognition of specific facts. Teaching methodologies to engage the cognitive domain include lecture, discussion, and assigned readings. In 1984, Benjamin Bloom described six levels of cognitive learning to categorize the level of abstraction of educational objectives. The levels of thinking proposed by Bloom follow a sequential profile. Thus, one must learn new content using the "lower" thinking skills (knowledge, comprehension, and application) before moving on to the more difficult responsibilities of the "higher" thinking processes (analysis, synthesis, and evaluation).

- **Knowledge:** Recall information, understand major themes or principles.
- **Comprehension:** Interpret facts, compare, contrast, and predict.
- **Application:** Use information, methods, concepts in new situations to solve problems.
- **Analysis:** See patterns, connections, and organization of components to make inferences, sort evidence, and identify causes.
- **Synthesis:** Generalize from old ideas to create new ones.
- **Evaluation:** Compare and discriminate among evidence to make reasoned choices based on sound conclusions.

The *affective domain* involves feelings, attitudes, values, and motivation. Attitudes are generally learned more gradually and benefit from a sensitive teacher who actively explores the values and feelings associated with the presented content. The affective domain is the most difficult to measure objectively. Teaching methodologies to engage the affective domain include role-playing, case studies, modeling, and exercises to develop self-awareness.

The *psychomotor domain* involves the use of motor skills and requires practice for mastery. The psychomotor domain focuses on precision of technique, imitation, and manipulation of objects. Psychomotor practice of skills reinforces and builds on cognitive knowledge. Teaching methodologies to engage the psychomotor domain include demonstrations, simulations, role-playing, and skills practice. When skills and information are presented at the same time and the learner has an opportunity to practice the skills with immediate feedback, learning is more effective.

Applying the Three Domains of Learning

▸ Health materials are easily readable and contain relevant images and designs.

▸ Use common (lay), simpler but concrete terms instead of medical jargon (e.g., instructing the patient to take one pill at 8 a.m. and another pill at 8 p.m. is generally more helpful than advising the patient to take one tablet twice a day).

▸ Use colorful pictures to illustrate concepts.

▸ Use "teach-back" formats, for example, with dialogue such as, "Let's review the next steps. Could you show me how you would …?" or "How would you be able to tell if you were beginning to feel a little manic?"

Sensory Learning Style Preferences

According to adult learning theory, learners display an inherent preference for one sense versus another for sending and receiving information. *Neurolinguistic programming* (NLP), developed by Bandler and Grinder (1975), is based on the premise that people create representational models of the world and use language to symbolize them. This concept can be applied to the teaching-learning process. Listening carefully to the language a learner uses makes it possible to determine whether a person learns better through use of visual, auditory, or kinesthetic (sensory) means. Although teaching to a person's preferred learning style is useful, incorporating more than one sense helps most learners retain information better. Learning is reinforced when appealing to several senses, and even more when learners are able to put their learning into practice while receiving feedback. Matching styles of teaching communication (human modeling) to the person's representational system makes it easier for the learner to comprehend information.

▸ **Visual learners** respond better to learning environments in which there are written materials, graphic illustrations, electronic slide presentations, or other projected presentations. Visual learners may respond, "That looks good to me" or "I see what you mean." The visual learner may also look up to the ceiling as if looking for the answers (visual processing).

▸ **Auditory learners** search for oral cues, stories, and words to help them learn material. They appreciate having group discussions and an oral presentation of new material. Auditory learners may say, "That sounds like an interesting topic" or "I hear what you are saying." The auditory learner may also look toward the side as if listening for the answer (auditory processing).

▸ **Kinesthetic learners** learn best with hands-on experiences and psychomotor practice. It is easier for them to learn material with demonstrations and when they have an opportunity to role-play or practice a skill. Kinesthetic learners may appear more active, with movements such as foot-tapping or shaking a leg during a lecture (sensory processing).The kinesthetic learner needs to be able to take frequent breaks.

Developing Teaching Plans: Know Your Audience

A comprehensive teaching plan is designed to improve overall literacy. Teaching plans provide guidelines for the effective implementation and evaluation of a teaching session. They may be developed as specific psychoeducational tools to be used with individuals or groups. Whether the teaching format is designed for an individual or group session, or is presented in a formal or informal way, learner objectives need be developed for the content. Learning objectives are clear and concise statements about what content the teacher intends for the learner to know and achieve after the particular teaching session. Specific patient-focused, measurable learning objectives helps to ensure that pertinent content that it is deliverable in the allotted time frame is included.

It is usually not possible to teach patients all they need to know in the increasingly limited time nurses have with patients. Thus, it is critical to establish priorities and to differentiate between what is essential and what is nice to know but not critical to treatment goals. The nurse can also plan for sequencing important content in over time, if possible.

In addition to the objectives, goals are developed considering the outline of content material. Content can focus on particular nursing diagnoses, signs and symptoms of disorders, treatment options, or other categories. Examples of NANDA-International nursing diagnoses that patients with mental health problems may need to address include:

▸ Risk of injury or violence

▸ Noncompliance (with medication or therapy)

▸ Self-care deficits

▸ Ineffective individual coping

▸ Ineffective family coping

Teaching strategies and learning activities, time frame for planned activities, including time for questions and discussions, and evaluation measurement using established criteria are necessary components of a complete teaching plan. Although the teaching session should follow the teaching plan, it is important to view health teaching plans as guides or aids to instruction with enough flexibility to allow different delivery methods and learner participation. When standardized teaching plans are used, they should be tailored to the patient's learning needs and abilities. The art of teaching will require that the individualized needs of the learner, some of which may not become clarified until after the session starts, are fully addressed. Every effort should be made to match teaching strategies with learner developmental levels and individualized needs. It is also important to view the patient education process as an integral component of the nurse-patient interaction that is not limited simply to the presenting of content or developing a skill.

Maximizing Teaching Interventions

Structuring the environment (milieu therapy is a standard of psychiatric–mental health nursing practice) to maximize learning is essential. The ideal patient teaching environment is one in which the patient feels comfortable, the environment is quiet and private, and the nurse is able to establish a bond with the patient. It also is important to explain why the teaching is important, even if you think the patient knows this already. Incorporating mental organizers can help patients remember complex concepts. A *mnemonic* is a useful shortcut for remembering unfamiliar terms or concepts. It consists of using letters or familiar words to represent a complex, unfamiliar term or key concept and help the learner remember it. For example, the mnemonic "I WATCH DEATH" (Chapter 4, Box 4–4) helps the nurse remember the important causes of delirium. At the end of the teaching, the nurse can provide a short summary or ask the patient to provide a summary of what he or she learned. When presenting complex material, it is important to

- Break the material down into manageable chunks,
- Deliver key points in sequential order so patients logically can follow the material,
- Encourage questions,
- Present one idea at a time,
- Provide frequent feedback,
- Provide opportunities for supervised practice,
- Use clear, precise language (be aware that many English words have multiple meanings), and
- Provide transitional cues to help link one set of ideas to another (Arnold & Boggs, 2007).

Formative and Summative Evaluation Styles

Two types of evaluation are typically used to evaluate professional learning. Formative evaluations are process-oriented and provide ongoing feedback on performance during an educational process as it is actually occurring. The purpose of formative evaluations is to improve or refine a course or educational program. For example, providing formative evaluations about clinical performance at frequent intervals allows nursing students to make performance corrections before final evaluation, and to have honest, clear feedback during the learning process. Formative evaluations given by students to instructors provide information about corrections needed to make instructional materials or presentations more effective and efficient. Formative evaluations typically are internal evaluations to improve program or course content and teaching methodologies.

Summative evaluations provide information assessing the results or outcomes of the learning process. Summative evaluations are given at the end of a course or formal learning process, and are outcome-oriented. They can be completed as an individual process between educator and student, for example, in the form grades and promotion, or as a group process involving numerical ratings. When students evaluate faculty teaching effectiveness at the end of a course or semester, numerical ratings can be used as evidence for tenure, promotion, and merit decisions. It is critical in all summative evaluations, whether of student learning or faculty teaching, that the same consistent, fair, explicit criteria be used to evaluate all faculty and similar program offerings, and that these criteria be uniformly applied. The process and criteria should be known to both the evaluators and those being evaluated.

Teaching Strategies

Teaching strategies for more formal and professional presentations:

▸ Select a topic of interest; people rarely forget a presentation by a passionate teacher.

▸ Set presentation goals and objectives to guide you in planning content and save preparation time. (A general rule of thumb is to plan 4 hours for preparation of the material for each 50 minutes of presentation). Establish clear and measurable goals and objectives for the presentation. Determine in advance what you hope the learner(s) will take from the presentation.

▸ Complete a literature search and get necessary materials together before developing the content. This can save time in the long run.

▸ Organize the material in a systematic fashion; ordering of information increases the ease with which learning takes place.

▸ Know your audience and gear the presentation to them.

▸ Select appropriate teaching strategies (e.g., lecture and discussion, case study presentations, role-play, role modeling, seminars, speaker panel, use of relevant examples from clinical practice, gaming or simulation, peer and group discussions).

▸ Use a variety of teaching aids (e.g., slides, handouts, simple overhead transparencies, electronic slide presentations, illustrations, audio- and videotapes, chalkboard or dry-marker board, songs, posters, webinar formats). Variety greatly enhances and complements a presentation and will keep learners actively engaged.

Effective presentations are those in which

▸ Presentation purpose is clear and consistently demonstrated throughout the presentation;

▸ The amount of material is appropriate to the allotted time;

▸ The content is related to the learner's abilities and interests;

- Appropriate instructional strategies clearly augment and support the content;

- Learners feel that assignments, content, and presentation are matched to personal or professional goals;

- The environmental climate is conducive to learning (e.g., comfortable temperature, frequently spaced breaks, refreshments, directions to local restaurants, nearby restrooms); and

- Written summative evaluations of presenter effectiveness, degree to which objectives were met, and relevance of content to learner needs collected at the end of the presentation are determined to be positive and accurate.

Evaluation of the Teaching and Learning Engagement

Evaluation of the teacher-learner engagement effort considers the appropriateness, accuracy, efficiency, and effectiveness of the teaching content and process. A formal evaluation tool that may collect both quantitative (numerical rankings) and qualitative (comments section) evaluation provides the teacher with necessary feedback through which needed enhancements to the teaching plan many be identified and addressed. The nursing staff development office can assist with preparation of relevant and timely presentations that incorporate all the necessary elements, whether designed for peers or patients. After each patient teaching engagement, the psychiatric–mental health nurse considers the following in evaluating patient teaching effectiveness:

- Patient feedback

- Achievement of identified educational outcomes

- Necessary modifications if outcomes were not achieved

- What went well; what could be improved

- Required follow-up

The Joint Commission (2012) requires documentation of patient teaching to include

- Initial assessment of teaching need and nursing diagnosis,

- Teaching interventions linked to nursing diagnosis and patient's individualized learning needs,

- Patient response to teaching interventions, and

- Additional referrals or modifications of teaching plan.

AGE-APPROPRIATE PATIENT EDUCATION STRATEGIES

Patient education strategies that are structured with consideration of individual patient needs for accurate information, targeted to the patient's developmental level, optimizes the effort. All patients, from womb to tomb, benefit from understanding the recommended screenings that are outlined based on age and individual risk factors (e.g., mammography, prostate examinations, immunizations). All patients need information about safe sex practices, quitting tobacco use, avoiding substance use, universal health precautions, and proper handwashing techniques.

- **Infants and toddlers** need stimulation of all senses; object manipulation repetition in a safe environment surrounded by emotional security.

- **Young children** want and need guidance; are naturally inquisitive and want to learn; are easily bored so need information delivered in short sessions. Encourage independence, active participation, and a sense of "good job!"

- **Adolescents** want an opportunity to explore, test concepts and ideas; value peer approval; need relevant information tailored to their belief and value system. Use peers to help promote health messages. Negotiate, avoid authoritarian strategies.

- **Adults** value self-directed learning at their own speed, pace, and style; want previous life experiences respected and integrated into new learning processes; want guidance without authoritarian styles; are motivated to learn what they view will help with efficient functioning; want to apply new learning immediately; respond best to pragmatic, problem-solving styles.

- **Older adults** want to learn, but may process information more slowly; explanations should be kept brief and concrete; speech may need to be delivered slower, yet with distinct clarity; distractions need to be minimized and information relevant, built from past life experiences and understandings. May need more repetition and reinforcement. Consider potential visual or hearing loss.

Screening and Prevention

Health screening is the identification of persons who possibly have a problem, and might aid in prevention of more serious illness. Screening tools can be helpful, although generalized screening for problems is not recommended owing to the potential of screening results to be false positives or false negatives. In diagnosis, we want the correct answer, so false positives are not acceptable. In screening, false positives are acceptable because it is better to refer the person for more intensive work-ups than to miss a case completely. In both diagnosis and screening we want to avoid false negative conclusions, missing something important. For this reason, general screenings are recommended by age. For adults, general recommended screenings includes:

- ▶ **Periodic Screenings**
    - ▸ Blood pressure, height, weight, labs
    - ▸ Alcohol, drug, tobacco use
    - ▸ Vision, hearing
- ▶ **Every 1 to 2 Years**
    - ▸ Women: Pap smear after age 18 or when sexually active
    - ▸ Women: Mammogram after age 40 (or based on individual risk factors)
- ▶ **Colonoscopy every 10 years**

Messages that promote safe sex behaviors:

- ▶ Use protection at each encounter.
- ▶ Practice monogamy.
- ▶ Know your sexual partner.
- ▶ Discuss sexual and drug-use histories with partner.
- ▶ Don't allow drugs or alcohol to influence decisions about engagement or use of protection.
- ▶ Get tested for sexually transmitted infections and HIV if sexually active.
- ▶ Get vaccinated for human papillomavirus (HPV).

As stated in Chapter 4, the Agency for Healthcare Research and Quality (AHRQ; 2012) recommends that all healthcare providers address tobacco cessation messages at each patient encounter using the 5 A's format:

1. Ask about use.
2. Advise to quit.
3. Assess willingness to quit.
4. Assist with quitting.
5. Arrange follow up with counseling or tobacco treatments

The National Institute on Drug Abuse's (NIDA) *Mind Over Matter Teaching Guide and Series* (2015) outlines how drugs, including tobacco, specifically affect organ brain at the neurotransmitter and structural levels.

FOCUS: INDIVIDUAL THERAPIES

Individual counseling in mental health settings represents a goal-directed, theory-based, interpersonal process between a qualified clinician and patient, provided in a skilled, organized way to achieve identified mental health goals. Individual counseling can be provided as a vital component of inpatient treatment, or as a primary form of behavioral treatment in outpatient settings. Most models of individual counseling are time-limited, with a focus on helping patients develop more effective coping strategies.

Psychodynamic therapy is informed by psychoanalytic theory, but differs from psychoanalysis in that it is an interactive treatment modality requiring a therapeutic alliance between the patient and therapist, with face-to-face contact. The focus is on helping patients discover the unconscious motivation from the past driving their maladaptive behaviors in the present, thereby allowing them to make realistic choices that separate the past from the present. Therapy emphasizes exploration of the patient's resistance and expressions of emotion as they occur in the therapy session.

Interpersonal therapy (IPT) is an evidenced-based, brief form of psychodynamic therapy in which the treatment goal is to improve a patient's interpersonal skills through clarification of feeling states and identifying areas of conflict or dysfunctional patterns of behavior. The emphasis is on working with patients on one or two key issues most closely related to the patient's symptoms and interpersonal deficits. It is based on the premise that corrective action in one sphere of life can have a ripple effect on other aspects of interpersonal functioning. Insight is an important therapeutic factor in the experiential development of more effective interpersonal behaviors. The therapist is active in offering encouragement and support for new behaviors.

Systematic desensitization is an example of a classical conditioning behavioral treatment methodology. It is used to help patients cope with unrealistic fears or phobias. With *systematic desensitization*, patients are gradually exposed over time to a situation they fear through graded assignments, which are then combined with counterconditioning relaxation techniques provided at the same time. The pairing of relaxation with the presence of the feared object or situation allows the associated fear to decrease because it is not possible for a person to be relaxed and fearful at the same time. With practice and over time, patients are able to experience less anxiety when thinking about the feared situation. The imagery is made more intense until patients are able to actively confront their fears in real-life situations. With therapeutic support and repeated, gradual exposure to the actual fearful situation, the patient is gradually able to control the pervasive fear of a previously avoided situation.

Flooding is an accelerated, more intense version of systematic desensitization in which the patient is exposed directly and repeatedly to the anxiety-provoking situation that she or he fears most. By deliberately facing the fear through real-life contact, patients are able to feel confident about their efforts to control their fear response. Therapist support encourages the patient to continue, despite fear.

Eye Movement Desensitization and Reprocessing (EMDR)

EMDR is an integrative approach that combines psychodynamic, cognitive, behavioral, interpersonal, experiential, and body-centered therapies to address various levels of trauma and to treat sexual predators (Ricci & Clayton, 2008). It uses a dual stimulation process involving series of bilateral eye movements, tones, or taps to access insight, changes in memories, or to make new associations. (See http://www.emdr.com/general-information/what-is-emdr.html for more information.) Initiated by Francine Shapiro, it has particular utility in patients with posttraumatic stress disorder.

Behavioral Theory

Behavioral theory, sometimes referred to as behaviorism, is based on the concept that reinforced behaviors are more likely to reoccur than behaviors that had not been reinforced in some way. Rather than considering underlying conflicts hidden in the subconscious, behavioral theorists propose that, by changing the environmental cues that reinforce a behavior, one can change the behavior. The patient's internal state or frame of reference is *not* a focus of treatment. Changing the environmental cues in a systematic manner is referred to as *conditioning*. There are two types of conditioning: classical conditioning and operant conditioning.

1. **Classical conditioning** refers to a process developed by Ivan Pavlov (Catania & Laties, 1999), and first pairs a naturally occurring stimulus with a response, and then pairs a previously neutral stimulus with the naturally occurring stimulus. Over time, the previously neutral stimulus will evoke the same response (*conditioned response*) without the naturally occurring stimulus. Classical conditioning frameworks have relevance as therapeutic approaches for the treatment of phobias (flooding, desensitization).

2. **Operant conditioning** is a method of learning that occurs through rewards and punishments for behavior. B. F. Skinner (Catania & Laties, 1999) proposed that changes in behavior occur when a stimulus response is reinforced and the person is "conditioned" to respond. Operant conditioning associates a behavior with a consequence for that behavior (reinforcer), thereby strengthening, attenuating, or extinguishing the behavioral response as a consequence of the reinforcement. Operant conditioning concepts are the foundation for behavior modification strategies often used in inpatient settings and for children with behavior problems.

Behavioral therapists believe that all behavior can be modified through systematic manipulation of environmental variables. The focus of behavioral therapy is on measurable behavior, observed in the "here and now." Insight, motivation, and past life experiences are not considered in applying behavioral strategies. Behavior modification programs are highly effective for children with developmental disabilities, attention deficit disorders, conduct problems, phobias, or addictions. They are incorporated as a structural treatment modality in many residential treatment facilities and the juvenile justice system. Behavioral strategies also are used quite successfully with adults presenting with anxiety issues. Treatment outcomes focus on helping patients create new, more productive patterns of behavior and reducing or extinguishing undesired behaviors and behavioral patterns.

To effectively modify undesired behaviors, it is essential to describe all parts of a particular behavior. Behavioral approaches are based on established principles of learning that can be systematically applied to help patients modify dysfunctional behaviors. Stuart (2009) defines behavior as "any observable, recordable, and measurable act, movement, or response" (p. 561). Following a detailed, narrowly focused assessment of a patient's targeted problem, treatment goals are identified, and action-oriented behavioral techniques are used to help patients achieve those goals.

Behavioral Treatment Sequence

▸ Collect baseline data, including information about the current conditions under which the targeted behavior occurs (stimulus response chains) and unintentional reinforcement of undesired behaviors.

▸ State the problem in behavioral terms, as a targeted behavior for intervention.

▸ Take baseline measures (frequency, duration, stimuli antecedents, specific actions, and consequences).

▸ Mutually identify behavioral treatment goals in terms of the desired behaviors to be achieved.

▸ Collaboratively specify concrete actions required to change the maladaptive behavior.

▸ Jointly and deliberately connect the reinforcer with performance of the desired behavior.

▸ Use behavioral strategies (reinforcement, shaping, modeling, discrimination, etc.) to achieve behavioral treatment goals.

▸ Gradually modify reinforcement schedules from continuous to variable interval or variable ratio as patients improve.

▸ Monitor changes in behavior from baseline data.

Behavioral Concepts and Strategies

▶ **Reinforcement:** Specific reinforcement is used to increase desired behaviors and to decrease undesired behaviors. A *reinforcer* is defined as anything that increases the probability and frequency of a desired behavioral response, and decreases the frequency of undesired behaviors, when presented as a consequence of a patient's behavior. To be effective, the reinforcement must always follow the target behavior as soon as possible. The reinforcement should fit the targeted behavior, and should be something the patient desires. Using more than one reinforcer is more effective than using only one. The *Premack Principle* describes that the chosen reinforcers or rewards should be meaningful to the patient. Unless the reinforcer has meaning to the patient, it is unlikely that the patient will work for it. *Reinforcers* can be given as a primary reward (e.g., candy, toy, privilege) or a secondary reward (e.g., tokens or points that can be exchanged for primary reinforcers); can be positive (something the person wants) or negative (response the person dislikes, which decreases the probability of the stimulus behavior). Examples of positive reinforcement include verbal praise and giving a child a desired object or activity. Examples of negative reinforcement include withholding of a desired object, activity, or privileges ("Unless you agree to take your medication by mouth, I will have to give it to you by injection."

▶ **Contingency contracts:** Used particularly with children, contingency contracts specifically identify the behaviors requiring change, conditions under which reinforcement will occur, and any specific time periods for achieving desired behaviors.

▶ **Token economy:** This is reinforcement designed to increase or decrease behavior with the use of tokens, which have no intrinsic value. Patients receive them at the time the behavior is displayed, and can later exchange them for a meaningful object or privilege. It is useful for children with developmental disabilities, attention-deficit hyperactivity disorder (ADHD), behavioral disorders, and in hospital inpatient treatment and juvenile justice settings.

▶ **Punishment:** Inhibiting an undesirable response by making negative consequences contingent upon it (e.g., grounding an adolescent). We do not punish patients.

▶ **Shaping:** Start with a small component of the desired behavior and gradually add more parts to a task behavior, like learning a dance routine by adding a few more steps to the combination each time. Initially, the approximations of desired behavior are successively rewarded until the final desired behavior is achieved (successive approximation).

▶ **Modeling:** Learning a desired behavior by observing competent models performing it, and imitating their behavior. Related strategies include behavioral rehearsal, in which a patient practices a new behavior with the therapist, and coaching, in which the therapist gives the patient constructive feedback.

▶ **Discrimination:** Teaching the child or patient to act one way under one set of circumstances, but not in another, by rewarding the behavior response only in the desired set of circumstances.

▶ **Extinction:** Decreasing a behavior by removing rewards that maintain the behavior, such not laughing when a child misbehaves. The learned behavioral response decreases because it is no longer being reinforced.

Varying the reinforcement schedules can be used to strengthen and increase desired behaviors and are given:

▶ **Intermittent:** Either based on the rate of the person's response (ratio schedules) or as determined by time factors (interval schedules).

▶ **Continuous:** Behavioral reinforcement given for every response.

▶ **Fixed interval:** At distinct time intervals, and a certain amount of time must elapse before the reinforcer is given.

▶ **Variable interval:** For the first response after a variable amount of time has elapsed (e.g., 30 minutes).

▶ **Fixed ratio:** After a fixed number of responses and every nth response is reinforced (e.g., every 5th response).

▶ **Variable ratio:** Initially very frequently, and then less frequently as performance improves; produces the highest response rate.

Cognitive-Behavioral Theory

Cognitive-behavioral therapy (CBT) draws from both behavioral and cognitive theories. The prototype for cognitive therapy is cognitive behavioral therapy, developed by Aaron Beck (Butler & Beck, 1995). Cognitive models of emotional response propose that our thoughts strongly influence our feelings and behaviors. It is not *how* the situation actually is, but how the person *perceives* it, that is the focus of CBT. Helping patients to change maladaptive thought patterns helps them begin to feel differently about themselves and their situations even though the situation itself remains unchanged. This is an evidenced-based therapeutic approach that may use the *Socratic method* to challenge dysfunctional thinking and broaden a person's perspective to consider alternative explanations for a situation. The approach uses an inductive format and requires the person to develop alternative hypotheses that can be questioned, challenged, or supported. The goal of therapy is to help patients become aware of the distorted thinking patterns that interfere with functional living and personal satisfaction. CBT techniques are designed to refute "stinking thinking."

Cognitive-behavioral therapy draws upon several different therapies that share some common elements; for example, rational emotive behavioral therapy (Albert Ellis, http://www.rebtnetwork.org/whatis.html), and cognitive-behavioral therapy developed by Aaron Beck. CBT is an evidence-based, time-limited form of psychotherapy, based on the premise that the way a person perceives and thinks about a situation influences how he or she feels about it and responds behaviorally. Thus it is not the situation itself, but how a person thinks about it, that creates distress and counterproductive behavior. For example, if someone steps on your foot, your reactions will be quite different depending on whether it was done purposefully or was an accident—or your perception as to whether it was on purpose or accidental. Beck contends that people often base their cognitive assessments on basic core beliefs, which were learned early in life. These core beliefs (schemata) continue to color people's thinking patterns throughout life, affecting how they think about themselves and others, if their validity is not challenged. Cognitive therapy helps people to first to identify their maladaptive thoughts, and then to challenge their validity. Changing thoughts will also change feeling and consequent behaviors; therefore, the implementations are designed to "refute stinking thinking;" modify dysfunctional perceptions and corresponding thoughts that negatively affect their emotions and behavior. As people learn to think more realistically, and to change their distorted thinking, they feel better emotionally and this, in turn, affects their behavior in a constructive manner.

Many CBT strategies used for adults can also be used with school-aged children and adolescents, with consideration given to their developmental levels and levels of cognitive processing. Children can be taught to recognize unrealistic thought patterns, and to assess factual information about the validity of these thought patterns. Putting events in perspective, accepting uncertainties as a part of life, ceasing to catastrophize situations (thinking in terms of worse-case scenarios), and replacing them with "What could I do to handle this situation?" provides alternative ways of looking at (perceiving) things.

If a child cannot use Socratic questioning because of attention, developmental stage, or learning difficulties, it may be possible to learn calming self-talk as a way of replacing negative, anxious self-talk. Referred to as self-instruction training, this can be an effective methodology in helping impulsive children learn self-control skills, and anxious children to reduce their anxiety.

The therapeutic process for CBT can include the following:

▸ Educating the patient about the CBT model and process of behavioral analysis (antecedents, behavior, consequences)

▸ Setting an agenda for each session, focusing on a problem identified by the patient for that session

▸ Examining core beliefs and cognitive distortions that are feeding the current problem

▸ Engaging the patient in Socratic dialogue to test beliefs and challenge dysfunctional thoughts

- Helping patients learn to monitor their negative automatic thoughts and recognize connections among cognition, affect, and behavior

- Keeping an activity record or mood check

- Consistently assessing for changes from baseline

- Using guided imagery, role-playing, and behavior rehearsal to help patients think about and develop different ways of doing things

- Coaching and supporting patients in making positive changes

- Capsule summaries after the agenda is set and, at the end of the session, helping patients make cognitive connections between the agenda of the current session and overall treatment goals

Processes of Concern to CBT

- **Cognitive distortions:** Automatic harmful thoughts that people can have in response to stressful situations.

- **Cognitive triad:** Cognitive distortions related to a person's negative view of him- or herself, the world, and the future. Beck viewed this triad as being influential in the development of depression.

- **Schemas:** Certain ingrained biases or core beliefs that cause people to interpret basically neutral situations in a personalized, negative way; are shaped by early life experiences and are difficult to dislodge.

- **Socratic questioning:** Teaching patients to examine their thoughts and to reflect on their potential for having drawn erroneous conclusions, through deliberate logical thinking. Socratic questioning makes it possible for patients to think critically about the validity and consequences of their behaviors. Helping patients develop alternative explanations (also referred to as guided discovery) for dysfunctional thoughts makes them better able to come to different conclusions, and to devise more realistic solutions to their problems.

- **Cognitive restructuring:** Teaching patients to challenge their irrational beliefs and to substitute positive self-statements for these negative thoughts.

- **Thought-stopping:** Teaching patients to intentionally detach from maladaptive thoughts, setting aside irrational and false beliefs, and using opposing internal self-talk to make self-made rules less absolute.

- **Homework assignments:** Giving patients a homework assignment—a task to accomplish outside the therapy session—reinforces the idea that the patient needs to continue to work on problems between sessions. A mutually agreed-upon homework assignment should be connected with the session agenda. The results of the homework assignment should be reviewed as an early agenda item in each subsequent session.

Dialectical Behavioral Theory

Developed by University of Washington in Seattle Professor Marsha Linehan, Ph.D., dialectical behavior therapy (DBT) is a comprehensive psychosocial treatment geared toward intervening with chronically suicidal persons, patients with borderline personality disorder (BPD), bipolar disorder, depressed older adults, and nonsuicidal adolescents (Shives, 2012). Dr. Linehan herself is diagnosed with BPD. The goal of this type of therapy is to help people build personal conceptualizations that life is worth living. Treatment strategies focus primarily on aspects of CBT, combined with interventions that focus on unconditional acceptance and validation.

Play Therapy With Children

Play therapy is a treatment approach that uses child's play as a medium of expression to enhance communication between the child (aged 3 to 12 years old) and the therapist. Landreth (2002) suggests that play is a child's language and that children can more effectively express their thoughts, feelings, and what is troubling them through play activities than they can through direct speech.

Children can use toys to express feelings verbally and behaviorally in the immediacy of the present, and in a safe environment. Manipulation and positioning of toys and playing games can give the therapist important information about a child's relationships, problems, and ways of coping. Implementing play sessions builds on children's natural inclination to learn about themselves and their environment and can be directive (therapist sets up particular toys, manipulatives) or nondirective (therapist observes child's selection and self-determination with the manipulatives or toys). Different cultures may have different expectations for play, which need to be taken into consideration with the choice of toys, setup of the playroom, and conduct of the play therapy process. Culturally relevant play materials will seem more natural to the child. Treatment goals for play therapy include outcomes that help children experience and express their emotions and concerns in a constructive way, develop respect, self-efficacy, and acceptance of self and others in their environments, and develop pro-social and interpersonal skills with school, family, and peers. Play therapy sessions provide a:

- ▸ Safe and natural environment for children to express their feelings verbally or behaviorally,

- ▸ Way to learn social and problem-solving skills and adaptive behaviors, such as taking turns, working out problems, creating one's own fun, and getting along with others, and

- ▸ Medium to uncover clues to the root of the child's problem.

EDUCATION STRATEGIES AMONG POPULATION GROUPS: FAMILY, GROUP, AND INTEGRATIVE

Theoretical Frameworks in Preventive Psychiatry

Gerald Caplan (1964) is generally acknowledged as the father of preventive psychiatry in the United States. He was one of the first clinicians to adapt public health principles to mental health care and to insist on population-focused prevention as a methodology for preventing mental disorders and promoting mental health. His work in identifying biopsychosocial hazards that contribute to the risk of future mental disorders; his efforts in analyzing the patterns of crisis, which can lead to positive growth or development of symptoms associated with mental disorders; and his insistence on the importance of enhancing competence and social supports as primary prevention strategies were significant forerunners of current primary prevention models.

FOCUS: FAMILY AND FAMILY-CENTERED THERAPIES

Having a theoretical understanding of family dynamics and structure is a critical basic skill for the psychiatric–mental health nurse. The psychiatric nurse understands that the provision of support for the family unit as the "patient system" may promote improved outcomes by helping each member enhance communication and learn to identify and meet individual needs within and among family members.

Families form an important environmental context for patients emotionally, and in many instances financially, socially, spiritually, and politically. Family members caring for members with persistent mental illness often are called upon to provide substantial caregiving, monitoring of their care, and advocating for community mental health services. Family caregivers often need support themselves to cope with the sometimes-lifetime care that family members with mental illness need to maintain their independence outside of acute or long-term-care settings. Health teaching and psychoeducation are particularly important interventions for improving family outcomes. Referral of the family to National Alliance for Mental Illness (NAMI), Mental Health America (MHA), the Substance Abuse and Mental Health Services Administration (SAMHSA), and other community networks or agencies to assist with psychological and practical social support can be helpful and hopeful.

Family is defined as a unit consisting of a defined group of persons connected by blood or emotional ties or both who, over time, have developed distinct patterns of interaction and relationship (Boyd, 2007). A family unit can describe two parents and their children, a single-parent family, a same-sex couple with or without children, step or blended family, common-law family, three-generational family, or a dyad couple without children. A family may self-define as LGBTQI (lesbian, gay, bisexual, transgender, queer, questioning, or intersex). "Emo," a term that means "emotional," is another commonly used self-descriptor.

Each family has a unique history, predictable ways of interacting, and a shared vision of the future. Within each family system are interpersonal subsystems of dyads, triads, and so on, with defined emotional bonds and common responsibilities. A *nuclear family* is a family consisting of one or two parents and their children living under one roof, such as mother, father, and their daughter living in one household. An *extended family* consists of second- and third-generation relatives (by blood or marriage) of the nuclear family. They may or may not live together or function as a family unit. Examples include grandparents, aunts, uncles, and cousins. Family stages of development can be identified according to its construction; that is, newlyweds, new-parent families, empty nesters, families without children, same-sex households, blended constructions, transgender families, unrelated members, mixed-race, and so on.

Families are dynamic rather than static organisms, and demonstrate a variety of response patterns ranging from dysfunctional to resilient coping with stressful family situations. In highly stressful situations, family members may need assistance in coping. The role of the nurse is to promote effective family functioning by enhancing family strengths, helping families to realistically understand and cope with a family member's illness, and linking them with appropriate community supports. Characteristics of healthy family functioning include the following:

- Maintaining clear, but permeable boundaries
- Maintaining social integration and collaborative relationships with the community
- Open and honest communication
- Appropriate division of labor
- Earning and spending abilities
- Parenting skills and education about development
- Appropriate sexual relationships and parent-child boundaries

Family counseling can be primary interventions or adjunctive to effective child and adolescent individual or group therapy approaches. Encouraging changes in family functioning can have a profound effect on the level and intensity of behavioral symptoms in children. The parent's ability to provide emotional support and appropriate parental monitoring is an important dimension of treatment for most children and adolescents with behavioral, psychiatric and mental health, or substance abuse problems. Planning for family health care necessarily encompasses a knowledge base of family social and financial circumstances, and the support networks available to the family.

Family System Concepts

Family systems theory applies a systems model to families, viewing the family as a complex, organized, interactive, and holistic organism. Rather than focusing on each separate family member as the phenomenon of interest, family theory emphasizes the connectedness and interdependencies occurring among family members. How they come together defines the uniqueness of a family unit. From a family systems perspective, the entire family is viewed as the "patient," so the focus of treatment is on the relationships among family members. The functioning of each family member is best understood by looking at the family unit as a whole. A family system is one in which the organism is more than, and different from, the sum of its parts, and each part mutually influences the others. Family values and rules have a tendency to shape individual member behaviors. Boundaries differentiate what is included in the family system and what is external to it. They regulate the flow of information into and out of the family. The family can be conceptualized as an emotional system or unit in which family members are emotionally interdependent, and function in reciprocal relationships with one another (Kerr, 2000). A family systems perspective is based on the following concepts:

- **Morphogenesis:** All family systems are in a constant state of flux as they adapt to changing family needs.
- **Morphostasis:** All family systems seek stability in the midst of these changes.
- **Homeostasis:** As individual family members change, the family seeks to restore and maintain a steady state of equilibrium or balance.
- **Equifinality:** Family systems can achieve the same goals or outcomes through different routes.
- **Circular causality:** Emotional problems can best be understood contextually, as part of ongoing feedback loops that maintain a problem.

Murray Bowen's Family Systems Theory (Kerr, 2000) is perhaps the best known framework of family systems therapy. His theory consisted of eight interconnected concepts:

1. **Triangles:** Three-person relationship systems in which a two-person system becomes unstable and involves a third party to reduce the tension.

2. **Differentiation of self:** Occurs when a person can think reflectively and can stay calm and clear-headed in the face of family conflict rather than responding emotionally.

3. **Nuclear family system:** Identifies four relationship patterns—marital conflict, dysfunction in one spouse, impairment in one or more children, and emotional distance between significant family members—that tend to occur when the level of tension rises in a family.

4. **Family projection process:** Parents transmit their emotional fears or issues onto one of their children, adversely affecting the child's normal development and behavior. The child may take on caretaker roles, for example.

5. **Multigenerational transmission process:** Relationship patterns can be transmitted from generation to generation, so behaviors and emotional issues in one generation will tend to repeat themselves in future generations.

6. **Emotional cutoff:** Occurs when people reduce the tension of unresolved emotional issues with family members by reducing or totally cutting off emotional contact with them.

7. **Sibling position:** Birth-order position in the family has an effect on individual development and expression. Common characteristics are associated with each birth-ordered sibling position, although children occupying the same position in different families may exhibit differences in functioning.

8. **Societal emotional process:** Bowen's assertion that each of his concepts applied to family therapy can also be applied to larger social groups such as work, social organizations, and society itself.

Structural theorists "join" with the family, mirroring their way of speaking (mimesis). They restructure and reframe family processes to create processes that are counterproductive to the identified pathological ways of relating used within the family. The structural model of family therapy, developed by Salvador Minuchin (1974) emphasizes:

▶ **Family structure:** Interactional patterns that exist within a family (e.g., time spent together, family rules [spoken and unspoken], automatic transactional responses).

▶ **Subsystems** are the subgroups with the family, which are based on generation, gender, or family function (e.g., spousal, parental, sibling subsystems, men or women).

▶ **Boundaries** are the invisible barriers that surround each family subsystem, protecting each from other subsystems and the external world. Boundaries can be diffuse or rigid. In an enmeshed family, the boundaries are so relaxed or diffuse that family members become overly involved in each other's affairs. The opposite of an enmeshed family is a *disengaged* family, in which the boundaries are so rigid that family members remain isolated from each other and the larger society.

Strategic family therapy, developed by Jay Haley and Cloe Madanes (Madanes, 1981), is based on the premise that symptoms and problem behaviors serve a function in the family system. Strategic therapists maintain that symptoms are also attempts to control a relationship. As nurses, we are all too familiar with the recognition that the "identified patient" may not be the person needing the most help. Families may scapegoat members to a "sick role" that serves to distract other family members from focusing on their dysfunctions. A family can change when the therapist works with the family to uncover the interactions that maintain the symptom and change them by creating therapeutic double-binds. A double-bind clinical strategy might provide conflicting messages or directives, so that the message the patient chooses to respond to would negate the contradictory message. The therapist might also reframe a deviant behavior as being a protective one for the family, or ask an angry family member in denial to pretend to be very angry. Strategic therapists also hypothesize what function a dysfunctional behavior might have for the family. The goal of strategic family therapy is to help family members act in ways that are counterproductive to the problem behavior.

Multi-Systemic Therapy (MST) is an evidence-based form of family-oriented, home-based therapeutic services for adolescents age 12 to 17 who are involved with the juvenile justice system. It is individualized to work with the family, and incorporates a network of interconnected extra-familial community systems (e.g., peer, school, neighborhood) that can provide intervention in one or more settings, using the strengths of each system to facilitate change. The goal is to work with the multiple factors associated with juvenile offenders to decrease behavioral problem, antisocial tendencies, substance use, the number of out-of-home placements because of delinquency, and to improve overall family functioning. This approach fosters appropriate parental involvement, clear rules and expectations, and behavior change in the adolescent's natural environment of home, school, and neighborhood.

Tools for Family Assessment

The genogram is a simple-to-use assessment tool that displays the family history over three generations in a straightforward schematic diagram (Figure 8–1). Included on the diagram are the ages; dates of marriage, divorce, and death; significant illnesses and mental disorders or chemical dependencies; immigration and geographic moves; occupations; and conflictual or close relationships between family members. Males are represented by squares and females by circles, with ages identified within the square or circle (Varcolis, Carson, & Shoemaker, 2006).

FIGURE 8-1. FAMILY GENOGRAM

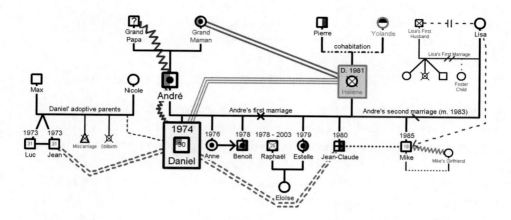

Reprinted from Intro to the Genogram by Genopro.com, n.d., retrieved from http://www.genopro.com/genogram/.

Ecomaps display important relationships occurring between different family members and the larger community-based systems, such as work, school, church, or healthcare system. Ecomaps are useful for identifying the intensity and frequency of contact between the family and external resources and other significant persons who can provide support for patients and other family members. Lines are drawn from the family members inside the larger family circle to those significant persons and institutions with which the family interacts on a regular basis. Straight lines indicate positive relationships, whereas slashes through the line indicate stressful relationships (Arnold & Boggs, 2007).

Wright and Leahey (2007) suggest focused implementations designed to identify and build family strengths and improve family problem-solving and coping strategies. These interventions can include offering information, commending family and individual strengths, validating and normalizing emotional responses, encouraging the telling of illness narratives, encouraging respite, promoting self-care for individual family members and the family as a unit, promoting family cohesiveness, supporting family subsystems, reinforcing functional subsystem boundaries, encouraging open communication, and devising rituals.

Solution-focused therapy is a pragmatic, short-term, strength-based collaborative treatment approach to individual and family issues. The goal of treatment is to enhance effective resolution of problems through cognitive problem-solving and by incorporating the creative use of personal resources and interpersonal strengths as a methodology. Solutions lies within the patient and can be accessed with the therapist's support. The solution-focused therapist helps patients think in terms of solutions rather than problems. Strategic techniques used include:

- ▶ **Miracle questioning:** "If someone waved a magic wand and your problems were resolved, what would be different in your life?"

- ▶ **Scaling questioning:** Ask patients to rate their current perception of a situation, and their progress towards their treatment goals, on a scale of 1 (lowest) to 10 (highest).

- ▶ **Exception-finding questioning:** Based on the premise that bad behaviors do not happen all the time. Asking patients to recall a time when a behavior did not occur broadens a patient's perspective and allows the patient to consider other options.

Attachment Theory proposed by John Bowlby (1958) avows that if a child receives sensitive and responsive parenting, they themselves are more likely to become sensitive and responsive parents.

Human Ecology Theory proposed by Urie Bronfenbrenner (1979) holds that one's behavior may differ in different settings, that is, school or work, in comparison to what we present amongst various contexts "This context includes relationships with other family members, friendship networks, neighborhoods, communities, and cultures."

FOCUS: GROUP THERAPIES

Psychiatric–mental health nurses participate in and support therapeutic groups with patients. Group therapy was developed during World War II as a serious treatment modality for persons with mental health issues when there were not enough psychiatrists to treat the large number of soldiers requiring psychological assistance. The results were so successful, and the cost so much more effective, that group therapy was extended to nonmilitary settings.

Group work offers other special considerations, depending on group membership and the stage of development of the group itself. Group composition is an important component of effective group therapy, and should be intimately connected to a specific group's treatment goals. For this reason, a person who is not a good candidate for one group may benefit from joining a group with different treatment goals. The size of the group is also important. Traditional psychotherapy groups function best with 6 to 8 members; groups with fewer than 5 or more than 8 members may not provide the optimal level of interaction needed for deep exploration of feelings.

Group therapy formats can be particularly helpful for children with mild to moderate mental disorders or situational crises, such as loss of a parent. Support from peers of similar age and interests offer the most important and influential relationships for this age group. The significance of "peer pressure" that is capable of promoting positive behaviors and encouragement in developing alternative behaviors cannot be overemphasized. Group therapy for younger children focuses on play activities; for school-age children, there is a joint focus on the play activity and talking about it (Varcolis, Carson, & Shoemaker, 2006).

Groups for children and pre-adolescents should be well structured, with clearly understood but flexible rules and expectations for group member participation. Activities should be consistent with developmental and age-appropriate expectations. Group discussion can focus on the application of social activity behaviors to group member situations. Seriously disruptive or aggressive children usually are not good candidates for activity groups if they cannot modify their behavior well enough to participate; including such children could sabotage group goals.

Group therapy for adolescents also can help strengthen the adolescent's ability to resist negative peer pressure in the community by providing constructive feedback about progress or lack of progress, and modeling appropriate responses. Theme-centered groups for children coping with the death of a parent or sibling or major violence threat or reality often offer needed critical support in schools and other settings. The psychiatric–mental health nurse is well-positioned to offer groups on various topics and in multiple settings. The following factors are important considerations in group composition:

- Group members must have the capacity to engage in the primary activities of the group, and enough functional similarity to be able to communicate with each other.

- Therapy groups can have a heterogeneous composition, i.e., a mix of persons with different diagnoses, or be homogeneous with regard to age, gender, type of emotional problems, personal characteristics, or diagnosis.

- In closed groups, members are identified before group treatment, and membership stays relatively constant. Most outpatient psychotherapy groups are closed groups. In open groups, membership fluctuates and group membership can change from session to session (e.g., bereavement groups, psychoeducation groups).

Tuckman (1965) identified five stages of group processing that are applicable to group development in psychotherapy:

1. **Forming stage:** This is the orientation phase. Acceptance, trust, and inclusion are major group issues. The leader is most active in this stage. Universal norms such as confidentiality, attendance, communication, and rules for participation are addressed.

2. **Storming stage:** Control and power issues emerge in the group, in the form of testing and acting-out behaviors (transitioning). Working through these issues helps create an interpersonal climate in which members feel free to disagree with each other.

3. **Norming stage:** Group members develop group-specific standards (cohesiveness), such as disapproval of late-arriving members or the level of levity or anger members will accept.

4. **Performing stage:** Most of the work of the group related to individual growth, team productivity, and effectiveness takes place during this stage.

5. **Adjourning (termination) phase:** Closure for the group as a whole or for individual members takes place during this phase. The task is to review goal achievement and explore feelings about termination at both individual and group levels. Introducing new areas of psychological concern or beginning new initiatives is not appropriate.

Irvin Yalom (Yalom & Leszcz, 2005) identified eleven curative or therapeutic factors that result from successful group therapy experiences. The psychiatric nurse, as group facilitator, can identify these processes occurring over time within groups, especially if there are sequential meeting opportunities. These eleven factors are:

1. **Instillation of hope:** Members see other members at different levels of growth and feel they can change too.

2. **Universality:** Members realize that they are not alone, and that others have similar problems, thoughts, and feelings.

3. **Altruism:** By helping others in the group, individual members gain more self-esteem.

4. **Impart information:** Members share their experiences.

5. **Development of new socialization skills:** Ability to correct maladaptive social behaviors through feedback from other group members.

6. **Imitating behaviors:** Members are able to increase adaptive interpersonal skills.

7. **Interpersonal learning:** Members learn from each other.

8. **Group cohesiveness:** Sense of belonging, identity, and social acceptance members get from their membership in the group.

9. **Catharsis:** Members become able to share their pain, successes, and progress achievements.

10. **Existential factors:** A new sense of personal meaning can develop through group therapy experiences.

11. **Corrective opportunities:** Members can have choice to rework issues in new and more productive ways.

In successful groups, different members typically display task and maintenance functions. These functions are complementary and both are needed for maximum therapeutic effect. Specific task functions help keep the group focused on the task and directed toward achieving group goals:

▸ Initiating

▸ Information- or opinion-seeking

- ▸ Clarifying or elaborating

- ▸ Consensus-testing

- ▸ Devil's advocate

- ▸ Summarizing

Maintenance functions help keep the group members connected and interested in working with each other to achieve group goals:

- ▸ Encouraging

- ▸ Expressing group feelings

- ▸ Compromising

- ▸ Gate-keeping

- ▸ Standard-setting

Disruptive or self-functions occur when individual group members are more concerned about their own agendas than in contributing to or learning from other group members. This can be a form of resistance or the member may simply be unaware of the impact his or her behavior has on the group. Depending on the level of disruption, the nurse facilitator may ask the offending patient to leave the group. The psychiatric–mental health nurse observes whether this disruption is used by the patient as a secondary gain; that is, avoidance of group work. In this case, the skilled nurse might enlist patient peers to call attention to

- ▸ Blocking or diverting discussion,

- ▸ Power-seeking,

- ▸ Recognition-seeking,

- ▸ Dominating,

- ▸ Attention-seeking, and

- ▸ Clowning or constant joking.

Types of Therapeutic Groups Facilitated by Psychiatric–Mental Health Nurses

- ▸ **Therapeutic Activity Groups:** Most common type of group therapy for children and pre-adolescents. They take advantage of a child's natural tendency to express feelings through play activities, and their preference to talk about what they are doing rather than about themselves. Activity groups are particularly effective with children between 5 and 12 years of age to help them learn competition, ground rules, getting along with others, goal-setting, and pro-social behaviors.

▸ **Psychoeducation groups:** Offered to teach patients, families, and community groups about specific mental disorders; patient medications; behaviors such as anger management, social skill development, coping with mental illnesses, vocational skills, risk factors, crisis intervention, symptoms, treatments; and related issues. These groups are usually time-limited and focused on one topic. Participants can learn from each other and often feel freer to ask questions in psychoeducation groups than in one-to-one patient teaching.

▸ **Family psychoeducation groups:** Offered to help improve patient outcomes. The goal of these groups is to assist families in promoting compliance with medication and successful re-entry of patients back into the community. The topics of these groups include information about the mental disorder and co-occurring disorders, if indicated, and the coping skills members can learn to provide the appropriate environment for their mentally ill family member.

▸ **Reality orientation groups:** Offered to confused patients or those out of contact with reality. The goal is to help patients maintain contact with their environments. Props such as calendars, clocks, and common objects are used to stimulate recognition.

▸ **Socialization or resocialization groups:** Offered to persons who are withdrawn or isolated and regressed psychotic patients. The goal is to improve the patient's basic social skills by providing patients with an opportunity to establish simple social relationships and to introduce healthy patterns of relating that can be reinforced and strengthened in a group format.

▸ **Reminiscence groups:** Offered to cognitively impaired older adults who may lack short-term memory, but still have access to long-term memory. A simple object is used to stimulate discussion. A form of reminiscence group is also sometimes used for higher-functioning patients to stimulate life review.

▸ **Support or self-help groups:** Offered to reinforce coping strategies and offer practical suggestions. Examples include Alzheimer's disease caregiver support groups and self-help groups, such as Alcoholics Anonymous, where a member has a "sponsor" who may provide support. Support groups provide a high level of success and are usually not led by professionals.

▸ **Psychodrama:** Highly structured form of group psychotherapy in which individual group members can explore, through enacted scenarios, conflictual relationships with significant others. Members play out the roles of others, and in the process, the participant can experience and clarify issues that otherwise would not be addressed. The format is experiential and enacted in the here and now, as though the situation were currently happening.

▸ **Assertive training:** Learning to use "I" language to express needs and wants.

▸ **Relaxation training:** Performing yoga, or listening to ambient music while counting breaths.

- ▶ **Medications management:** Discussing explicit schedules for taking medications independently.

- ▶ **Modeling:** Demonstrating how to stop and listen to one person at a time, or learning empathy.

- ▶ **Communication skills groups:** Focus on hearing tone of one's own voice and content of verbalizations.

- ▶ **Problem-solving groups:** Focus is on particular problems, such as how to navigate to the pharmacy by public transportation.

- ▶ **Special populations groups:** Offered to focus on specific needs, such as discussing menses with young women.

FOCUS: INTEGRATIVE THERAPIES

Human beings are infinitely complex; therefore, the treatment of persons with behavioral, emotional, or mental health problems and illnesses is multifaceted. In approaching patients as biopsychosocial-spiritual beings, we strive to be open to whatever therapies or interventions help to restore functionality and homeostasis in the person and family system. Alternative therapies such as hypnosis and biofeedback, and expressive therapies of music, play, art, dance, and relaxation, are sometimes used in lieu of (or to augment) more traditional approaches to treatment. They can be effective ways to connect with and heal a patient when other approaches fail or cannot be used. A child who cannot speak may be approached with art, music, or dance in addition to play therapy. A person in a psychotic state can be helped with relaxation techniques or music until the psychosis can be controlled. Anxiety disorders respond to relaxation techniques and the use of art, play, music, and dance to relieve anxious feelings. Expressive therapy works by stimulating the senses and different pathways in the brain. There are special training programs in these types of therapeutic interventions. Adaptability, flexibility, sensitivity, regard for human dignity, a sense of humor, and knowledge of therapeutic needs are all essential components of psychiatric–mental health nurses working with alternative and expressive therapies in the clinical setting.

Dance and movement therapy is a form of expressive therapy in which feelings are expressed through rhythmic body movements. Through this medium, rigid, nonverbal, or repressed patients are sometimes able to express what they cannot express in other ways. Dance, Tai-Chi, and Qigong are examples. Done regularly, it can also be an aerobic exercise with all the accompanying benefits that such exercise entails. Movement therapy can help both energize and calm persons with dementia.

Music therapy involves listening to music, playing in rhythmic bands, singing, moving to music for relaxation and enjoyment, and getting in touch with feelings evoked when different types of music are heard. Music crosses over many diverse barriers—intellectual, cultural, and linguistic. Rhythm is the energizer of music. Music integrates the left- and right-brain hemispheres. It operates at a subliminal level. It is capable of producing a trance-like state, which, in turn, promotes relaxation and the ability to focus. Music combined with guided imagery is effective because it continues subliminally where the verbal message leaves off. Music has been used successfully as a distracter for dental patients and persons with chronic pain. Music can also be effective with chronically mentally ill and dementia patients.

Ambience Medical Systems, Inc., provides a novel application that has demonstrated efficacy through clinical trials to show positive effects with hospitalized patients. Hospitalization recognizably creates stress and anxiety, and persons who require an inpatient stay in a behavioral health setting may have difficulty articulating feelings or expressing emotions in appropriate manners. The Ambient Therapy System's special dosing and timing capabilities help guide emotional perceptions by evoking "psychoacoustical flooding" through sensory-neural brain pathways. This implementation could help provide a relaxed venue by promoting a sense of calmness in the therapeutic milieu and holds promise as a potential de-escalation tool (Benson, Hutchinson & Melcher, 2010; Hutchinson & Melcher, 2009).

Art therapy uses a person's artwork (drawing, painting, sculpting) as a means of communication and expression, rather than relying primarily on verbalization. The artistic creations and use of color can contain clues or insights into the stressors experienced by a person. It is the process and content of the art produced that is important to therapeutic change, not the end product. Art therapy can be appropriate for a wide range of people, from sophisticated adults to nonverbal, developmentally delayed children or psychotic patients. It provides an acceptable and controlled outlet for emotions and conflicts that otherwise might remain unexpressed in verbal therapy. The expression of dreams, fantasies, and conflicts through images is encouraged. The goals of art therapy can be ego-strengthening, catharsis, uncovering emotions, developing impulse control, and developing an ability to integrate and relate, depending on patient need.

Animal-assisted therapy (AAT) provides opportunities for motivational, educational, and recreational benefits to enhance a person's quality of life. Animal-assisted therapy is a goal-directed intervention using animals as in integral part of the treatment process. As a comforting agent, AAT assists in coping with hospitalization and effects of diagnosis, and can otherwise help patients become more amenable to a therapeutic environment of care.

Relaxation techniques are behavioral strategies used primarily to assist patients with stress management, performance enhancement, and pain control. They also are used in conjunction with other forms of psychotherapy to reduce anxiety. Relaxation techniques can be accompanied by music or art images and can be used in conjunction with behavioral therapies, such as systematic desensitization and biofeedback. Many of these relaxation techniques are used for pain management and in childbirth. The simplest forms of relaxation techniques emphasize teaching patients to reduce tension in their bodies by learning to recognize its presence and then to release the tension or anxiety with special autogenic methods, such as:

- Meditation or centering techniques

- Guided imagery, in which a person mentally visualizes relaxing images or situations

- Progressive muscle relaxation, a method developed by Benson (2000) in which a person tenses then relaxes muscles one at a time, progressively throughout the body

- Deliberate, deep breathing

Hypnosis involves inducing a state of very deep relaxation that facilitates openness to suggestion and changes in perception (Varcolis, Carson, & Shoemaker, 2006). Some people erroneously associate hypnosis with mind control, but they are not the same. People will typically only follow suggestions that would conceivably be within their range of normal behavior. The therapist uses guided relaxation and intense, focused concentration to help a patient achieve a heightened state of awareness, referred to as a *hypnotic state* or *trance*. In this state, healing suggestions related to specific tasks or thoughts are given to the patient.

Hypnosis can be useful as a form of suggestion therapy for pain control and breaking habits such as smoking or excessive nail-biting. It is also used as an adjunct to psychodynamic therapy to help patients uncover painful thoughts and feelings that otherwise would not surface spontaneously. For this reason, hypnosis is sometimes used with treatment-resistant anxiety, phobias, sleep disorders, sexual abuse, and posttraumatic stress disorder.

A caution about using hypnosis is that it can sometimes provoke the presentation of false memories. Patients need to be motivated to engage in hypnosis, and only a therapist who is clinically trained and licensed to perform hypnosis should use it as a therapeutic technique. Patients with psychotic hallucinations or dissociative disorders would not be good candidates for hypnotic suggestion therapy methods.

Biofeedback uses electronic equipment to reveal unconscious physiologic processes associated with anxiety, generalized stress, high blood pressure, chronic headaches, certain types of epilepsy, or pain. Biofeedback is used as a complementary mind-body therapy. It is particularly effective as a noninvasive adjunctive treatment for pain. Through a biofeedback unit, which measures processes such as breathing and heart rates, muscle tension, and skin temperature, the patient receives immediate feedback in the form of visual and auditory signals. Types of feedback include the galvanic skin response, heart rate, blood pressure, temperature, electromyogram (EMG), and electroencephalogram (EEG). The goal of biofeedback is to teach a person to alter his or her physiological processes from a status suggesting nervous arousal to a state of relaxation. The desired outcome is that the patient will be able eventually to produce the relaxed state associated with a decrease in symptoms without the equipment.

Biofeedback is commonly used for general health and stress management. Most forms of biofeedback, such as EMG (muscle activity) or thermal (hand-warming) require expensive equipment and extensive training. One form of biofeedback, called *cardiac coherence training*, uses a finger probe to pick up the heartbeat and a computer algorithm to log heart rate variability (HRV) and calculate the coherence of the signal or how smooth and regular it is.

The HeartMath Institute is a company that has developed programs for a PC or Mac, as well as a small hand-held unit that can be used in a counseling setting or by a person for self-training. They have written educational material and conduct training on this technique. This group has conducted research finding benefit of the program for stress reduction, hypertension control, and enhanced work performance. A variant of this approach, called resonant frequency biofeedback, has shown benefit for asthma and anxiety disorders (Glick, 2010).

PROFESSIONAL PERFORMANCE STANDARD 15: RESOURCE UTILIZATION FOCUS: COMMUNITY AND NATIONAL EFFORTS

Mental healthcare community services can vary from state to state and from county to county within a state. Information about specific public and nonprofit mental health services can be found on county government websites. Most counties have mental health and alcohol and drug abuse advisory committees composed of providers, consumers, legal, religious, school, and law enforcement representatives. These advisory boards advocate for persons with mental illnesses, advise the county government on community needs (e.g., third-shift crisis center coverage), and make recommendations for enhancing the public mental health system and local community resources.

The **PRECEDE-PROCEED model** is a well-established community-based health promotion assessment model designed as a structural process to identify community needs by examining nine phases. The model identifies predisposing, enabling, and reinforcing factors that influence community education success.

- **Predisposing factors** are previous experience, knowledge, beliefs, and values that can affect the teaching process (e.g., culture, prior learning).

- **Enabling factors** are environmental factors that facilitate or present obstacles to change, such as transportation, scheduling, and availability of follow-up.

- **Reinforcing factors** include the positive or negative effects of adopting the new learned behaviors including social support, fear of recurrence, and avoidance of health risk.

The first five phases relate to the community needs assessment required to address the most appropriate need. Compiled data are referred to as the PRECEDE component, which includes the following:

- **Phase 1:** Social diagnosis—people's perception of their health needs and current quality of life

- **Phase 2:** Epidemiology diagnosis—epidemiology of the health problems in the target population

- **Phase 3:** Behavioral and environmental diagnosis—specification of the health-related actions most likely needed to change the problem behavior, and systematic assessment of the environmental factors that would influence health outcomes

- **Phase 4:** Educational and policy diagnosis—assessment of priority factors needing change to initiate or sustain desired health outcomes.

- **Phase 5:** Administrative and policy diagnosis—assessment of the actual educational objectives and type of teaching program needed to achieve identified outcomes.

Phases 6 through 9, PROCEED to focus on the logistical, administrative, and evaluative components of the program needs to achieve successful outcomes.

- **Phase 6:** Implementation—the process of converting program objectives into the actions to be taken at the organizational level

- **Phase 7:** Process evaluation—assessment of resources, personnel, quality of practice, and services offered

- **Phase 8:** Impact evaluation—assessment of intermediate objectives occurring as a result of the training

- **Phase 9:** Outcome evaluation—assessment of final outcomes in terms of changes in health status, well-being, and quality of life

NATIONAL AND COMMUNITY SUPPORTS

Assertive Community Treatment Model

The Assertive Community Treatment (ACT) Model is an evidence-based practice initially developed in the late 1960s. This multidisciplinary and comprehensive team-based approach to mental health and psychiatric care provides initial and ongoing assessments, case management, employment and housing assistance, medication management, family support and education, substance abuse counseling, and other supports that promote successful residency in the community. ACT services are highly individualized and are intended to be long-term engagements because of the severe disability associated with serious and persistent mental illness (SPMI) and work to reduce recidivism rates of patients back into hospitalization. The ACT service delivery model provides comprehensive, immediate treatment for persons with serious and persistent mental illness within their home environments. These services are available to persons with mental illnesses and their families 24 hours a day, 7 days a week.

Wellness Recovery Action Plan

A Wellness Recovery Action Plan (WRAP) represents a person's road map for recovery. Each plan is individualized to reflect a person's needs, preferences, values, and culture. The plan includes personally defined goals, realistic objectives, and a strengths-based orientation, with services and interventions needed for success clearly identified. Although a WRAP is driven and managed by the person who is receiving services, a WRAP should identify and embrace the support of other persons and services who can help patients with mental illness achieve personal goals. Key elements of a WRAP should include the following:

- ► Developing a wellness tool box
- ► Creating a daily maintenance plan
- ► Identifying triggers and an action plan
- ► Identifying early warning signs and an action plan
- ► Planning for a crisis, and the time after a crisis

Wrap-Around services are a form of community-based, intensive mental health services available to families with children and adolescents with multiple psychological and social issues. Such a program is designed to provide families with a variety of supports to prevent the need for more restrictive levels of care. The purpose of providing these home- and school-based supports is to enhance the capacity of families to cope with difficult issues in both home and school settings. With Wrap-Around services, child or adolescent and his or her family are considered important parts of the treatment team.

Substance Abuse Brief Intervention, Referral, and Treatment (SBIRT)

Some communities offer the evidence-based Substance Abuse Brief Intervention, Referral, and Treatment (SBIRT) service that provides communication and aspects of motivational interviewing in outpatient settings. The idea is that at each encounter or meeting, patient substance use behaviors should be discussed, and support for treatment engagement offered.

Head Start Programs

Head Start preschool programs provide comprehensive developmental and social services for low-income preschool children ages 3 to 5 years. The purpose of Head Start programs is to stimulate the social and cognitive development of children by providing health, nutrition, and social services to build self-esteem and promote school readiness. Head Start programs are used to provide comprehensive developmental services for preschool children and their parents. This type of community support is available in most states. Developmental pediatricians are not available in all communities.

Shelters and Other Crisis Centers

Many communities provide temporary shelters for homeless mentally ill persons, although the need far exceeds availability. The public mental health system has case management capabilities for qualified persons to help serious and chronically mentally ill persons navigate the public health and social services systems. Crisis and detox centers exist in most larger and urban communities. Depending on the jurisdiction and available funding, these can operate on a 24-hour basis. Again, the need exceeds availability. Outreach programs are a crucial link for those with serious and persistent mental illnesses or homelessness. Outreach services employ formerly homeless persons to make connections for the purpose of linking case management, health, substance abuse, and other stability-oriented services. Considering Maslow's hierarchy of needs theory, persons served may initially be focused on meeting basic needs. Persistent mental illness or homelessness often results in poverty, which creates a downward spiral resulting in psychiatric patients dying 25 years sooner than those in the general population (DeHert et al., 2011). Experiences associated with impoverished living conditions:

▸ Reduced housing options; overcrowded or substandard housing

▸ Lack of access to health care

▸ Lack of access to quality schools and educational services

▸ Dangerous and toxic environments

▸ Lack of access to information technology services

- Increased experience with crime

- Food desert communities

- Greater overall life stress

Therapeutic Community Model

The Therapeutic Community Model provides an example of an environment that incorporates safety, structure, norms, limit-setting, and balance. The Therapeutic Community is a "living-learning situation," where everything that happens between members (staff and patients) in the course of living and working together. Pioneered by Maxwell Jones (Center for Nonviolence and Social Justice, n.d.), the Therapeutic Community Model is an important component of milieu therapy in many settings (inpatient psychiatric, addiction centers, psychiatric long-term residential settings, jails, shelters). Central to a Therapeutic Community Model, staff and patients join together to become a unified agent of change and rehabilitation. The community supports the concept of patient self-governance. The Therapeutic Community offers practical learning opportunities that are designed to enhance personal development of more effective social skills and social responsibility. The Therapeutic Community acts as a microcosm of the larger society in which a person is supported through peer influence to re-establish healthy social functioning. They are not available in all states.

Characteristics of a Therapeutic Community that incorporate a partial self-governance format for the unit:

- Daily community meetings in which patients review goals and functional rules, and participate with staff in decision-making regarding issues affecting the hospital unit

- Patients and staff mutually creating the structure, overall guidelines, and social controls needed to maintain the environment as a safe milieu

- All clinical activities, including attendance at unit community meetings, treatment groups, job assignments, and other educational or vocational activities considered as elements of successful participation in the therapeutic community

- Privileges, disciplinary pass approvals and disapprovals, and discussion of unit matters needed to maintain the physical and psychological safety of the environment are managed by the therapeutic community as a whole.

Nurse-Family Partnership Programs

Nurse-Family Partnership (2011) programs are evidence-based supports that exist in many states to pair a registered nurse home visitor with a first-time mother during pregnancy and until the child reaches two years of age. The relationship is designed to foster positive regard and attachments between the infant and mother and offer coaching, knowledge and support to create a better life for mother and child.

Nurse-Managed Healthcare Centers

Nurse-Managed Healthcare Centers exist in some communities. Along with free community-run health clinics, they provide first-level triage for some communities where access is difficult or community members do not have funds or routine primary care providers. Family Psychiatric Nurse Practitioners (FNPs) are pivotal links in closing the access gaps and provision for primary and mental health care in many communities.

Forensic Nursing

Forensic Nursing is a specialized model of nursing practice when issues of health and the legal system intersect. Forensic nursing certification is available to nurses who obtain training and education in trauma care, identification, and management whether the violence is precipitated by physical, sexual, or emotional abuse and assault. Forensic nurses may function as Sexual Assault Nurse Examiners (SANEs), or Forensic Nurse Examiners (FNE), with responsibilities as medical examiners in death scene and crime investigation permitted in some states. The International Association of Forensic Nurses (www.iafn.org) provides resource information and conferences.

Disaster Psychiatry

Disaster Psychiatry has an important role in community preparedness efforts in the event of widespread disasters that may result from climatic extremes or individual or group violence. Psychological first-aid training and curricula are provided to mental healthcare workers and others by way of field operational guides. Mental healthcare first responder support may be requisite to save lives and facilitate appropriate grief responses.

Grassroots Peer Support Efforts

Grassroots peer support efforts exist as community resources. Support groups and organizations, such as the NAMI, mental health associations, Narcotics Anonymous (NA), Alcoholics Anonymous (AA), On Our Own, Sante Group, Survivors of Suicide, and so on are available in some communities. The National Alliance for Mental Illness (NAMI) is such a self-help, support, and advocacy organization of persons with severe mental illnesses and their families and friends. These groups are part of a network of support that helps maintain persons in need of mental health services in the community and their families. In this patient and family advocacy organization, peer-to-peer counseling and recovery support is led by persons living with mental illness. Church-affiliated mental health services are often offered at a reduced rate or sliding scale (e.g., Ephesians for drug abuse and comorbid mental health problems).

The Agency for Healthcare Research and Quality

The Agency for Healthcare Research and Quality (AHRQ; http://www.ahrq.gov/qual/nurseshdbk) and other national agencies are working to accelerate the impact of health services research on direct patient care, and helps professionals keep abreast of new developments in the field of psychiatric care.

The Substance Abuse and Mental Health Service Administration (SAMHSA)

The Substance Abuse and Mental Health Service Administration (SAMHSA) works to improve the quality and availability of substance abuse prevention, alcohol and drug addiction treatment, and mental health services. The SAMHSA website (www.promoteacceptance.samhsa.gov/campaigns/Program_aspx?ID=194) assists with locating mental health care providers, and provides information about grants, anti-stigma campaigns, mental health initiatives, and other programs. SAMHSA has created a center for integrated health solutions that updates information relevant to integrated primary and behavioral healthcare (http://www.integration.samhsa.gov/about-us/what-is-integrated-care).

SAMHSA also maintains the **National Suicide Prevention Hotline** (1-800-273-8255), which connects callers to its toll-free hotline to trained crisis counselors in their area to prevent suicide. The hotline is always staffed.

Silver Ribbon Campaign for the Brain

Silver Ribbon Campaign for the Brain (http://www.silverribbon.org/) is an anti-stigma initiative developed by the Brain and Behavior Research Foundation (formerly NARSAD) to raise "public awareness of the need for emotional, social, governmental, and research support" for those affected by a brain disorder or disability. Since 1999, the organization has collected signatures requesting the creation of a first class postage stamp depicting a silver ribbon.

PROFESSIONAL PERFORMANCE STANDARD 16: ENVIRONMENTAL HEALTH

The psychiatric–mental health nurse practices in an environmentally safe and healthy manner by analyzing and critically evaluating the impact of social, political, and economic influences on the environment and human health exposures. In advocacy roles, the nurse voices concern and support for principles of safety, such as appropriate and adequate personal protective equipment and garb. Additional actions include:

▸ Practice reducing environmental health risk.

▸ Communicate about environmental health risks and exposure reduction strategies.

▸ Assess sounds, odors, noises, lights that threaten health.

▸ Advocate for judicious and appropriate use of healthcare products.

▸ Use scientific evidence to determine whether product or treatment is an environmental threat.

▸ Strategize to promote healthy communities.

▸ Promote sustainable environmental health policies and practices.

FOCUS: MENTAL HEALTH, DISEASE PREVENTION, AND HEALTH PROMOTION

Because "health is a state of complete physical, mental, and social well-being and not merely the absence of disease or infirmity" (WHO, 2012), mental health is considered to be much more than the absence of mental disorders. Mental health is an integral part of the general health of every person. Mental health promotion and disease prevention theoretical frameworks, principles, and strategies are primary ways to address health optimization at the individual, community, national, and global levels. To this end, interventions support psychosocial functioning and facilitate lifestyle, community, and environmental changes. Interventions can include various types of counseling, behavioral therapy, cognitive therapy, communication enhancement, coping assistance, patient education, and psychological comfort promotion. The family may be included in some of the counseling and education interventions.

Health promotion is conceptualized as a basic human right that emphasizes supporting and enhancing health-related self-management skills needed to achieve maximum functioning and well-being. Mental health issues of concern range from awareness of personal attitudes towards mental disability, parity, and access to care to behavioral problems in children and adolescents, physical or relationship circumstances with a mental health component, and specific clinically diagnosable mental or addictive disorders.

Disease prevention refers to activities that prevent the incidence and reduce the prevalence of mental disorders. Disease prevention efforts in mental health are aimed at keeping a mental health disorder from appearing, delaying its onset, stopping or slowing its progression, or minimizing its impact on a person's life. Former U.S. Surgeon General David Satcher, MD, in his ground-breaking Surgeon General's report on mental health (U.S. Department of Health and Human Services, 1999), stated: "Americans assign high priority to preventing disease and promoting personal well-being and public health; so, too, must we assign priority to the task of promoting mental health and preventing mental disorders" (p. 5).

Preventing the development of mental disorders and minimizing their impact on persons, families, and society through patient and community education is an important health promotion emphasis in today's mental health care. In addition to creating a significant emotional and financial burden for these persons and their families, mental health issues can be extremely costly in terms of reduced or lost productivity because of mental illness. The 65th World Health Assembly (2012) estimates that approximately 13% of the global burden of disease worldwide are mental disorders, with depression considered the leading cause of disability worldwide (World Health Organization, 2012). Specifically, in the case of autistic spectrum disorder, the U. S. incidence is noted to be rising to afflicting 1 in 68 children (CDC, 2014).

Healthy People 2020 (CDC, 2015) presents the health promotion and disease prevention agenda for the nation and is updated every 10 years. This document sets forth health objectives related to preventive health care and identifies outcome benchmarks to verify their achievement. *Healthy People 2020* goals and objectives are a principal resource used to develop goals, objectives, and actions for the CDC. Specific objectives and health indicators related to tobacco and substance abuse, responsible sexual behavior, mental health, injury and violence, and access to health care are of special interest to the psychiatric and mental health nurse. The psychiatric–mental health nurse can access reports through the CDC's website (http://www.cdc.gov/nchs/healthy_people.htm) as they become available to remain abreast of foci and progress.

The overarching mental health goal of *Healthy People 2020* is to improve mental health through prevention and by ensuring access to appropriate, quality mental health services. Specific objectives for reaching this goal include mental healthcare improvement strategies and treatment expansion, as listed in Box 8.1. One of the objectives of *Healthy People 2020* is to increase early detection and intervention for mental health problems. Screening tools are one measure that can help practitioners detect persons who are at risk for specific mental disorders. Mental Health Awareness Day campaigns provide opportunities for free screening and information for the public.

BOX 8-1.
HEALTHY PEOPLE 2020 MENTAL HEALTH OBJECTIVES

▶ Reduce the suicide rate.

▶ Reduce suicide attempts by adolescents.

▶ Reduce the proportion of adolescents who engage in disordered eating behaviors in an attempt to control their weight.

▶ Reduce the proportion of persons who experience major depressive episodes.

▶ Increase the proportion of primary care facilities that provide mental health treatment on site or by paid referral.

▶ Increase the proportion of children with mental health problems who receive treatment.

▶ Increase the proportion of juvenile residential facilities that screen admissions for mental health problems.

▶ Increase the proportion of persons with serious mental disorders who are employed.

▶ Increase the proportion of persons with serious mental disorders who receive treatment.

▶ Increase the proportion of persons with co-occurring substance abuse and mental disorders who receive treatment for both disorders.

▶ Increase depression screening by primary care providers.

▶ Increase the proportion of homeless adults with mental health problems who receive mental health services.

Source: http://www.healthypeople.gov/2020/topics-objectives/topic/mental-health-and-mental-disorders/objectives

The CDC is the nation's premier health promotion and disease prevention agency. The CDC is responsible for tracking actual and potential health problems and morbidity and mortality rates. The CDC takes a holistic view of health, providing guidelines for basic health and wellness and preparedness goals to deal with health hazards and challenges. To this end, a toolkit for promoting positive mental health among populations residing in nursing homes (http://www.nursinghometoolkit.com/) has been developed. The CDC (Roy, et. al., 2009) has identified four health protection and promotion goals according to five life stages (infants and toddlers birth to 3 years; children 4 to 11 years; adolescents 12 to 19 years; adults 20 to 49 years; older adults and seniors more than 50 years) to help focus its work:

1. Healthy people during every stage of life

2. Healthy people in healthy places

3. People prepared for emerging health threats (e.g., hepatitis C endemic, Ebola virus crisis, personal protective equipment (PPE) protocols)

4. Healthy people in a healthy world

FOCUS: PUBLIC POLICY AND THE PSYCHIATRIC– MENTAL HEALTH NURSE

The integration of therapies, healthcare providers, and psychopharmacological treatments addresses a variety of risk factors across the life span. Primary care service providers are required to integrate mental health services in all practices, and in all specialty areas. Consider how office-based questionnaires all now have at least one question asking something along the nature of "Have you ever felt depressed or suicidal?" or "Do you feel sad or depressed now?" These contemporary multisystem strategies represents the movement for assessment and treatment of the whole person, and not just the chief complaint.

Serious disparities still exist in gaining access to public mental health services, particularly for minority and migrant populations and undocumented immigrants. Many agencies, such as some emergent care centers and drug store chain clinics, expect up-front payment. Migrant health centers can provide mental health care for persons who qualify. Other sources include public housing programs or waivers, which can help persons with mental illnesses achieve enough economic self-sufficiency to survive in the community; community food banks and gardens; support groups; hospice and respite care; transportation assistance, long-term care centers; and clubhouse programs. This type of assistance is essential because it is estimated that 30% or more of homeless persons have serious mental disorders. The juvenile justice system serves as an alternative funding source for the many children who receive initial mental health treatment within the legal system. More recently, mental health courts in several states are using forced treatment for offenders with a mental illness as an option in lieu of prosecution or as a condition for reduced charges.

Advocacy: Public Policy

Advocacy, public policy, and community supports are designed to reduce recidivism and promote overall health and wellness. With deinstitutionalization starting in the 1960s and the advent of the community mental health model, patients began transitioning to community residences and outpatient care and follow-up. Transitional group housing was developed in some areas, but not others. Funding streams were not adequate to increase service provision and patients who were not accustomed to independence were released without sufficient or appropriate life skills training. In some cases, families were also ill-prepared and unable to cope with returning, formerly institutionalized family members.

As a result of this and other *social determinants of health* factors, many with SPMIs are homeless. Social determinants of health shape personal health behaviors. They include disparities in economics; neighborhoods; food quality, access, and cost (food deserts); healthcare quality, access, and cost; educational quality, access, and cost; and community-based passive health promotion strategies (e.g., walking trails, parks, public transportation, gyms and exercise facilities). The growth in homelessness is attributed to deinstitutionalization, job losses (and related loss in insurance), low incomes, bankruptcies (personal or medical). Today, it is estimated that more than 250,000 homeless people have an SPMI, and 600,000 people are estimated to be homeless (Johnson, 2014); unaccompanied homeless youth comprises almost 8% (46,924) people in 2013 (National Alliance to End Homelessness, 2014). Homelessness often follows job and welfare entitlement loss. Homeless populations are without residences for longer periods of time, and are increasingly visible in subway stations, parks, and on the streets. At least half are estimated to have a co-occurring substance use disorder. Overall they tend to be in poorer physical health than the general population. Most are eligible for, but fewer receive, income assistance, including from the Social Security Administration and public assistance. Minorities, especially people of color, are overrepresented among the SPMI population, and most are willing to accept treatment, but initially are more likely to want help in meeting basic needs. The fastest growing homeless population is children and youth. Family and community-based treatments to prevent youth out-of-home placements are an example of an effective evidence-based strategy.

President Bush's New Freedom Commission on Mental Health called for a fundamental transformation of the mental health delivery system (Executive Order of the White House, 2002). It endorsed language to eliminate inequality for Americans with disabilities, and fix the fragmentation in mental health services. The overall mission is to break down existing barriers among public and private service providers that affect children with serious emotional disturbances, and adults with serious mental illnesses to live, work, learn, and participate fully in their communities. Targeted arenas include health, educational, rehabilitative, housing, and technology sectors.

The idea that recovery is possible provides the overarching framework. Recovery does not necessarily mean "cure"; rather, it points to the ability of persons with mental illnesses to live fulfilling and productive lives despite the disability. Self-determination is an important component of recovery. In the context of recovery-based care, the nurse involves patients and their families in healthcare decision-making to set mutually agreeable goals and to develop a realistic plan of care. The model takes a holistic view of a person with a serious mental illness, considering him or her from a strengths-based perspective. A recovery-oriented mental health framework addresses self-esteem and self-actualization needs by treating patients with dignity and respect, including them as essential partners in the healthcare team, and empowering them to regain control over their lives and return to previous higher levels of functioning. Self-determination includes giving people the freedom to choose where and with whom to live, as well as how one organizes other important aspects of one's life with freely chosen assistance as needed. Patients have the authority, support, and responsibility to make choices about how healthcare dollars are spent on their behalf. The recovery model focuses on helping people live in the community as productive citizens leading satisfying lives despite having a mental disability. Fundamental characteristics of the recovery model:

- ▶ Self-determination and self-advocacy

- ▶ Hope and empowerment

- ▶ Viewing relapse as a temporary setback, with continued expectations of personal success

- ▶ Resiliency drawn from personal strengths, personalized support systems, and ongoing education about each person's clinical picture

- ▶ The person with a mental illness as the teacher; the nurse as the student

- ▶ Hope is the fundamental message

Laws that affect psychiatric and mental health nursing practices as they pertain to the 0.federal protection and rights of persons with mental illnesses and disabilities are described below.

- ▶ **Protection and Advocacy for Mentally Ill Individuals Act (1986):** Mandates that all states must designate an agency responsible for protecting the rights of mentally ill patients.

- ▶ **Americans With Disabilities Act (ADA) of 1990:** Protects persons with physical or mental disabilities from discrimination related to their disabilities and requires reasonable accommodations, based on disability.

- ▶ **Patient Self-Determination Act (1990):** Protects the rights of mentally ill patients whose mental symptoms result in alternating periods of competence and incompetence; bipolar disorder is one example. Advance directives for mental health are written documents that specify how the patient wishes treatment decisions—for example, medications, choice of hospital facility—to be made during episodic periods of incompetence.

- **Drug Treatment Act of 2000** limits prescription of buprenorphine to physicians with American Society of Addictions Medicine (ASAM) certification.

- **Patient Protection and Affordable Care Act (2011):** Informally known as the Affordable Care act or "Obamacare," it requires persons to maintain minimal essential health insurance coverage or pay a penalty.

- **The Wellstone-Domenici Mental Health Parity and Addiction Equity Act of 2009 (Final Rule 2013):** Requires that group health and insurance benefits ensure that co-pays, deductibles, or treatment limitations applicable to mental health and substance use disorder treatments are no more restrictive than the requirements or limitations applied to medical and surgical benefits. The law outlaws health insurance discrimination against persons with mental illnesses and substance use disorders in employer-sponsored health plans. It bans employers and insurers from imposing stricter limits on coverage for mental health and substance use conditions than those set for other medical conditions.

Advocacy: Psychiatric–Mental Health Nurses

The psychiatric–mental health nurse has a profound role in advocating for those with mental illnesses. After all, as Halter (2008) found, psychiatric nurses are stigmatized as a result of our association with stigmatized populations. As we know and understand, persons with mental illnesses enrich our lives. The ensuing stigma, discrimination, and criminalization is counterproductive to the aims and principles of the recovery model. Although thought to be more violent, and often treated as though they are, persons with mental illnesses are no more violent than the average population. Violence risk is increased, however, in a small subset: persons with mental illness experiencing control and command hallucinations who are not medicated. Otherwise, if there is not a co-occurring substance use disorder, persons with mental illness are no more violent than those without mental illness. Substance abuse, however, seems to increase the risk for violence among persons with mental illness.

The psychiatric–mental health nurse has a role in modeling appropriate language when referring to a person with any illness. Person-centered language describes the person with the disorder, not the disorder. Hence, "Mary has schizophrenia," not "the schizophrenic in room 5." We need to also refrain from pejorative, discriminating, and stigmatizing language such as, "the alcoholic," "junkie," "psycho," "crazy one," "lunatic," and similar pejorative terms. Such terms do not demonstrate a professional nurse's understanding of psychopathology. When among lay people, the psychiatric–mental health nurse has an obligation to model and inspire an appreciation for the fact that organ brain, too, can be impaired (like the heart, liver, or any other organ). Finally, additional ways that the psychiatric nurse can advocate for patients with mental disorders would be to

- Work for legislation change that supports healthcare rights for those with mental illnesses; stay abreast of local and national politics;

- Lobby for mental health and substance abuse funding support;

- ▸ Empower patients and others to speak up and speak out about stigma, discrimination, and criminalization;

- ▸ Challenge systems that are not supportive;

- ▸ Sponsor and participate in mental health awareness events and services (e.g., Out of Darkness Walks, suicide hotlines, World Suicide Prevention Day events, National Alliance for Mental Health walks, October Is Depression Awareness Month, Silver Ribbon Campaign for the Brain, Tobacco-Free Nurses);

- ▸ Provide community education to reduce stigma, discrimination, and criminalization of those with mental illness; and

- ▸ Advocate that treatment works and recovery is possible.

The American Psychiatric Nurses Association (2014) posits a position advocating for the reduction and ultimately, the elimination of restraining patients. More evidence based research is needed to examine the variables associated with the prevention of and safe management of behavioral emergencies.

Global Health Perspectives

The World Health Organization (2014) estimates that between 35% and 50% of people who live in high-income countries and between 76% and 85% of people in low- and middle-income countries receive no treatment for mental disorders. The burden of depression and other mental health conditions is also on the rise. Suicide is among the top 20 leading causes of death globally for all ages; annually there are nearly 1 million suicides. World Mental Health Day is recognized annually on October 10th.

FOCUS: MENTAL HEALTHCARE PAYMENT DELIVERY SYSTEMS

Mental healthcare services for both adults and children are financially directed by managed behavioral health organizations. Managed care refers to a broad category of health insurance plans designed to provide persons and families with a range of healthcare services at a reduced cost. The goal of managed care services for mental health and substance dependence disorders is to provide the best, individualized, cost-effective care to patients. They differ in cost, degree of provider choice, and flexibility of service area. Reimbursement for mental health and substance abuse services is handled as "carve-outs," meaning that insurance payments are financially separated from those provided for other clinical services, and are managed under a separate contract. Carve-outs have separate provider networks. These carve-outs were designed as a way to restrict the potential high costs of long-term psychotherapy and extended hospital stays associated with some forms of mental illness. The impact of managed care on mental health care delivery has been to foster short-term treatment and to cut the cost of mental health services. Ideally, these cost-cutting measures will not lower the quality of care or prevent access to necessary treatment. (Most carve-out options had separate, lower annual and lifetime limits on care per person and per episode, but limits are no longer allowed for mental health care or substance abuse services under the Affordable Care Act.) Primary forms of managed care consist of health maintenance organizations (HMOs), point-of-service (POSs) plans, and preferred provider organizations (PPOs).

HMOs are closed healthcare systems in which the primary care physician coordinates the patient's specialty care and most mental health services require a primary care provider referral or direct authorization from the HMO carve-out management company. Although the most restrictive, HMO coverage is usually the least costly. As an HMO subscriber, a person pays a monthly premium with a small co-pay for primary or specialty care, and all necessary care is provided through the HMO contracted or group practice healthcare providers. There are exceptions for emergency treatment or medically necessary treatment not obtainable through the HMO, with HMO approval. Components of major HMOs include:

- **Utilization review:** Cases are reviewed to ensure appropriate length of stay, medical necessity, and suitable level of care.

- **Case authorization and referral:** Patients must receive authorization for mental health treatment. The HMO oversees the mental healthcare and monitors level of treatment for the behavioral healthcare program.

- **Quality assurance or improvement:** Patients are followed from intake through the treatment process, with treatment plans required for authorization of further treatment. The purpose of this monitoring and follow-up is to ensure that the benefit dollar is spent in providing quality care throughout the mandated mental healthcare program.

Point-of-service (POS) plans offer subscribers a choice to select an HMO, PPO, or out-of-network provider. Depending on the choice of provider (i.e., in or out of network), the person can pay a larger or smaller share of the cost and typically has higher deductibles. POS plans offer the most flexibility for persons traveling beyond the designated service area and needing care.

Preferred provider organizations (PPOs) are service plans in which the insurance organization contracts with care providers who then are reimbursed at a discounted service rate for their professional services. This type of plan usually has higher monthly premiums, and an annual deductible must be met before coverage begins.

The Centers for Medicare and Medicaid Services (CMS) is the federal agency that administers Medicare, Medicaid, and the Child Health Insurance Programs (CHIP). Medicare is a federal health insurance program providing coverage for persons 65 years and older and persons younger than 65 with long-term disabilities. Medicaid is a jointly funded state–federal health insurance program for eligible low-income persons. Certain requirements apply, such as age, disability, pregnancy, or blindness. Persons applying for Medicaid must meet other requirements related to financial resources and citizenship or legal residency. Coverage for Medicaid varies by state and is subject to federal requirements, and benefits still only reach portion of those in need—not most of the poor. The working poor often make too much money for entitlements, although coverage has expanded in some states under the Affordable Care Act. The same law eliminated Medicaid and Medicare financial restrictions on long-term care of mental disorders.

The Protection and Advocacy for Mentally Ill Individuals Act of 2010 and The Affordable Care Act heralded by President Barack Obama established mandatory insurance options for formerly uninsured, uninsurable, and low-income households. This initiative called for Medicaid expansion and the formation of Patient-Centered Medical Homes. It also outlines more directives for integrative care models in which both mental (behavioral or emotional) care could be provided in the same practice as physical care services. Patient-Centered Medical Homes are an outgrowth of the Affordable Care Act.

Accountable care organizations (ACOs) are voluntary participation programs that propose rules to help coordinate care for Medicare patients. Defined in 2011 by the U.S. Department of Health and Human Services, ACOs are patient-centered networks of providers and suppliers of services that work together to improve health and slow cost growth. Quality standards and performance outcomes are tied to specific metrics defined by CMS (U.S. Department of Health and Human Services, 2011).

Social Security Disability Insurance (SSDI) and Supplemental Security Insurance (SSI) funds may be available to persons with documented psychiatric problems who are unable to survive financially in the community.

REFERENCES

Abele, M., Brown, J., Ibrahim, H., & Jha, M. K. (2014). Teaching motivational interviewing skills to psychiatry trainees: Findings of a national survey. *Academic Psychiatry (May 15).* doi: 10.1007/s40596-014-0149-0.

Agency for Healthcare Research and Quality. (2012). *Five major steps to intervention (the "5 A's").* Retrieved from http://www.ahrq.gov/professionals/clinicians-providers/guidelines-recommendations/tobacco/5steps.html.

American Nurses Association, International Society of Psychiatric–Mental Health Nurses, and American Psychiatric Nurses Association. (2014). *Psychiatric–mental health nursing: Scope and standards of practice, 2nd ed.* Silver Spring, MD: Nursesbooks.org.

Arnold, E., & Boggs, K. (2007). *Interpersonal relationships: Communication skills for nurses, 5th ed.* Philadelphia: Saunders/Elsevier.

Bandura, A. (1977). Self-efficacy: Toward a unifying theory of behavioral change. *Psychological Review, 84,* 191–215.

Bandler, R., & Grinder, J. (1975). *The structure of magic.* Palo Alto, CA: Science and Behavior Books.

Benson, H. (2000). *The relaxation response.* New York: Harper Paperbacks.

Benson, K., Hutchinson, K., & Melcher, S. (2010). Abstract: Adolescent experiences with ambient therapy. *Journal of the American Psychiatric Association, 16*(6), 368.

Bloom, B. (1984). *Taxonomy of educational objectives.* Boston: Allyn & Bacon.

Bowlby, J. (1958). The nature of the child's tie to his mother. *International Journal of Psychoanalysis, 39,* 350–373.

Boyd, M. A. (2007). *Psychiatric nursing: Contemporary practice, 4th ed.* Philadelphia: Lippincott Williams & Wilkins.

Bronfenbrenner, U. (1979). *The ecology of human development.* Cambridge: Harvard University Press.

Butler A. C., & Beck, A. T. (1995). Cognitive therapy for depression. *The clinical psychologist, 48*(3); 3–5.

Caplan, G. (1964). *Principles of preventive psychiatry.* New York: Basic Books.

Catania, A. C., & Laties, V. G. (1999). Pavlov and Skinner: Two lives in science. *Journal of the experimental analysis of behavior 72*(3): 455–461.

Center for Nonviolence and Social Justice. (n.d.) Maxwell Jones. *The Sanctuary Model.* Retrieved from http://www.sanctuaryweb.com/maxwell-jones.php.

Centers for Disease Control and Prevention. (2015). *Progress reviews for Healthy People 2020.* Retrieved from www.cdc.gov/nchs/healthy_people/hp2020/hp2020_progress_reviews.htm.

Centers for Disease Control and Prevention. (2014). *Facts about ASD.* Retrieved from http://www.cdc.gov/ncbddd/autism/facts.html.

Centers for Medicare and Medicaid Services. (2010). *Patient's bill of rights.* Retrieved from http://www.cancer.org/treatment/findingandpayingfortreatment/understandingfinancialandlegalmatters/patients-bill-of-rights.

Copeland, M. E. (2007). *About WRAP [Wellness Recovery Action Plan].* Retrieved from http://www.mentalhealthrecovery.com/aboutwrap.php.

DeHert, M., Correll, C. U., Bobes, J., Cetkovich-Bakmas, M., Cohen, D. Asai, I., & Leucht, S. (2011). Physical illness in healthcare consumers with severe mental disorders. I. Prevalence, impact of medications and disparities in health care. *World Psychiatry 10*(1), 52–77.

Executive Order of the White House. (2002). President's new freedom commission on mental health. Accessed February. Retrieved from http://govinfo.library.unt.edu/mentalhealthcommission/20020429-2.htm.

Genogram Analytics. (n.d.). Homepage. Retrieved from http://genogramanalytics.com/index.html.

Genopro.com. (n.d.). Intro to the Genogram. Retrieved from http://genopro.com/genogram.

Goodman, R. & Scott, S. (2005). *Child psychology, 2nd ed.* Hoboken, NJ: Wiley-Blackwell.

Glick, R. (2010). Cardiac coherence training. [PowerPoint Webinar].

Halter, M. J. (2008). Perceived characteristics of psychiatric nursing: Stigma by association. *Journal of the American Psychiatric Nurses Association, 22*(1): 20–6.

Hutchinson, K. & Melcher, S. (2009). *Ambient therapy project with hospitalized children and adolescents.* Paper presented for Sigma Theta Tau, Rho Lambda Chapter; School of Health Sciences, Winston Salem State University, Winston Salem, NC.

Institute of Medicine. (2004). *Report on Health Literacy: A Prescription to End Confusion.* Retrieved from https://www.iom.edu/Reports/2004/Health-Literacy-A-Prescription-to-End-Confusion.aspx.

Johnson, S. R. (2014, March 22). Shelter for convalescence: Hospitals link with respite programs to aid homeless patients through recovery. *Modern Healthcare.* Retrieved from http://www.modernhealthcare.com/article/20140322/MAGAZINE/303229937.

The Joint Commission. (2012). *Patient education and training standards.* Retrieved from http://www.mghpcs.org/eed_portal/Documents/PatientEd/JC_Standards_PatientEd.pdf.

Kerr, M. (2000). One family's story: A primer on Bowen theory. *The Bowen Center for the study of the family.* Retrieved from http://www.thebowencenter.org.

Knowles, M., Holton, E., & Swanson, D. (2005). *The adult learner.* London: Butterworth-Heinmann.

Kymissis, P., & Halperin, D. A. (Eds.). (1996). *Group therapy with children and adolescents.* Washington, DC: American Psychiatric Press.

Landreth, G. L. (2002). *Play therapy: The art of the relationship.* New York: Brunner-Routledge.

Landreth, G., Sweeney, D., Ray, D., Homeyer, L., & Glover, G. (2005). *Play therapy interventions with children's problems, 2nd ed.* Northvale, NJ: Jason Aronson.

Lazarus, A. A. (2008). *Multimodal Therapy: Systems of Psychotherapy Video Series.* Washington, D.C.: American Psychological Association. Retrieved from http://www.apa.org/pubs/videos/4310817.aspx.

Madanes, C. (1981). *Strategic family therapy.* San Francisco: Jossey-Bass.

Miller, W. R. & Rollnick, S. (1991). *Motivational interviewing: Preparing people to change addictive behavior.* New York: Guilford Press.

Minuchin, S. (1974). *Families and family therapy.* Cambridge, MA: Harvard University Press.

Motivational Interviewing Network of Trainers. (2013). *Welcome to the Motivational Interviewing Website!* Retrieved from http://www.motivationalinterviewing.org/.

National Alliance to End Homelessness. (2014). National Alliance to End Homelessness in America: Author: 1–86.

National Assessment of Adult Literacy. (2006). *The health literacy of America's adults: Results from the 2003 National Assessment of Adult Literacy.* Retrieved from http://nces.ed.gov/pubsearch/pubsinfo.asp?pubid=2006483.

National Cancer Institute. (2014). *American Cancer Society recommendations for colorectal cancer early detection.* Retrieved from http://www.cancer.org/cancer/colonandrectumcancer/moreinformation/colonandrectumcancerearlydetection/colorectal-cancer-early-detection-acs-recommendations.

National Institute on Drug Abuse. (2015). *Mind Over Matter Teaching Guide and Series.* Retrieved from http://teens.drugabuse.gov/educators/nida-teaching-guides/mind-over-matter.

New Freedom Commission on Mental Health. (2003). *Achieving the promise: Transforming mental health care in America. Final report.* DHHS Pub. No. SMA-03–3832. Rockville, MD: U.S. Department of Health and Human Services.

Nurse-Family Partnership. (2011). *The theories that support Nurse-Family Partnership nursing.* Retrieved from http://www.nursefamilypartnership.org/nurses/nursing-theory.

Patient Self Determination Act of 1990. Retrieved from http://thomas.loc.gov/cgi-bin/query/z?c101:H.R.4449.IH:

Pender, N., Murdaugh, C., & Parsons, M. A. (2006). *Health promotion in nursing practice, 5th ed.* Upper Saddle River, NJ: Prentice Hall.

Prochaska, J. O., & Velicer, W. F. (1997). The transtheoretical model of health behavior change. *American Journal of Health Promotion, 12,* 38–48.

Protection and Advocacy Act of 1986. Retrieved from http://www.gpo.gov/fdsys/pkg/STATUTE-100/pdf/STATUTE-100-Pg478.pdf.

Rankin, S., Stallings, K., & London, F. (2005). *Healthcare consumer education in health and illness, 5th ed.* Philadelphia: Lippincott Williams & Wilkins.

Ratzan, S. C., & Parker, R. M. (2000). Introduction. In C. R. Selden, M. Zorn, S. C. Ratzan, & R. M. Parkers (Eds.), *National Library of Medicine current bibliographies in medicine: Health literacy.* NLM Pub. No. CBM 2000–1. Bethesda, MD: National Institutes of Health.

Ricci, R. J., & Clayton, C. A. (2008). Trauma resolution as an adjunct to standard treatment for child molesters: A qualitative study. *Journal of EMDR Practice and Research, 2*(1), 41–50.

Roy, K., Haddix, A.C., Ikeda, R.M., Curry, C.W., Truman, B.I., & Thacker, S.B. (2009). Monitoring progress toward CDC's health protection goals: Health outcome measure by life stage. Public Health Reports, March-April, 124: 304-316.

Rusch, N., & Corrigan, P. W. (2002). Motivational interviewing to improve insight and treatment adherence in schizophrenia. *Psychiatric Rehabilitation Journal, 26,* 23–32.

Shives, L. R. (2012). *Basic concepts of psychiatric mental health nursing, 8th ed.* Philadelphia: Lippincott Williams & Wilkins.

Schyve, P.M. (2014). Violence in the health care setting. *JC Physician Blog.* Retrieved from http://www.jointcommission.org/jc_physician_blog/violence_in_the_health_care_setting/.

Simmons, J. E. (1981). *Psychiatric examination of children, 3rd ed.* Philadelphia: Lea & Febiger.

Sixty-fifth World Health Assembly. (2012). The global burden of mental disorders and the need for a comprehensive, coordinated response from health and social sectors at rhe county level. WHA65.4; 1–4.

Stuart, G. (2009). *Principles and practice of psychiatric nursing (9th ed.).* St. Louis: Mosby.

Substance Abuse and Mental Health Services Administration. Drug Treatment Act of 2000. Retrieved from http://buprenorphine.samhsa.gov/fulllaw.html.

Tuckman, B. (1965). Developmental sequence in small groups. *Psychological Bulletin, 63,* 384–399.

U.S. Department of Education. (2004). *The Individuals with Disabilities Education Act.* Retrieved from http://idea.ed.gov/.

U.S. Department of Health and Human Services. (2014). Mental health and mental disorders. In *HealthyPeople 2020.* Retrieved from http://www.healthypeople.gov/2020/topics-objectives/topic/mental-health-and-mental-disorders/objectives

U.S. Department of Health and Human Services. (2011). *Press release: Affordable Care Act to improve quality of care for people with Medicare.* Retrieved from http://www.cms.gov/Newsroom/MediaReleaseDatabase/Press-releases/2011-Press-releases-items/2011-10-24.html?DLPage=1&DLFilter=Affordable%20Care%20Act&DLSort=0&DLSortDir=descending.

U.S. Department of Health and Human Services. (n.d.) *Surgeon General's family history initiative.* Retrieved from http://www.hhs.gov/familyhistory/.

U.S. Department of Health and Human Services. (n.d.). *Your rights under section 504 of the rehabilitation act:* Fact sheet. Retrieved from http://www.hhs.gov/ocr/civilrights/resources/factsheets/504.pdf.

U.S. Department of Health and Human Services. (1999). *Mental health: A report of the surgeon general.* Retrieved from http://profiles.nlm.nih.gov/ps/retrieve/ResourceMetadata/NNBBHS.

U.S. Department of Justice—Civil Rights Division. Americans with Disabilities Act. Retrieved from http://www.ada.gov/.

Varcolis, E., Carson, V., & Shoemaker, N. (2006). *Foundations of psychiatric mental health nursing: A clinical approach, 5th ed.* St. Louis: W.B. Saunders.

Wellstone-Domenici Mental Health Parity and Addiction Equity Act of 2009 (Final Rule 2013). Retrieved from http://webapps.dol.gov/federalregister/HtmlDisplay.aspx?DocId=27169&AgencyId=8&DocumentType=2.

World Health Organization. (2012). *Depression: fact sheet no 369.* Retrieved from http://www.who.int/mediacentre/factsheets/fs369/en/.

World Health Organization. (2014). *Mental disorders. Fact sheet.* Retrieved from http://www.who.int/mediacentre/factsheets/fs396/en/.

Wright, L. M., & Leahey, M. (2007). *Nurses and families: A guide to family assessment and intervention, 4th ed.* Philadelphia: F. A. Davis.

Yalom, I. D., & Leszcz, M. (2005). *The theory and practice of group psychotherapy, 5th ed.* New York: Basic Books.

APPENDIX A

REVIEW QUESTIONS

1. A global assessment tool used by healthcare providers that identifies multiple and major risk areas among adolescent populations is the:

   a. Hamilton Anxiety Rating Scale

   b. Johari Window

   c. Global Assessment of Functioning Scale

   d. HEEADSS Assessment

2. A form of therapy that focuses on helping the patient resolve unconscious conflicts through dream analysis and free-association of thoughts is:

   a. Systematic desensitization

   b. Psychoanalysis

   c. Behavior modification

   d. Dialectical behavioral therapy

3. Which of the following was developed as an appropriate and sensitive therapy for patients with borderline personality disorder?

   a. Benzodiazepine administration as needed

   b. Neuroleptics daily

   c. Dialectical behavioral therapy

   d. Flooding therapy

4. Socratic questioning is a technique used in which type of therapy intervention?

   a. Multimodal therapy

   b. Family therapy

   c. Cognitive behavioral therapy

   d. Play therapy

5. Which of the following is a tricyclic antidepressant?

   a. Marplan

   b. Oxazepam

   c. Tofranil

   d. Buspar

6. Which of the following is a long-acting benzodiazepine?

   a. Alprazolam (Xanax)

   b. Triazolam (Halcion)

   c. Clonazepam (Klonopin)

   d. Lorazepam (Ativan)

7. Which neuroleptic is available in a sublingual form?

    a. Paliperidone (Invega)

    b. Asenapine (Saphris)

    c. Iloperidone (Fanapt)

    d. Olanzapine (Zyprexa)

8. Glioblastoma is a tumor that specifically affects:

    a. Astrocytes

    b. Cytoplasm

    c. Myelin metabolism

    d. Glia

9. Symbyax is a unique psychopharmaceutical in that it combines a:

    a. Benzodiazepine and a neuroleptic

    b. Selective serotonin reuptake inhibitor and a neuroleptic

    c. Anticonvulsant and an antiemetic

    d. Tricyclic antidepressant and an anxiolytic

10. Severe damage to Broca's area of the brain results in:

    a. Inability to express speech

    b. Inability to understand speech

    c. Difficulty with executive functions

    d. Memory impairment

11. The Scope and Standards of Psychiatric–Mental Health Nursing represents a collaboration between:

    a. Robert Wood Johnson Foundation and the Institute of Medicine

    b. International Society of Psychiatric Nurses, the American Nurses Association, and the American Psychiatric Nurses Association

    c. American Psychiatric Nurses Association and the American Nurses Association

    d. National League for Nurses and the American Association of Colleges of Nursing

12. The *Future of Nursing* publication report is a collaboration between:

    a. Robert Wood Johnson Foundation and the Institute of Medicine

    b. International Society of Psychiatric Nurses and the American Psychiatric Nurses Association

    c. American Psychiatric Nurses Association and the American Nurses Association

    d. National League for Nurses and the American Association for Colleges of Nursing

13. Professional Performance Standards set forth by the *2014 Scope and Standards of Psychiatric–Mental Health Nursing* acknowledges that the nurse understands:

    a. Principles related to resource utilization

    b. Need for a BSN degree by the year 2020

    c. Civil involuntary commitment laws

    d. Specialty certification as a requirement

14. An important finding drawn from the Institute of Medicine's (IOM) 1999 *To Err is Human* report revealed:

    a. Upwards of 98,000 patients die annually while in hospitals.

    b. Nurses are seen as the most trusted healthcare providers.

    c. Healthcare settings must set independent standards according to the community population demographics.

    d. Root cause analyses should be implemented whenever there is a near miss event.

15. Clinical ability to view blood flow throughout the brain is achieved by:

    a. Transcranial Magnetic Stimulation

    b. Functional MRI

    c. Electroencephalogram

    d. Elicitation of cranial nerve X reflex

16. Clinical decision-making at the point of care is best demonstrated in which nursing activity?

    a. Bedside reporting

    b. Enlisting assent from a minor

    c. Storage and labeling personal items in a space that is separated from the medication room

    d. Obtaining report from the emergency department for a new transfer

17. Which of the following initiatives is considered a useful evidence-based intervention in any outpatient or community mental health facility?

    a. Screening, brief intervention, and referral services

    b. Wrap-around services that include provisions for shelter

    c. Standardized recommendations to quit tobacco first, if that is an issue

    d. Contingency reinforcement schedules when collecting urine drug screens

18. What is the best definition of a Magnet-designated work environment?

    a. Nurse-initiated protocols are to be used before physician-initiated protocols.

    b. Bedside nurses have baccalaureate degrees.

    c. Leadership is authentic and autocratic.

    d. Nurses are excellent.

19. The most current publication used by psychiatrists that outlines criteria for diagnosing psychopathologies is the:

    a. Diagnostic and Statistical Manual of Mental Disorders IV

    b. Diagnostic and Statistical Manual of Mental Disorders IV-TR

    c. Diagnostic and Statistical Manual of Mental Disorders 5

    d. Diagnostic and Statistical Manual of Mental Disorders 6

20. The nurse is giving report on a newly admitted patient with schizophrenia. The nurse states that the patient has predominantly negative symptoms. Which symptoms would you expect?

    a. Nihilistic delusions

    b. Commanding voices

    c. Paranoia about taking medications

    d. Impaired motivation to perform self-care

21. Patients with psychotic disorders have a 20% shorter life expectancy than the general population. Which factor highly contributes to this shorter life expectancy?

    a. Metabolic syndrome due to long-term neuroleptic use

    b. Cardiac irregularities, notably QTc prolongation

    c. Antipsychotic medications are metabolized by the kidneys, so renal failure may compromise healthy elimination

    d. Medication nonadherence

22. A patient says "There's a copperhead snake" while pointing to the computer cord that is attached to the medication scanner. This perceptual anomaly is referred to as a(n):

    a. Delusion of persecution

    b. Déjà vu experience

    c. Illusion

    d. Visual hallucination

23. Inability to perform a voluntary purposeful movement is referred to as:

    a. Alexithymia

    b. Anhedonia

    c. Alogia

    d. Apraxia

24. A synthetic drug that is structurally related to endorphins is:

    a. Morphine

    b. Amphetamines

    c. Benzodiazepines

    d. Guanfacine

25. Which clinical laboratory measure can help substantiate a diagnosis of chronic alcohol dependence?

    a. Serum prolactin levels

    b. Serum albumin levels

    c. Serum AST levels

    d. Serum RPR levels

26. A clinical measure to determine whether a patient is continuing to use nicotine may be assessed by results from the:

    a. Polysomnography

    b. Salivary cotinine

    c. Serum cortisol

    d. Gamma-glutamyl transaminase (GGT)

27. What features characterize qualitative research methods?

    a. Randomized samples are invited to participate.

    b. Half the participants are in the control group.

    c. The researcher seeks verbatim understanding of themes.

    d. The research participants have consented and assented.

28. The statement "Health is a state of complete physical, mental, and social well-being and not merely the absence of disease and infirmity" is proposed by the:

    a. National Institutes of Medicine

    b. American Psychiatric Association

    c. American Medical Association

    d. World Health Organization

29. According to Maslow's Hierarchy of Needs Theory, the highest level that can be achieved is:

    a. Self-esteem

    b. Self-transcendence

    c. Love and belonging

    d. Safety and security

30. Optimized learning situations are facilitated when the education process:

    a. Invokes affective, behavioral, and cognitive domains of learning

    b. Holds attention and provides hourly breaks and small group discussions

    c. Is presented to groups who are seated in semi-circular arrangements

    d. Evokes a sense of safety and security in the audience and participants have chosen to be there

31. Medical record formats that use charting by exception templates address:

    a. Subjective, objective, and assessment components

    b. Deviations from within normal limits

    c. Situation, background, and response sections

    d. Assessment, diagnoses, planning, implementation, and evaluation segments

32. The first atypical antipsychotic proposed for the treatment of psychotic disorders was:

    a. Chlorpromazine

    b. Clozapine

    c. Imipramine

    d. Aripiprazole

33. The therapeutic effects associated with the reduction of positive and negative symptoms are due to blockage of:

    a. Dopaminergic receptors

    b. GABA receptors

    c. Serotonergic receptors

    d. Norepinephrine receptors

34. Pharmacogenomics involves:

    a. Selective action of medications on different persons

    b. Adverse effects caused by pharmacodynamics

    c. Genetic mutations that result from taking pharmacologic agents

    d. Teratogenic potential of psychopharmaceuticals

35. Psychopharmaceuticals that block muscarinic receptors cause which side effects?

    a. Agitation, nausea, elevated temperature

    b. Akathisia, wry neck, stiffness

    c. Cogwheel rigidity, pupil dilation, hypotension

    d. Urinary retention, dry mucous membranes, constipation

36. Which topical psychopharmacologic preparation may be indicated for a patient who expresses helplessness and hopelessness?

    a. Nicotine patch

    b. Selegiline patch

    c. Daytrana patch

    d. Voltaren gel

37. What physical signs of recent cocaine intoxication would the nurse expect to find in a 56-year-old man being admitted to the inpatient unit?

    a. B/P 190/100; P 135; R 30; loquacious, muscle twitching evident, paranoid

    b. B/P 90/50; P 100; R 22; withdrawn, insists on "getting to a bed to come down"

    c. B/P 142/102; P 86; R 26; alogia; flat affect; keeps eyes closed because of "seeing God looking at me"

    d. B/P 100/70; P 99; R 16; marked tooth decay; multiple lesions and needle prick venous tracks

38. Which of the following professional performance standards are expectations of the psychiatric–mental health nurse?

    a. Maintaining competency in the field of nursing

    b. Learning psychology and psychiatry

    c. Sitting on Institutional Review Boards (IRBs)

    d. Willingness to engage in extended shift-work for patient continuity of care

39. Which cognitive development theorist proposes a characteristic schema wherein a person gradually learns that significant others in their lives are permanent, although out of sight?

    a. Sigmund Freud

    b. Erik Erikson

    c. John Bowlby

    d. Jean Piaget

40. Which nursing theorist proclaims that if a person believes that an action has positive consequences, he or she is more likely to engage in lifestyle modifications to improve health?

    a. Barbara Johnson

    b. Dorothy Orem

    c. Jean Watson

    d. Nola Pender

APPENDIX B

ANSWERS TO THE REVIEW QUESTIONS

1. **Correct Answer: d.** The HEEADSS assessment scale is particular for assessing issues of concern within adolescent populations. HEEADSS looks at these specific areas: **H**ome and environment, **E**ducation and employment, **E**ating, **A**ctivities, **D**rugs, **S**uicide, and **S**exuality. The Hamilton Anxiety Rating Scale is used to evaluate for the presence and degree of subjective anxiety; the Johari Window is an assessment tool that helps a person become more self-aware, by considering perceptions of others; the Global Assessment of Functioning Scale provides a measure from 100 (highest functioning) to 1 (lowest functioning) when making a psychiatric diagnosis.

2. **Correct Answer: b.** Psychoanalysis is an old yet relevant technique, developed by Freud. It prompts patients to tap into unconscious experiences that may be affecting current perceptions and behaviors. Systematic desensitization is a technique that gradually exposes a person to a feared stimulus to help him or her control that fear; behavior modification uses operant and classical conditioning concepts to shape more adaptive, less maladaptive behaviors; dialectical behavioral therapy was designed as a specialized approach for patients with borderline personality disorder.

3. **Correct Answer: c.** Dialectical behavioral therapy was designed as a specialized approach for patients with borderline personality disorder. Benzodiazepines are medications that work to induce relaxation and are used in alcohol withdrawal; neuroleptics target positive and negative symptoms found in psychotic conditions; flooding is an intense type of systematic desensitization therapy that directly and repeatedly exposes a person to a feared stimulus.

4. **Correct Answer: c.** Socratic questioning is a technique proposed by cognitive behavioral therapists as a means of logically challenging one's perception about a belief. In multimodal therapies, variants of different theories are used to facilitate positive change. Family therapy has many variations, but in all the family is at the center of psychotherapeutic intervention; and play therapy is a specialized form of practice that illuminates issues of concern within children who, because of developmental ages or issues, have not attained sophisticated language skills.

5. **Correct Answer: c.** The only tricyclic antidepressant listed is Tofranil. Marplan is an MAOI, oxazepam is a benzodiazepine, and Buspar is a nonaddicting anxiolytic.

6. **Correct Answer: c.** The only long-acting benzodiazepine listed is clonazepam (Klonopin). Lorazepam (Ativan) and alprazolam (Xanax) are intermediate-acting; and triazolam (Halcion) is a short-acting GABA enhancer.

7. **Correct Answer: b.** Saphris is the sublingual preparation; Invega, Fanapt, and Zyprexa are oral formulations.

8. **Correct Answer: d.** Glioblastoma is technically a tumor of the glial cells. These "glue-like" cells hold neuronal circuits in proper spaces, thereby affording proper transportation of electrical stimuli within neuronal networks. Astrocytes provide nutrients to glial cells, whereas the cytoplasm is the fluid-filled cellular content and myelin is the protective shell-like coating surrounding neurons.

9. **Correct Answer: b.** Symbyax combines pharmaceutical elements of the antidepressant type—selective serotonin reuptake inhibitor—with the properties of neuroleptics, making it a unique brand. The pharmaceutical pairings named in the other three choices may not even exist.

10. **Correct Answer: a.** Broca's aphasia is commonly defined as difficulty or inability to express speech; the person cannot get intelligible words out. This aphasia may be seen in cardiovascular accidents or other forms of severe head trauma when Broca's area has suffered assault.

11. **Correct Answer: b.** This important document that addresses professional nursing practice for the psychiatric–mental health nurse is contained in the International Society of Psychiatric Nurses, American Nurses Association, and American Psychiatric Nurses Association's specialty designed publication. It provides a basis for consistency of patient-focused care. The other listed choices provide relevant but more generalized guidance.

12. **Correct Answer: a.** This important publication represents a collaboration between the Robert Wood Johnson Foundation and the Institute of Medicine, two organizations that are critically examining the healthcare environment and workforce to identify elements where structural improvements need to be made. Expertise offered by the other listed choices provides relevant and specific guidance within nursing itself.

13. **Correct Answer: a.** The only professional performance standard listed is related to resource utilization. The other choices have selective validity and applicability.

14. **Correct Answer: a.** Analyses of the self-reported data disseminated in the 1999 IOM report revealed that 98,000 patients die annually in U.S. hospitals. This and subsequent findings outlined the charge for quality assurance changes that are driving issues of safety in the workplace, enhanced education among healthcare providers of all levels, and close examination of error occurrences and near-misses.

15. **Correct Answer: b.** The functional magnetic resonance imaging technique (fMRI) provides a much enhanced visualization of the brain's circulation networks. Transcranial magnetic stimulation is a new technique that uses magnets to polarize and depolarize ionic particulates in the brain to treat depression; the electroencephalogram provides graphic images of brain wave motility; eliciting cranial nerve X identifies functional indices of the heart and digestive systems.

16. **Correct Answer: a.** Bedside reporting strategies provide nursing professionals an opportunity to determine the patient's status and needs level, at the point of care when being transferred from one nursing professional to another. At this point, all parties can come to a collective understanding of recent past condition, and be able to collectively identify future care needs.

17. **Correct Answer: a.** Screening, brief intervention, and referral services (SBIRT) is an evidence-based model of care for addressing and intervening when patients enter a healthcare system. Providers are recommended to screen, intervene, and refer patients to a higher level or expert level of care and treatment in the case of uncovering substance use disorders, in particular.

18. **Correct Answer: d.** In its most direct and simple form, Magnet-designated facilities validate that their nurses are excellent. It is a statement that nurses are engaged at all levels of the healthcare enterprise—interprofessional committees, task forces, research endeavors, continued education. Nurse-initiated protocols are expected, but not necessarily before physician-initiated protocols; BSN degrees are a recommendation, not necessarily a mandate; leadership strives to be authentic, not necessarily autocratic.

19. **Correct Answer: c.** The *Diagnostic and Statistical Manual of Mental Disorders,* 5th edition, was published in 2013 and describes the latest diagnostic criteria endorsed by the American Psychiatric Association.

20. **Correct Answer: d.** Negative symptoms are those that are evidenced by alogia, amotivation, withdrawal, and a general tendency to refrain from self-care concerns. Positive symptoms, such as nihilistic delusions, commanding voices, and paranoia, may respond to neuroleptic medication intervention; the negative symptoms are not as responsive to neuroleptics in general.

21. **Correct Answer: a.** Metabolic syndrome, evidenced by hyperlipidemia, abdominal adiposity, and glucose intolerance, can be problematic side effects that result from psychopharmaceuticals, particularly the typical neuroleptic classes (e.g., Zyprexa, Geodon), and with many of the antiepileptic and anticonvulsant mood stabilizers. These side effects accelerate cardiac disease, the number one cause of death in the United States, among patients in treatment for psychiatric disorders. Coupled with risky behaviors, suicides, and substance use co-occurrence, patients with psychiatric disorders die sooner than others in the general population.

22. **Correct Answer: c.** An illusion is the misinterpretation of a stimuli; a hallucination is a perception in the absence of any stimuli. A delusion of persecution is a specific belief that someone or something wants to harm a person; and déjà vu experiences describe a phenomenon wherein a person believes or perceives that he or she "has been here before," or "knows you from somewhere."

23. **Correct Answer: d.** Apraxia, a neurological condition, is the inability to execute purposeful movements. This phenomenon may result from neuroleptic therapy, neurological disorders, or basal ganglia impairment. Alexithymia defines a condition of absence of feelings; anhedonia is the absence of finding pleasure in things or experiences previously found pleasurable; alogia is the inability to express language.

24. **Correct Answer: a.** Morphine is a synthetic drug that is structurally similar to endorphins, neurotransmitters synthesized in the brain. Amphetamines are more similar to adrenalin, benzodiazepines target GABA receptors, and guanfacine is a hypertensive agent.

25. **Correct Answer: c.** Chronic alcohol dependence produces elevations in enzymes such as AST (aspartate aminotransferase) and ALT (alanine aminotransferase). Serum AST and ALT levels are used to detect liver damage. Prolactin is a hormone that may be elevated as the result of neuroleptic therapy; albumin is a measure of serum protein; and the serum RPR (rapid plasma regain) screens for syphilis.

26. **Correct Answer: b.** Salivary cotinine levels are a biomarker for whether nicotine has recently been used. Cotinine is a metabolite of nicotine. Polysomnography is a sleep study test, serum cortisol indicates depression, and GGT (gamma-glutamyl transaminase) is a liver enzyme.

27. **Correct Answer: c.** Qualitative research designs seek to understand the lived experience of research participants; this type of research usually will engage the participant in answering open-ended questions while the researcher tape records the responses and transcribes the recordings verbatim. The goal is to uncover specific themes that occur in the participants' descriptions. All participants over the age of 18 years have provided consent for participation; if younger than age 18, assent is also required for participation. Randomization and control groups are selected in comparison-type studies.

28. **Correct Answer: d.** The World Health Organization (WHO) provides this definition of health. The IOM provides evaluations of healthcare outcomes and future needs; the APA publishes the DSM5; the AMA is the licensing body for physicians.

29. **Correct Answer: b.** According to newer resources, Maslow described a level of self-transcendence as the highest personal attainment in the hierarchy of needs theory. Self-transcendent persons seek to give back efforts to others, a further reach than self-actualization, which describes reaching a pinnacle for self.

30. **Correct Answer: a.** Optimized learning situations invoke affective ("how do you feel about this learning"), behavioral (show-and-tell type activities), and cognitive ("what do you know; need to know") domains. These invocations use different parts of brain reservoirs, thereby facilitating retention and understanding. The other three answers offer aspects of the teaching-learning environment that should be considered as well.

31. **Correct Answer: b.** The charting by exception format of medical recordkeeping offers the options to select "within normal limits" or "not within normal limits" categories when assessing body systems or other clinical findings. The exception, therefore, is the "not within normal limits" categorization—which when selected, opens to opportunities to elaborate on that particular issue. Subjective, objective, and assessment charting reviews "what patient said; what nurse or clinician sees; what nurse or clinician thinks about it." SBAR communication invokes the situation, background to the situation, and response (patient) parameters of a presenting problem. The assessment, diagnosis, planning, implementation, and evaluation segments define the areas of concern in the nursing process.

32. **Correct Answer: b.** The first atypical antipsychotic was clozapine; first typical antipsychotic was chlorpromazine; a later atypical antipsychotic is aripiprazole; imipramine is a TCA-type antidepressant.

33. **Correct Answer: a.** Dopaminergic receptor blockage is responsible for reducing the positive and negative symptoms in psychotic disorders. GABA receptor effects have affinity for inducing a calming and relaxed state; serotonergic effects work to reverse experiences of depression; norepinephrine effects arousal, concentration, and learning experiences.

34. **Correct Answer: a.** Pharmacogenomics is a new field that primarily examines pharmacodynamics and pharmacokinetic expressions among a diverse constituency in the population. It addresses effects based on gender, ethnicity, genetics, and other variables. Secondary data derived may contemplate genetic mutation expressions, adverse pharmacological effects, and teratogenic potential.

35. **Correct Answer: d.** Muscarinic blockage results in the classic anticholinergic side effects commonly seen with the administration of psychopharmaceuticals. These side effects are classically urinary retention, dry mouth, and constipation.

36. **Correct Answer: b.** Selegiline patch is classified as a monoamine oxidase inhibitor (MAOI) antidepressant that may be indicated for the symptoms of helplessness and hopelessness. Nicotine patch may be used for assisting with reducing cigarette smoking; Daytrana patch may be used to quell symptoms of attention-deficit hyperactivity disorder; Voltaren gel is a topical anesthetic typically indicated for arthritis pain relief.

37. **Correct Answer: a.** With cocaine intoxication, the central nervous system is stimulated, therefore the expected signs would be increased blood pressure, pulse, and respiration, in addition to muscle twitching, increased talking, and paranoia. A flat affect is more apparent with opioids and inhalants that may or may not be accompanied by psychotic features.

38. **Correct Answer: a.** It is expected as one of the professional performance standards that the psychiatric–mental health nurse maintain competency in this specialized area of nursing. Sitting on the IRB board would exponentially elevate the nurse's understanding of the research process and ethics, integrity, and rights associated with research engagements. An adjunctive field for learning would be the study of psychology and psychiatry, but is not a requisite part of the scope and standards of psychiatric–mental health nursing practice.

39. **Correct Answer: d.** Jean Piaget, a Swiss psychologist, proposed the theory of cognitive development in which infants learn an important concept known as object permanence. Object permanence is recognized when the infant develops awareness that, although a caregiver may be out of sight, the caregiver still exists—evidenced by his or her returning at intervals. Freud characterizes development through 5 psychosexual stages; Erikson conceptualizes emotional and psychological development as commencing at birth and continuing throughout life in stages characterized by particular mastery or nonmastery of opposing emotional and psychological obstacles; Bowlby is noted for proposing the theory of attachment, which is central to infant-parent dyads.

40. **Correct Answer: d.** Nurse theorist Nola Pender proposes cues to action and other factors associated with health beliefs that prompt a person to be more likely to engage in health-promoting lifestyle behaviors. Dorothy Johnson proposes the behavioral system model of nursing care that fosters effective and efficient patient functioning; Dorothy Orem proposes a model of self-care for nurses; Jean Watson speaks of nurses as the proponents of the human caring model.

INDEX

INDEX

Note: Page numbers followed by *f* indicate figures; *t* tables; and *b* boxes.

M

ABOUT THE AUTHOR

Kim M. Hutchinson, EdD, PMHCNS-BC, CARN

Over my 36 years in nursing, I received scholarships and grants from the National Institute of Mental Health, American Association of University Women of Fairfield County, American Nurses Association's Ethnic and Minority Fellowship Program, Robert Wood Johnson Foundation, and the National Cancer Institute to support my baccalaureate nursing education (Fairfield University), graduate education in child and adolescent mental health nursing (Lehman College of City University of New York), postgraduate education in tobacco epidemiology and health services research (Wake Forest University Graduate School), and graduate education in educational and health psychology with a secondary concentration in gerontology (Northern Illinois University) to further pursue my educational interests. Drawing from this background as a psychiatric–mental health nurse faculty, clinician, mentor, and educator, my views fully encompass the life span developmental trajectory. From this lens, I continue to gain appreciable exposure to expansive views of human complexities and potentials.

CERTIFICATIONS

American Nurses Credentialing Center

- Board certified clinical nurse specialist in child and adolescent mental health nursing (PMHCNS-BC)
- Board certified psychiatric mental health nurse (RN-BC)

International Association of Forensic Nurses

- Sexual Assault Nurse Examiner (SANE)

International Nurses Society on Addictions

- Certified Addictions Registered Nurse (CARN)

American Lung Association

- Tobacco Cessation Specialist

Review and Resource Manual

Addendum to Psychiatric– Mental Health Nursing

th Edition

NURSING CERTIFICATION REVIEW MANUAL

CONTINUING EDUCATION RESOURCE

CLINICAL PRACTICE RESOURCE

Kimberly Campbell, DNP, RN-BC

    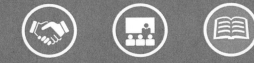

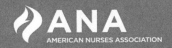

ANA
AMERICAN NURSES ASSOCIATION

Library of Congress Cataloging-in-Publication Data

The American Nurses Association (ANA) is the only full-service professional organization representing the interests of the nation's 3.1 million registered nurses through its constituent/state nurses associations and its organizational affiliates. The ANA advances the nursing profession by fostering high standards of nursing practice, promoting the rights of nurses in the workplace, projecting a positive and realistic view of nursing, and lobbying the Congress and regulatory agencies on healthcare issues affecting nurses and the public.

© 2020 American Nurses Association
8515 Georgia Ave., Suite 400
Silver Spring, MD 20910

Table of Contents

INTRODUCTION TO THE PSYCHIATRIC–MENTAL HEALTH NURSING REVIEW AND RESOURCE MANUAL, 5TH EDITION ADDENDUM

The requirements for Psychiatric–Mental Health Nurses and the needs of patients are constantly evolving alongside new research, techniques, policies, and technologies. The American Nurses Credentialing Center and American Nurses Association both recognize the importance of staying abreast of these changes. This addendum is based on ANCC's revised 2019 test content outline to ensure that the Psychiatric–Mental Health Nursing Review and Resource Manual is up to date. This additional information will assist you with successful completion of the certification exam and may be used as a guideline for your practice. While this addendum highlights these content areas, it is not meant to be all-inclusive. For detailed information, we encourage you to explore the topics, using the Psychiatric–Mental Health Nursing reference list. We hope you will find this content useful as a study guide and a source of information for your practice.

Questions regarding this addendum should be sent to publications@ana.org.

CATEGORY I

ASSESSMENT, DIAGNOSIS, AND PLANNING

ASSESSMENTS ACROSS THE LIFE SPAN: PHYSICAL, DEVELOPMENTAL, EMOTIONAL, MORAL, AND PSYCHOSOCIAL

BASIC COMPETENCIES AND PERFORMANCE SKILLS OF PSYCHIATRIC AND MENTAL HEALTH NURSES

Nurses have been ranked as the most trusted profession by the U.S. public (Brenan, 2018), and have held this distinction for 17 consecutive years.

INTRODUCTION TO THE SCOPE AND STANDARDS OF PSYCHIATRIC–MENTAL HEALTH NURSING PRACTICE

PMH Practice Standard 1. Assessment

Current medical status and history should include height and weight rather than BMI as well as recent weight loss or gain.

COMPONENTS OF THE PHYSICAL EXAMINATION AND REVIEW OF SYSTEMS (ROS)

Critical Assessment Priority Areas

Clinical Standardized (Evidence-Based) Measures: Vital Signs and Laboratory Values

TABLE 3-4.
OVERVIEW OF PHYSICAL FINDINGS RELATED TO MENTAL DISORDERS
OR TREATMENTS AND POSSIBLE ETIOLOGIES

FUNCTIONAL SYSTEM	SYMPTOMS	POSSIBLE MECHANISM
Head	Progressively severe headache (potentially affecting eyes and vision)	Hypertensive crisis due to ingested tyramine interacting with monoamine oxidase inhibitors (MAOIs)
Eyes (vision)	Nystagmus	Substance intoxication, brain lesions
	Oculogyric crisis	Neuroleptic-induced dystonia
Ears (hearing)	Diminished hearing	Poor hearing acuity may be misinterpreted as cognitive impairment in older adults
Throat and neck	High fever and sore throat	Agranulocytosis (greatest risk with clonazepam [Clozapine])
	Thyroid enlargement (goiter)	Hypothyroidism
Respiratory system	Anxiety	Hyperventilation, asthma, shortness of breath
Integumentary system	Rash	Possible allergic reaction
		Risk for Stevens-Johnson syndrome (toxic epidermal necrolysis) if on lamotrigine (Lamictal)
Neurological system	Tremors	Lithium: fine-motor
		Parkinson's disease: slow-resting
		Anticonvulsants: fine-motor
		Acute alcohol withdrawals: fine-motor
	Gait and balance disturbances	Encephalopathy, intoxication, cerebellar injuries
	Disorientation, confusion	Delirium, anticholinergic toxicity, serotonin syndrome
	Weakness, numbness	Cerebrovascular events, electrolyte imbalances
	Anxiety	Drug intoxication or withdrawal, stimulants, seizures

(CONTINUED)

TABLE 3-4.
CONTINUED

FUNCTIONAL SYSTEM	SYMPTOMS	POSSIBLE MECHANISM
Cardiovascular system	ECG changes	Tricyclics, anticholinergics, some antipsychotics (e.g., ziprasidone [Geodon])
	Orthostatic hypotension	Tricyclics, antipsychotics, antihypertensives
	Tachycardia	Anxiety, stimulants, anorexia
	Hypertension	Antipsychotics (metabolic syndrome)
		MAOI-induced hypertensive crisis
	Bradycardia	Beta-blockers, anorexia, Parkinson's disease
	Anxiety	Angina, congestive heart failure, mitral valve prolapse, tachycardia
	Hypercholesterolemia	Antipsychotics (metabolic syndrome)
	Hyperlipidemia	
Gastrointestinal (GI) system	GI distress, nausea	Lithium: recommend taking with food
		SSRIs: especially early in treatment
Endocrine system	Abnormal glucose metabolism	Antipsychotics (metabolic syndrome)
	Hyperprolactinemia	Antipsychotic dopaminergic blockade
	Depression	Hypothyroidism, chronically elevated cortisol (prolonged stress response)
	Anxiety	Hyperthyroidism, hypoglycemia, premenstrual syndrome
Genitourinary system	Polyuria, polydipsia	Lithium
		Renal disease or drugs that reduce renal clearance (e.g., NSAIDs) may increase serum concentration of drugs that are excreted by the kidneys (e.g., lithium)
	Unusual pattern of bruises or trauma	Rule out sexual or physical abuse
	Sexual dysfunction	Can be side effect of antihypertensives, antidepressants, antihistamines, or antispasmodics
	Delirium	Kidney failure
		Liver failure
Musculoskeletal System	Body asymmetry	Dystonias (muscle spasms as a result of Parkinsonian side effects), CVAs, lesions
	Abnormal movements: dyskinesia, dystonia, bradykinesia, akathisia	Parkinson's disease and Parkinsonism related to antipsychotic extrapyramidal side effects (EPS)
	Gait disturbances	Cerebellar dysfunction such as seen with alcoholic encephalopathy (Wernicke's disease), substance use disorders
	Swallowing problems	Parkinson's disease, advanced dementia, antipsychotic-induced dystonias
Hematological system	Easy or excessive bruising	Thrombocytopenia secondary to anticonvulsants (e.g., divalproex sodium [Depakote])

SUICIDE RISK ASSESSMENT

According to the Centers for Disease Control and Prevention, in 2017, suicide is the second leading cause of death among individuals between the ages of 10 and 34, the fourth leading cause of death among individuals between the ages of 35 and 54, and the eighth among persons aged 55 to 64 years (National Institute of Mental Health, 2017). Rates are higher among lesbian, gay, bisexual, and transgender (LGBT) youth than among non-LGBT youth. White men have the highest risk, followed by Native Americans and Alaskan Natives; firearms are implicated in 56% of all cases (National Institute of Mental Health, 2017, para. 11).

VIOLENCE AND ASSAULT RISK ASSESSMENT

In 2017, homicide was the third leading cause of death among 15- to 34-year-olds, the second leading cause of death for 1- to 14-year-old black males, and the number one leading cause among 15- to 34-year-old black males (Centers for Disease Control and Prevention, 2019).

Although people of any age can be abused, children aged 4 or younger are the most vulnerable with the highest rates of fatal child abuse in this age range (WHO, 2002, p. 1).

SUBSTANCE USE SCREENING

Examples of Specific Treatment Regimens for Alcohol Withdrawal Monitoring:

▶ Symptom-triggered regimens

▶ Monitor patients every 4 to 8 hours by means of CIWA-Ar until score has been less than 8 for 24 hours

▶ Administer one of the following medications every hour when CIWA-Ar is 8 to 10:

   o Chlordiazepoxide,

   o Diazepam,

   o Lorazepam,

▶ Repeat assessment with CIWA-Ar 1one hour after every dose to determine need for further medication

(Mayo-Smith, 1997).

The Clinical Opioid Withdrawal Scale (COWS) is a clinical assessment for 11 medical signs and symptoms of opioid withdrawal (e.g., gastrointestinal distress), which are both objective and subjective in nature.

The American Society of Addiction Medicine (ASAM) National Practice Guideline 2015 is used to measure opioid withdrawal symptoms during the initial assessment to make the diagnosis of opioid withdrawal.

SUBSTANCE USE AND RISK FOR DEVELOPMENTAL DISABILITY

According to Shepard's Catalog (1995), there are more than 2,000 drugs, chemicals, and other physical and biological teratogenic agents that may adversely affect the newborn's development. Such effects to the mother and newborn may include chromosomal abnormalities, nonchromosomal congenital abnormalities and defects, low birth weight, altered fertility patterns, spontaneous abortion, developmental disabilities, behavioral disorders, childhood malignancies, and fetal, neonatal, or childhood death. Tobacco smoke, carbon monoxide, nicotine, alcohol, and polycyclic aromatic hydrocarbons can all adversely affect the fetus by causing increased bleeding during pregnancy, long-term birth disorders, spontaneous abortion, and rupture of the membranes. Drugs such as opiates, barbiturates, anesthetics, sex steroids, and food additives can produce developmental disabilities, congenital heart defects, and fetal death.

REFERENCES

Brenan, M. (2018). *Nurses Again Outpace Other Professions for Honesty, Ethics*. Retrieved from https://news.gallup.com/poll/245597/nurses-again-outpace-professions-honesty-ethics.aspx.

Centers for Disease Control and Prevention. (2019). *Web-based Injury Statistics Query and Reporting System (WISQARSTM) Leading Causes of Death Reports 1981–2017*. Retrieved from https://webappa.cdc.gov/sasweb/ncipc/leadcause.html.

Kampman, K., & Jarvis, M. (2015). American Society of Addiction Medicine (ASAM) National Practice Guideline for the Use of Medications in the Treatment of Addiction Involving Opioid Use. *Journal of Addiction Medicine*, 9(5), 358–367. doi:10.1097/ADM.0000000000000166.

Mayo-Smith, M. F. (1997). Pharmacological Management of Alcohol Withdrawal. Pharmacological management of alcohol withdrawal. A meta-analysis and evidence-based practice guideline. *JAMA*, 278, 144–51.

National Institute of Mental Health. (2017). *Suicide*. Retrieved from https://www.nimh.nih.gov/health/statistics/suicide.shtml.

Shepard, T. H. (1995). Catalog of Teratogenic Agents (Shepard's Catalog). *Children's Environmental Health Network*. Retrieved from http://cehn.org/catalog_teratogenic_agents_shepards_catalog.

World Health Organization. (2002). *Child abuse and neglect*. Retrieved from https://www.who.int/violence_injury_prevention/violence/world_report/factsheets/en/childabusefacts.pdf?ua=1.

CHAPTER 4

PROBLEM IDENTIFICATION, NURSING DIAGNOSES, AND PLANNING ACROSS THE LIFE SPAN

MAJOR PSYCHIATRIC MENTAL HEALTH PROBLEMS

Psychotic (Thought) Disorders

Schizophrenia Syndrome

According to the DSM-V: Late onset schizophrenia has been defined as onset of symptoms after the age of 44 and accounts for 15% to 20% of all cases of schizophrenia.

Anxiety Disorders

Generalized Anxiety Disorder (GAD)

▶ Onset for generalized anxiety disorder is later than other anxiety disorders. A meta-analysis study found that GAD "had the latest AOO [age of onset] at around 35 years" (Lijster et al., 2017).

SUBSTANCE USE DISORDERS

Alcohol

Psychiatric–Mental Health Practice Standard 4: Planning

See addendum for Chapter 3.

PROBLEM IDENTIFICATION ACROSS THE LIFE SPAN (CHILD AND ADOLESCENT FOCUS)

TABLE 4-4.
NEURODEVELOPMENTAL DISORDERS

Learning Disorders (Reading [Dyslexia], Mathematics [Dyscalculia], Written Expression [Agraphia or Dysgraphia], Drawing [Constructional Apraxia], Learning Disorder Not Otherwise Specified [NOS])	• In 2017–18, the number of students ages 3–21 who received special education services under the Individuals with Disabilities Education Act (IDEA) was 7.0 million, or 14% of all public-school students. Among students receiving special education services, 34% had specific learning disabilities (National Center for Education Statistics, 2019). • Nationally, about 5.9% of students drop out of high school. But among children with learning and attention issues, about 18% drop out of school (National Center for Education Statistics, 2019).
Autism Spectrum Disorders (Autism, Rett's Syndrome, Asperger's Syndrome, Childhood Disintegrative Disorder)	• Prevalence: In 2018, the CDC determined that approximately 1 in 59 children is diagnosed with an autism spectrum disorder (ASD). Boys are four times more likely to be diagnosed with autism than girls. Most children were still being diagnosed after age 4, though autism can be reliably diagnosed as early as age 2 (Baio et al., 2018). • One in 37 boys and 1 in 151 girls are diagnosed with an autism spectrum disorder (Baio et al., 2018).

REFERENCES

American Psychiatric Association. (2013). *Diagnostic and statistical manual of mental disorders, 5th ed.* Arlington, VA: American Psychiatric Publishing.

Baio, J., Wiggins, L., Christensen, D. L., Maenner, M. J., Daniels, J.,…Dowling, N. F. (2018). Pvalence of Autism Spectrum Disorder Among Children Aged 8 Years — Autism and Developmental Disabilities Monitoring Network. *Morbidity and Mortality Weekly Report Surveillance Summaries, 67*(6), 1–23. DOI: http://dx.doi.org/10.15585/mmwr.ss6706a1external icon.

Lijster, J. M., Dierckx, B., Utens, E. M., Verhulst, F. C., Zieldorff, C., Dieleman, G. C., & Legerstee, J. S. (2017). The Age of Onset of Anxiety Disorders. *Canadian Journal of Psychiatry. Revue Canadienne de Psychiatrie, 62*(4), 237–246. doi:10.1177/0706743716640757.

National Center for Education Statistics. (2019). Children and youth with disabilities. *NCES.* Retrieved from https://nces.ed.gov/programs/coe/indicator_cgg.asp.

CATEGORY II

IMPLEMENTATION AND EVALUATION

IMPLEMENTATION AND EVALUATION OF THE COMPREHENSIVE CARE PLAN ACROSS THE LIFE SPAN

The APGAR screening tool is used to evaluate a newborn's overall status and response to resuscitation immediately after birth (Committee on Obstetric Practice & AAP Committee on Fetus and New Born, 2015).

TYPICAL (OLDER OR CONVENTIONAL) ANTIPSYCHOTICS

Evaluation: Efficacy, Side Effects, and Adverse Effects of Typical (Older or Conventional) Antipsychotics (Neuroleptics or Major Tranquilizers)

Untoward or Adverse Effects and Treatments

Photosensitivity: In addition to a wide-brimmed hat and sunglasses, patients should wear a water-resistant, broad-spectrum sunscreen with an SPF of at least 30 to shield from harm incurred from the sun.

NONPHARMACOLOGICAL PAIN MANAGEMENT INTERVENTIONS AND EVALUATION

Electroconvulsive Therapy (ECT)

"Electroconvulsive therapy is the best studied brain stimulation therapy and has the longest history of use" (National Institute of Mental Health, 2016, para. 2).

The nursing care of a patient receiving ECT includes the following:

▶ Make sure that the patient does not eat or drink after midnight the night before treatment. Regular medications may be held and given after the treatment.

REFERENCES

Committee on Obstetric Practice & AAP Committee on Fetus and New Born. (2015). *Committee Opinion: The Apgar score*. The American College of Obstetricians and Gynecologists & The American Academy of Pediatrics, #644. Retrieved from https://www.acog.org/Clinical-Guidance-and-Publications/Committee-Opinions/Committee-on-Obstetric-Practice/The-Apgar-Score?IsMobileSet=false.

National Institute of Mental Health. (2016). *Brain Stimulation Theories*. Retrieved from https://www.nimh.nih.gov/health/topics/brain-stimulation-therapies/brain-stimulation-therapies.shtml.